WINDOWSILL WHIMSY:

Gardening & Horticultural Therapy Projects for Small Spaces

by

Hank Bruce & Tomi Jill Folk

Windowsill Whimsy: Gardening and Horticultural Therapy Projects for Small Spaces

Petals & Pages Press
860 Polaris Blvd SE
Rio Rancho, NM 87124
petals_pages@msn.com

Published by Petals & Pages Press 2008

ISBN 978-0-9797057-4-8

Cover photos, design and interior photos by Tomi Jill Folk and Hank Bruce

Dedication

This book is dedicated to Wilheminia V. Bruce and Donald Folk, Hank's mother and Tomi's father. These two gentle people taught us both so much about what really grows in the garden, the human spirit. They also taught us the adventure, discovery, joy and patience that also grows there.

Thank you

A horticultural therapy book doesn't just happen. Like a garden it is planted and nurtured by many helping hands. We want to thank all the senior citizens and children, all the troubled and challenged, all the clients who shared their time, wisdom, stories and smiles. We appreciate the fact that they also shared their fears, frustrations and failures with us in this adventure we call horticultural therapy. They may have been called clients, but each one of them was very much a teacher and a friend. We also want to thank all the other horticultural therapists, teachers, health care professionals, activity directors and so many others who willingly enrich lives every day. We wish to thank them also for sharing their time, thoughts, ideas and suggestions with us. Each of these people is a gift. And so are you. Thank you for reading and using this book.

WINDOWSILL WHIMSY:
Gardening & Horticultural Therapy Projects
for Small Spaces
by
Hank Bruce & Tomi Jill Folk

This book is written with the hope that it can in some small way help you, the reader, experience the joy of gardening, even when the space and resources are limited. It is our hope also that this book be used by families sharing the experience together, and by gardeners of all ages making discoveries and enjoying the opportunities to be with plants. Perhaps horticultural therapists, teachers, activity professionals, and counselors will also find these pages of value. The plants and projects explored in this text have all been used in horticultural therapy programs conducted by the authors at senior care facilities, with children in schools, home schooling programs and programs for those of us with special needs.

Gardening isn't age specific. From toddlers to centenarians the wonder of life itself holds a fascination for all of us. Each day is a new journey of discovery in the garden, even if that garden is only a couple of plants on the windowsill. The pleasure to be found in communion with plants isn't gender specific. Men and women, girls and boys can enjoy both getting their hands dirty and nurturing life. Gardening doesn't have to be backbreaking activity, it can be self paced exercise. The plants don't care what language you speak, what degrees you hold, whether it is cared for with the pudgy insecure hands of a two year old or the arthritic hands of a veteran of ninety years or more. The plants will respond to the care they receive, and reward the caregiver, regardless of who she or he is.

We have divided this book into several sections and tried to provide readable information while avoiding the appearance of a textbook. This is designed to be read and enjoyed, not only used as a reference when there is a need or a problem.

Above all, these projects and activities are only suggestions, points of departure for you as a gardener, educator, activity professional or horticultural therapist. You are encouraged to modify, change, or expand on any of these as you see fit, or as needed to accommodate the limitations of your clients or students, and such factors as time, space, season and finances. We also encourage you to engage all those who will be participating in the decision making process. It is empowering to make decisions about what plants will be used, how the container will be customized and how they will be grown. You and the participating gardeners are encouraged to set your imaginations free, have the courage to be creative, explore and experiment. Then it really is your garden.

Table of contents:

Introduction:

Part I: Whimsical Plant Projects, Just for the Fun of It

Part 3: Thinking Like a Plant

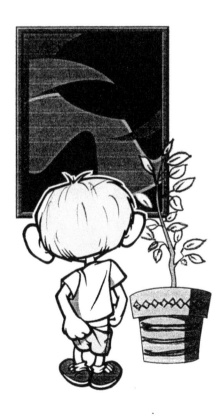

3

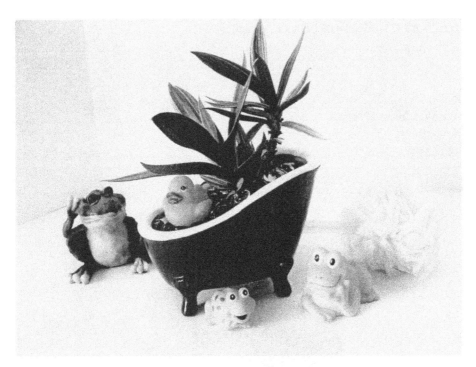

"Gardening is good clean fun,
Being green's good for everyone."

Notes from the windowsill

Hi, I just wanted to chat with you for a few minutes before you get started.

I'm over here on the windowsill. Didn't know plants could talk, did ya?

Well we do communicate in a number of ways. I asked Hank & Tomi to give me a couple pages of this book to talk to you about "thinking like a plant." It's easy, and if we are both on the same page you can have a green thumb and we can have green leaves. We both have the same goal. We want to live and grow, and that's exactly what you want us to do. So, let's get started.

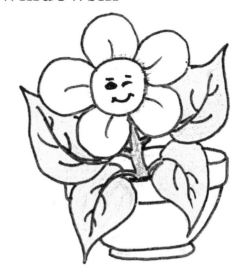

Please talk to us.

First of all, I want to encourage you to talk to your plants, whether they are in a garden or on a windowsill. We are your green friends and we enjoy hearing your voice. We breathe in Carbon Dioxide and "exhale" Oxygen. We call this transpiration and when you get close to us and chat for a little bit you give us an extra serving of CO_2. We give you an extra serving of Oxygen and this helps your circulation and more blood to the brain helps you think better. This is one of the reasons gardeners live longer. We particularly like it when you smile and laugh and tell us we are beautiful. But, you can also tell us your problems. We are patient and we don't scold, walk away or laugh at you. Like a good friend, we just listen.

We talk to you with our leaves.

With our new leaves we tell you we are getting enough light. If our leaves are pale, and twisted rather than bright green, and our stems are weak and flop over we are starving for light.

We are the pioneers in solar energy. You didn't know that? Well, we are. We take the sunlight and convert it into enough energy to grow and bloom. This is a process we call photosynthesis and it uses chlorophyl, the stuff that makes us green. We actually turn sunshine into carbohydrates that we can burn in our cells to feed ourselves and make new leaves, flowers, fruit, roots and our little green children.

Now us plant people are as diverse and varied as people. That's how we are able to live in the shade of a hemlock forest, the never ending sun of the Sonoran desert, the mountaintops of the Alps and the lakes and oceans. But this means that some of my friends need a lot more sunshine than others. If a plant that is accustomed to the forests of central Africa, like the African violet, is set out in the bright sun, just like you, it gets a sunburn. Even if your green friend was designed by Mamma Nature to live in the sunshine, but you had it growing in the shade for months, exposure to bright sun will give it a serious sunburn.

Us plants get hungry, too.

We also tell you when we need a snack or some minerals like Iron, Calcium, Manganese and Magnesium with our leaves. If they are pale with dark veins it may mean we need Iron, or Nitrogen. A good balanced fertilizer (dinner to us) specially cooked up for your friends on the windowsill, or other places indoors can be just what we need. It can be a snack like Miracle-Gro or any other liquid plant food. These don't last to long, but do give us a boost. Be very careful not to make it too strong though. This can make us sick, like eating to many hot dogs will make your tummy uncomfortable. Use the directions on the package, never make the mixture stronger than it says. Hank & Tomi give you feeding suggestions with each project in this book and they give good advice.

Another option is to use a slow release plant food like Osmocote about twice a year. Make certain that you are using the formula for indoor plants. Just a bit of advice from your green friend, some plants, like orchids and cacti are on a special diet and they will do much better of you can give them what they need. For my flowering friends you can use 'bloom booster" plant foods that give us what we need to produce more, bigger and brighter flowers.

Important! Don't over feed. This makes us weak and we can't defend ourselves against the bugs and diseases that can make us sick or even kill us.

Home, sweet home.
Home is where our roots are. You can call it a pot or a container. It can be something you found at a garage sale like a frying pan turned into a cactus condo, or a tin can you personally painted and decorated just for us, or even a coffee mug where a small plant can put down roots and raise a flower or two. It is important to us that there be enough room to grow. And if we are successful in this people-plant partnership, you may need to provide us with a larger apartment every year or two.

If it is possible to provide a drainage hole or two in this container it helps to prevent our roots from drowning. Healthy soil is about 25% air and if the soil is soggy, only the "Swamp Things" can grow there. You can put about ½ inch of aquarium gravel and charcoal in the bottom of a tea cup or coffee mug to help keep the soil from souring, but the real trick is to only water us when the soil is almost dry. The garden centers have this neat gadget called a moisture meter, and, in my humble opinion, no windowsill should be without one. It will tell you whether we need water or not. Some of us wilt when we get thirsty, but if the leaves turn brown and just hang on our stems, then, unfortunately we are ready for the compost pile.

We don't live in dirt.
Dirt is what you sweep under the rug. We plants live in soil. This is our home and we ask that you treat it with respect. Good soil is a mixture of organic matter, sand and often perlite or vermiculite to help aerate and hold moisture. Some soil mixes contain moisture retaining crystals, but most of my friends don't need this and will do better if you monitor our drinking habits.

Please make certain that you are using a potting soil for indoor use that doesn't contain animal manures. These can cause mold growth and other health problems for you and they may have a rather unpleasant aroma that even my most aromatic herb cousins can't cover up.

Soilless mixes are a blend of organic matter, the perlite or vermiculite I mentioned above and sterile sand. While this can help prevent soil borne diseases for both you and me, it also limits the microscopic soil organisms that I need to digest the vitamins and minerals that are in the soil. It's just like the special collection of similar organisms in your digestive system to help you digest your burger and fries. Usually we carry a few of these with us, just in case. The soilless mixes are great for our people friends that are cancer patients, or have immune system problems. We can still be friends and you aren't exposed to what might be harmful fungi or bacteria.

Please, I beg you, don't use the really cheap budget potting soils that are little more than black mud and will pack down into something like a brick. This is very hard for our roots to grow through and they contain almost none of the stuff we need to grow and make you happy.

Some of my cousins are heavy drinkers.
The question people ask all the time is, "How often do I water my plants." This isn't an easy question because there are so many things that make a plant thirsty. The temperature on our windowsill, the humidity, the amount of light and the time of year all play a part in how fast the water in the soil is either used up or evaporates. If we are cramped into a small apartment with little room for our roots we will need watered more often that if we have a spacious home with lits of room to grow. Even the kind of soil we are living in makes a difference. Some soils hold a lot more water than others.

Just like you people, us plants have different needs, so saying you will water twice a week or once a week doesn't mean we are getting the care we need. Remember, and this is difficult for me to say, but we are really at your mercy. We can be either prisoners in your pot, or guests in your home. This part of the people-plant connection is up to you.

All plants need water, but some drink a lot more than others. Many of the tropical plants want their soil kept evenly moist. Some of my really weird cousins, they ones that catch and eat bugs just for the fun of it, like to live in soggy soil. But, many of the plants that you will grow on your windowsill are at their best when the soil is allowed to become almost dry between waterings. These are the cacti and succulents that come from the exotic deserts of Africa, Asia, South and North America, even a few wander in from Australia.

The moisture meter I mentioned above is a great way to help determine when my cousins need water. If you group the plants that have similar needs together this make sit easier for you to keep us happy.

Save the windowsills.
While most of us plants don't really need for our containers to sit in a pan, tray or saucer, it can help to protect the windowsill we consider our neighborhood. When you give us a drink, sometimes the soil is a little too dry to absorb the water and it runs right through the pot. If our home is sitting in a saucer this will catch the water and let the soil soak it up slowly in a process called osmosis.

If you place our pots or containers in a tray or saucer that has a layer of gravel, decorative stones or even marbles and keep a little water in this tray it will help to increase the humidity for those of us who like our air on the moist side. I'm speaking of my cousins the ferns, and the begonias and many of the orchids and tropical plants. This can keep the tips of the leaves from turning brown. Cacti ans succulents are from the deserts of the world and they don't need the humidity.

There's something that's really bugging me.
We try as hard as we can to please you, to grow, bloom and sometimes even produce some fruit for you. But, sometimes we are attacked by bugs like aphids, mites, scale and mealybugs. They are mean vicious monsters that attack us from the undersides of our leaves where you don't see them until its too late. They are worse than mosquitoes are to you because they don't just hit and run. They set up housekeeping on our leaves and stems. They suck our life blood, you call it sap, from our veins and destroy us leaf by leaf, stem by stem. Mites are like miniature spiders except that they will spin webs, set up first colonies, then entire cities of thousands of mites. They have to be stopped and our only hope is you.

Visit with us every day. Talk to us, look under our leaves for signs of webs, salt and pepper spots on the leaves, little white or gray spots where our leaves join our stems, little white flies that flutter around us. You might want to use a small magnifying glass to check if you suspect one of these critters. If you spot any of

these horrible monsters, please don't give up on us. Help us fight them. There are organic house plant sprays that work if they are sprayed under the leaves where there blood sucking vampires are hiding.

You can wash our leaves with mild soapy water, but be certain that the soap is not anti-bacterial. That contains alcohol and this can destroy our leaves. You can also take a Que Tip dipped in vegetable oil or rubbing alcohol and dab the critters with it. They will stick to the Que Tip and can easily be discarded. Do not rub the leaf with this oil or alcohol, just dab the pests and get them away from us.

Keep checking every few days because new eggs may hatch and we still need your help.

"Care & Feeding" part of each project

Hank and Tomi have included a few notes at the end of each of the projects in this book to help you care for us after getting us started. They tell you what my cousins and I need to be successful in this people-plant partnership that we are both looking forward to. Please read what they have to say and try to follow these suggestions as best you can. They tell you about the light, soil and water needs, about what temperatures we most enjoy, what kind of home we are comfortable in and how to help us build a family, bloom and share the joy of simply being alive.

We plants also suggest that you get to know us better by visiting the library, or researching on the Internet to learn as much as you can about us. We will pose for photos, do our best to make you smile, and perhaps we can even inspire you to be creative. Best of all, as your plants, we encourage you to share our cuttings, seeds, pups and offsets with your friends so that they will also know the joy of the people-plant connection.

Getting started.

If you are doing a group program as a horticultural therapist, teacher or activity professional there are many ways to get started. I wanted to tell you a little about how Tomi & Hank do their programs. Keep in mind this is only one way to do these projects and make new green friends.

They start with options, because the opportunity to make decisions is empowering. Hummm. I don't think they gave us plants any options though. Must be a people thing.

1.   They set up two or three work stations, depending on how many people are in the group. Each work station is a table with a different color plastic table cloth. It's interesting to see which color table cloth is the most popular.

2.   The first station may offer a variety of pots or containers. They may be different colors or styles, or they may have paints, stickers or trims available so that each person can use to make our new home uniquely ours. This is great for both parts of what they call the people-plant connection, us plants get a customized place to call home and the people get to be creative. Sometimes preparing our new home is done ahead of time as a separate project. This give you an opportunity to be truly artistic.

3.   The next station may contain plastic tubs or storage totes filled with the potting soil. Putting the soil in our new home is sorta like carpeting your house. Once Hank forgot the trowels they used to fill the pots with soil. Tomi found a couple serving spoons, a measuring cup and an ice cream scoop.

Everyone laughed but they worked so well that this is what they have been using ever since. It is also empowering to pick the tools you are going to work with. By the way, the most popular is the ice cream scoop. People will stand in line to use it, even when there are other tools to use. Some people prefer to simply use their hands, and this works well too. After all good soil is something you can really get your roots into.

4. They also try to give the people choices in selecting the plants to be adopted. It may be as simple as selecting which cutting or baby plant to make friends with, or it may be a matter of choosing which species of plant they want on their windowsill. Some folks will pick the strongest, healthiest looking plantlet, while someone else might pick the weakest one that looks like it needs them to care for it.

5. Once the plants, cuttings or seeds are planted they offer different trims and decorations like a silk flower, colored stones or other items from a yard sale or junk drawer. These decorate our new home and make us feel welcome and cared for. Now we are ready to grow.

6. The main point is that everyone gets to do something different. This may be a little more work for you as the facilitator, but Tomi says, "The rewards are well worth the extra effort."

7. If some of the "Whimsy Gardeners" have limited mobility other gardeners or volunteers can either move the project materials to them or they can move wheelchairs from station to station.

8. Even when physical or mental limitations make it impossible for someone to actually pot or care for one of us, this doesn't mean we can't be friends. We can become sensory stimulation or memory triggers. Sometimes people will be inspired to ask really good questions, or share a great story. Remember, us plants really enjoy a good story, and we don't care how longs it takes to tell it, or even if someone forgets what they were going to say part way through. We enjoy being with them and swapping Oxygen for some CO_2. We have seen people smile and speak up about our colorful flowers or soft fuzzy leaves or delightful herbal scent when they haven't spoken for months. That's one of the nice things about us plants, we make people smile.

9. Take the time to enjoy our company, and don't worry about doing everything exactly right. We are adaptable and have a great will to live, and really fo want to be friends with you.

10. Relax and remember that it's you and me kid. "We're all in this together." When we become friends people and plants make an unbeatable combination. Let's grow together.

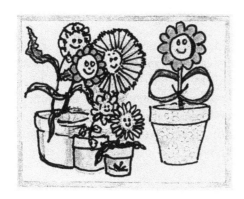

I want you to meet Buzz and Dottie,
a couple of our friends,
(*rock art can be a whimsy project too*)

Introduction:

Finding the Courage to Garden

Many of us are afraid to even attempt to grow plants. Often this is based on a fear of failure, and that may well be based on past experience. We are often told by reluctant gardeners, "I like plants, but I have a brown thumb," or "Every plant I touch seems to die." It does seem that some people are blessed with a GREEN THUMB and can do no wrong. Rachel had grown up in the heart of New York City and never so much as started an avocado pit. She was 87 years old and living in a nursing home when she planted her first seeds and struck her first cuttings. She insisted that she couldn't grow anything. After becoming a part of our horticultural therapy program at Leu Botanic Gardens in Orlando, Florida she soon had a windowsill filled with plants, not to mention the other plants that were thriving in the lobby and screen room. This only happened because she mustered enough courage to try, and face possible failure, or possible success.

We have had a long association with Walt Disney World and have taken great delight in the marvelous plantings that surround the guests and offer colorful surprises at every turn. We have also been backstage at Disney World and seen the loads of plants that were spent, in decline or could be viewed as downright failures. These plants, destined to become compost, were removed from public view but they were still proof that even the ultimate professional horticulturists of Disney World have failures. We all lose plants sometimes, but each plant that doesn't make it doesn't mean that we are miserable failures. In fact, it could be viewed as an opportunity to learn, to try again, or to try something new and different.

We were once told by an activity coordinator who was convinced that she was poison to plants, "For the last three years I have planted petunias and each year they die." After further questioning, it was found that she was purchasing them as soon as they were available at the garden center and planted them as soon as she got home. This was at least a month before the last frost of the season. Gardening, like much of life, is a matter of timing.

Life is a never-ending learning experience, and so is this thing we call gardening. It is important that we put everything in perspective. Each time we enter into a partnership with nature we have the opportunity to learn, to gain in understanding. We gradually learn to think like a plant. We gradually become more confident, and the successes become more frequent. All living things have a natural life span and many plants live to bloom once, set seeds then become compost for the next generation. Other plants are perennial and live for many years, until old age, severe weather, or other unfriendly conditions spell the end.

Spending time with plants is healthy; there is a natural, instinctive relationship between us and the green world. Charles Lewis eloquently explored this in his book, *Green Nature, Human Nature*. It is called by many, the people-plant connection. Regardless of what you call it there is much comfort and joy to be found in the company of plants. We can find beauty, curiosity, discovery, companionship and much more in this communion with green friends. However, none of this can happen until we enter into this partnership. We cannot succeed until we gather the courage to try. Even if the plants do die, we are still here, perhaps sadder, but a bit wiser. The plant died, we are doing fine. We can try again.

There is real therapeutic value in being with plants, cultivating and being partners with life. In fact, this is called horticultural therapy. This is a field that can, and does, make a monumental difference in the quality of life, rehabilitation and treatment of a number of physical and mental limitations.

The Garden as a Healing Place

Imagine a place of healing, a place where everyone is accepted, where stress can be lost and joy found. The garden, even if it is only a small windowsill, can be a powerful place of renewal and connection with your true self. Gardening is great therapy and a simple pathway to stress reduction. It's also a never-ending journey of discovery. Because your plants are living things, there is constant change, always something happening and a never ending parade of surprises. Experiencing the garden strengthens the body, comforts the mind and inspires the soul.

On the windowsill we can all embark on a journey of self-discovery as we explore how our senses can be stimulated by the simple act of being with living plants. We experience every plant with one or more of our five physical senses: sight, touch, smell, hearing, and taste. Then we go beyond that to a sense of being, sense of place, sense of purpose and a sense of belonging; and we cannot forget our sense of wonder and sense of adventure. Gardening is a partnership with nature, not a duel.

The Garden as Therapy
It's Called Horticultural Therapy

It's only logical. If the garden is a healing place, then working with the plants must be therapeutic. This is what horticultural therapy is all about. As professional horticultural therapists we use the garden and gardening activity as therapeutic tools. This experiencing of the people-plant connection can improve the social, educational, psychological, spiritual and physical adjustment of many people. This time in the garden, the time with plants, nurtures the mind, body and spirit, restores balance and improves the quality of life. This communion with plants is often classified as either active or passive, but there is almost always a response to the contact, so that for most of us, all people-plant contact is an active, or interactive, experience.

Gardening as a therapeutic tool has a long history that dates back to the gardens of ancient Egypt where both the physically and mentally ill took long walks or relaxed among aromatic plants, beautiful flowers and calming water gardens. One of the signers of the US constitution, Dr. Benjamin Rush, founded a healing farm in Eastern Pennsylvania in the early 1800's. Today professional horticultural therapists use plants and the gardening experience for many special populations ranging from the physically disabled to the mentally ill, the elderly and victims of abuse, at risk students and substance abusers, AIDS victims and cardiac patients, those suffering from depression and those in hospice programs, as well as the professional caregivers.

For all of us who experience the burdens of everyday living, including family caregivers and those who are undergoing the trauma of life change (death of a loved one, loss of a job, divorce) gardening is a means of momentary retreat and renewal. Those of us who find our stress in the workplace can also find comfort in the companionship of plants. There is a growing interest in workplace gardening programs to limit stress and increase productivity and creativity.

Individuals with physical or mental conditions that force them into dependent or passive roles can find in living plants a role reversal. Caring for plants puts this individual in a responsible, care giving position. This can not only bring pleasure, it can build confidence and a sense of purpose. The growth of these plants gives the gift of hope and a reason for tomorrow.

All too often our elders, our children and individuals with limitations suffer from depression and low self esteem. Working with plants provides the opportunity to be successful, to feel that each and every one of us does have value.

Horticultural therapy can provide opportunities for social interaction and cooperation. Participants in horticultural therapy programs are also presented with learning experiences.

The physical and mental activities that are a part of all horticultural therapy programs help hospital patients who have undergone surgery or are recovering from illness heal faster. Horticultural therapy can lower blood pressure, diminish depression, help lower blood sugar levels for many diabetics. Today many hospitals have horticultural therapy programs, or at least, garden courtyards where patients and families can stroll or sit and reflect in the midst of life and beauty. The garden both soothes the soul and stimulates the senses.

Horticultural therapy programs have proven very beneficial in nursing homes, assisted living facilities, schools, substance abuse and rehabilitation centers, prisons and juvenile detention centers, community centers and homeless shelters. Health care organizations, hospice programs, welfare agencies, shelters for victims of violence and abuse, programs and facilities serving the developmentally disabled and a multitude of others have been able to improve the quality of life through horticultural therapy.

> The garden is a safe place, a benevolent setting where everyone is welcome. Plants are non-judgmental, non-threatening and non-discriminating. They respond to the care given. It doesn't matter whether one is white or black, been to kindergarten or college, is poor or wealthy, been a victim of abuse or an abuser, is handicapped or blind, can call a plant by name, or only caress the leaves with arthritic hands.

A Bouquet of Benefits from Being with Plants

Mental stimulation: Growing, or simply being with plants, either in the great outdoors or on the windowsill, provides a multitude of opportunities to learn new skills and acquire new knowledge. Being with plants increases attention spans, raises concentration levels, improves our ability to work independently and make decisions. Gardening even helps us develop problem solving skills. The opportunity to learn about new plants, share wisdom and past experiences helps to keep the mind active.

Making friends: Plants are a great, safe topic to discuss with friends, total strangers and potential new acquaintances. Sharing wisdom, curiosity, stories and experiences about "green friends" past, present and future are safe topics for conversation. Engaging with others without focusing on today's pains and discomforts is beneficial. On the windowsill garden we can grow new friendships with both plants and other people. Working as a member of a group, such as a Green Thumb Club (see page 249), increases the opportunities even more.

Psychological benefits: The plants depend on the gardener for survival; they need us. Our compassion and nurturing needs are met through the care of something living. This sense of responsibility cultivates our sense of worth and improves self-esteem. Both the opportunity to be creative and the potential for success are present. In groups where depression is prevalent, an active horticultural therapy program can reduce the incidence of depression, and the need for anti-depressive medications. In senior care facilities it can reduce the number of complaints from residents, family members and staff. In a larger garden setting the physical acts of weeding, cultivating and pruning relieve, in a socially acceptable way, feelings of tension, anger, aggression, frustration and stress.

Physical rehabilitation: The activities of gardening can be adapted to our individual limitations. It also provides incentives to exercise both gross and fine motor skills, retain or strengthen muscles. Being actively involved with plants and gardening can lower blood pressure, improve circulation and respiration. Gardening provides meaningful exercise for stroke patients, those recovering from surgery, illness or accidents, and particularly, those of us with arthritis.

Reality connections: Recent studies seem to indicate that "nature deficit" a lack of contact with the real world may be one of the contributing causes of ADHD and other behavioral disorders and learning disabilities common with today's children. Perhaps school gardening programs can replace some of the medications now being used. Perhaps family gardening activities could reduce some of the tension and stress that divides families today. It's worth contemplating.

From the earliest of civilizations humanity has felt the need to be with plants, to be a part of the natural world, to sense the wonder and the beauty of which we are all a part. Being in the garden is not, cannot be, a passive experience. There is an ever present symphony for the senses, a senso-round experience twenty four hours a day, every day of our lives. The beauty of this never-ending concerto of life is that we are one of the musicians in this infinite orchestra.

Why We Enjoy the Companionship of Plants

Gardening answers a host of our instinctive needs. We are a part of the natural world. Before there was the computer, before television, before air conditioning, people lived in the real world and found comfort and enjoyment there. They were a part of the all encompassing, multi-dimensional experience that far exceeded the myth of reality TV. The garden is a connection with our ancestral past, a place where we can rediscover our instincts for survival. In our garden, in this living microcosm, we find the allegory of Eden, the African veldt, the forest, the jungle, the great plains, the mountains and the lakes of human history. Even when that garden is a single pot on a small windowsill, it is all still there, just waiting for us.

Security can be found in the garden. We are with nature yet not alone in the wilderness. We instinctively need to feel comforted by the living world, the connection with the soil, the energy of the earth itself.

Sustenance, the source of food for the body and the soul are found in the communion with live plants. The fruit, leaves, roots and fiber of many plants nourishes the body while the beauty, fragrance and life forces nourish the soul. Even on a windowsill, nature is the artist and we are the brush. There is always something new to witness, experience or do.

Beauty is such a primary need for us all that we sometimes fail to recognize it as one of our basic drives. The garden provides so rich and varied an array of the beautiful, from minute flowers to massive trees. Exploring the windowsill garden with a magnifying glass will open a whole new world to us.

Whimsy is the surprise that a sense of humor can give us. It's the laughable unexpected, the fanciful, the playful, the poetic incongruity of life. Whimsy is the counterpoint to the serious work of being human. Garden whimsy can take the form of an old shoe used as a planter, the statue of a cat watching the birdbath, or single white petunia in a bed of all red ones, or a flower bed inside an old bedframe. The garden doesn't always come with a laugh track, but you can provide one.

All Gardens Are Sensory

The people-plant connection is an instinctive link to our ancestral past, our semi-domesticated connection to the reality of nature. In the garden we can find security, adventure, mystery, intrigue, sustenance and beauty. Strolling through the garden soothes stressed emotions while stimulating all of our senses. The garden is an ever changing kaleidoscope of color. There's a constant teasing of scents and aromas. There's always something that calls to us to be touched or tasted; and the music of the garden is the impromptu harmony of nature. Even when the garden is only a pot on the windowsill there is sensory magic to be experienced there.

All gardens are sensory. The traditional English garden of a century or two ago was designed to dispel melancholy. The French gardeners designed elaborate patterns of color and form. Buddhist temples of the Orient and India are surrounded by gardens of flowers and herbs. The Mayans of Ancient Mexico had great floating gardens of flowers. All of these traditions, and many more, speak of the basic human need to experience beauty, involve the senses, and be a part of something beyond ourselves. When we are with beauty then we are beautiful ourselves.

Beyond what we call the "five senses" are the emotional senses that this communion with plants involves. Within all of us is the sense of beauty. Perhaps our cave artist ancestors gazed at the stars through the dancing leaves of a birch or willow and saw beauty, carried colorful wildflowers to their lovers and loved ones. Perhaps it is our sense of beauty that makes humanity possible.

We also need a sense of place and a sense of being. In the green world, with all the variety of life that can be found there, we can discover the joy of belonging to something greater than ourselves. With this connection life has meaning. In the companionship of plants we can sense that we are home.

There Is No Such Thing as Passive Gardening

Even sitting on a park bench we are actively aware of our surroundings. We are physically, mentally, emotionally and spiritually engaged as our senses are stimulated. Touching the wild and domesticated life, watching the clouds, simply smelling the flowers affects our blood pressure, stress level, even respiration and heart rate. We don't have to be constantly digging, pruning, spraying, planting or harvesting to benefit from the people-plant connection. Nor do we have to be in control of the landscape, or do battle with the forces of nature. The true victory is in being a part of this big picture, not in dominating it. Every action we take doesn't have to have a practical purpose. We don't have to always carry with us this stress inducing drive to be productive, to succeed. Nor do we need to be in control in the garden. Even the windowsill garden can be a comfort zone. There we can engage in one of the most important of all activities, resting, an activity that can both heal and renew. We can relax and let life happen around us. Sometimes it's ok to simply be along for the ride; we don't have to be the driver all the time.

Unfortunately, many of us are so compelled to make our relationship with the garden work that we never give ourselves time to truly experience it. Nowhere is it written that we must carry tools every time we visit green friends, nor are required to sweat to experience the garden. The garden is not our place to escape into some temporary world of non-reality; it is the place where we can truly connect with the ultimate reality of life itself. This is not, this cannot, be a passive experience.

Windowsill Landscaping for the Senses

It's both enjoyable and healthy to escape the confines of the sterile residence, which, in reality, is our cage. We can set ourselves free and play in the companionship of plants. When we can learn how to cooperate with nature rather than compete, accept what is happening around us rather than demand total and absolute control, then we can immerse ourselves completely in the moment and enjoy our place in the universe.

We can make this part of our home a place of retreat and renewal, a source of adventure and discovery, a space to share. When we do that we can have a lot more fun. The windowsill landscape should be a joy, and it should be a reflection of your tastes, lifestyle and interests. You can make your great indoors a living, multi-sensory experience.

☺ Our landscape can be multi-level. We can vary the heights at which the plants are viewed by using a variety of containers and hanging baskets.

☺ A garden is so much more than the plants living there. The whimsy of unusual containers, statuary, fountains, even the furniture, can be a part of your multi-sensory reality.

☺ When using aromatic plants we can space them out so that the scents don't clash with each other.

☺ We can use color, both in foliage and flowers, to create images and set moods.

☺ We can use containers of aromatic plants as a friendly welcome sign at the entrance to our space.

☺ We can plant for the view from the window and, by placing a few plants near by, we can create an invitation to experience the venue.

☺ We can make our windowsill landscape truly our own by growing plants that connect us to our past, and help us to cope with the present as we look toward the future.

The Whimsy is Up to You

Whimsy is the unexpected, the lighthearted, the stuff of life that makes us smile, chuckle or laugh out loud. It's the use of thrift store items, like old shoes as unconventional containers for your plants. It's the crafty use of beads or seeds, stamps or coins, clippings from comic books, or junk drawer treasures as the decor of your chosen botanical friend's residence. It's the wild and weird items we use as garden statuary, even when the garden is only a potted plant on the windowsill and the statuary is a rock, plastic Halloween insects or clay frogs and snails. It's an Easter Bunny sitting in the middle of your windowsill salad garden. The elements of whimsy are yours to choose and use.

Whimsy is your imagination, your creative energy at work. Or, perhaps it's the demented part of ourselves that has been held in check far too long. However you choose to view the element of whimsy, it is the incongruous, the joke that is planted in the garden to make others smile. The whimsy is the message that it's safe to relax, share thoughts and fire up the imagination. It is also the way that we communicate the simple message to ourselves and with others that life is far too serious and we all need to lighten up. And the garden, even the windowsill garden is a great place to grow smiles. It's the whimsy that lets us open up, engage in conversation with others and face the day ourselves.

Don't be shy about using whimsy. This is your opportunity to experiment, to try things, to engage in the most important aspects of being crafty or artistic. Every smile, yours, or the smile adorning friends or strangers, is a work of art. If you provided the inspiration for that smile, then you are truly an artist. If you are willing to use the garden as a place to play, rather than work, you possess a wisdom of great value.

Looking for the Surprise

The never ending parade of discoveries is one of the great adventures for the gardener. The surprise that lies in wait for us around the bend in the garden path is the whimsy, the punch line, the reason so many gardeners are able to smile at themselves and the world. Because a garden, even a windowsill garden, is filled with life, there will always be something new, changes expected and unexpected, good news and bad. Too much of our time is spent in the garden looking for the work to be done when we should be discovering the surprises and experiencing the wonder of it all.

Start each morning looking for the surprise and the rest of the day goes much better. This discovery might be as awesome as a flower bursting into bloom with an explosion of color, or as inspirational as a seed sprouting with new life. If we are willing to unleash our sense of beauty we can find art in the form of a fallen leaf casting morning shadows on the windowsill, or the dramatic technicolor visit of a passing butterfly.

Some of these discoveries can come with the aid of a magnifying glass looking at the architecture of an African violet flower. Others may involve binoculars to bring us closer to the joy of birds engaged in an aerial ballet outside the window. It may be in the texture of a sage leaf or a palm frond, the scent of a chocolate mint or the pungent aroma of a Swedish ivy. Sometimes the same discovery can be made day after day with subtle variations on a theme, as the fruit of the tomato ripens, the sprout grows, the cutting forms new leaves, as sunlit mornings and cloudy afternoons change the colors, and your mood changes and different thoughts, memories and new ideas form in your mind.

When you experience the surprise with your senses it is added to the essence of you. It becomes a part of you. It can be an even richer experience when yesterday's discovery is shared with today's friend. When it's mentioned in a letter or an e-mail, or recorded in a photograph, a sketch or a poem it becomes a part of your creative self. How can we not seek these surprises, and the joy they bring?

Keeping a Gardener's Journal

Because the gardener is dealing daily with life, there are the surprises mentioned above. There are also many expectations, logical and reasonable developments that we can all anticipate, even when the garden is on the windowsill. Gardening is itself a creative expression, a partnership with God and nature, the Creator and the creation. It is also a never-ending learning experience. It is only logical that we be inspired when in the presence of plants. We can feel safe as our minds are given the freedom to wonder, be inspired and intrigued.

This is why we encourage you to keep a Gardener's Journal. And it can include everything from weather notes and measurements to the musings of your creative spirit.

- We can wax poetic, preserving moments in verse as we think, imagine, remember and anticipate.

- Record moments of inspiration, sparks of insight, hopes found and memories relived.

- In a gardener's notebook you can record events like the germination of a seed, the opening of a flower bud or the taste of a new herb.

- Successes, failures and experiments can be recorded in your own words.

- Art, drawings, sketches, paintings by your own hand, or impressions of others can have a place in your chronicle of you and your green friends growing together.

- Research the library or the internet, learn all you can about the life, history, myth and lore of each plant you choose to adopt. Gradually, you become an expert and your journal can be your primary reference.

- Newspaper, gardening catalog and magazine clippings can also be a part of your notebook/journal.

- Even dried leaves and pressed flowers can find their way into this chronicle of the garden and the gardener.

- You can also include jokes, humorous observations, whimsical windowsill creations, and light moments.

- Take photos of your green friends, and your people friends too as they visit you and your plants.

Some call this a journal, other might refer to it as a scrapbook. It doesn't matter what you call it, it can be a valuable part of the gardening experience, as much a part of this experience as the pots, sunshine and the watering can. This can be a three ring binder, a formal scrap book, a blank journal, or a formal Garden Journal. You can use whatever you wish, after all, it is YOUR notebook.

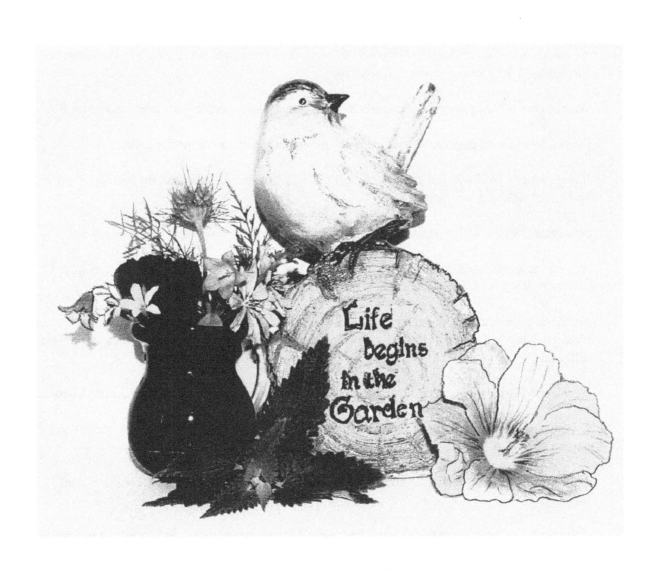

Part I

Windowsill Whimsy
Projects
Activities
Quizzes
&
Stories

Some basic information
to help select the right projects & activities for you

Adventures in Growing: Green and growing plant projects. Each entry begins with some basic notes. Such as:

Common or familiar name:	African Violet
Botanical name:	Example, *Saintpaulia ionantha*
Plant family:	Lily family, *Gesneriaceae*
Where this plant came from:	This is included to give participants an understanding of the global nature of gardening, even on the windowsill.
Safety factor:	This is important for many population groups where there may be a tendency to ingest plant parts. Ratings may include: All parts safe, leaves may be toxic, or do not ingest the sap.
Rating:	This refers to ease of culture: Very easy, Easy, Moderately easy, Difficult. Some plants are easier to grow than others. Some of these projects require more dexterity or coordination than others. This may also be noted here.
How long does it take:	Time frame: Time to initiate project, usually 1 hour (1 HT session).
Life span of the plant:	This can range from a month to a season, or years to generations.
Size:	How much space will this take? Small scale project is equal to a 4 inch pot or less. A medium scale project is equal to a 6 inch or 1 gallon pot. A large scale project means this is a big project and may not fit on the average windowsill. Often a small or medium project will grow into a large, or very large, specimen plant with time.

Activities:

These are the projects that can be done while waiting for the plants to grow. They are designed to serve as conversation starters and memory triggers. Many of these focus on creative containers or learning experiences.

Quizzes:

These are mostly trivia. These are designed to be fun as they provide conversation starters and memory triggers. These are NOT tests.

Stories:

These are included to entertain, to provoke thought, amuse, inspire and encourage the sharing of the stories each of us carries within ourselves. We are all storytellers at heart, and we all have great stories to tell. Sharing stories has been a part of the human experience from the cave entrance to the dinner table.

As you go through these projects, meet new green friends, and perhaps start an informal 'Green Thumb Club,' take time to laugh, share memories and ideas, enjoy the companionship of both the garden and fellow gardeners. This is what life is really about, smiles, laughter, friendship, sharing and learning.

Thrift Store Shopping Spree
Found Containers

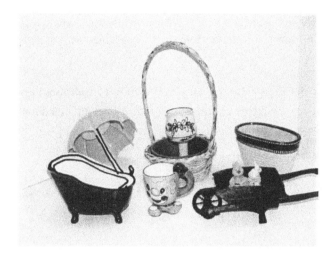

Gerald has muscular dystrophy. This means he has limited stamina and frequently lacks the strength to engage in much activity, but this disease has not put the brakes on his creative energy, or affected his warped sense of humor. During one of our horticultural therapy sessions the mission was to go through the closet and find a whimsical container for a windowsill plant. He found an old tin Jack-in-the-box. After carefully removing Jack he filled it with soil and planted several ivy cuttings. They rooted quickly and were soon clambering over the edge and across the windowsill as they enjoyed their place in the sun. He joked, "It's important to think outside the Jack-in-the-box, and that's what my ivy is doing."

Growing plants in small spaces is one of life's simple pleasures, but sometimes we can literally grow out of the box as we cultivate true whimsy on the windowsill.

Objective:
To create whimsy and stimulate the imagination by using found or discovered planters.

There is an unlimited diversity in what we can use as a home for our plants. Almost anything that will hold soil can be used. Some will last longer than others, but we are creating moments not eternities. Baskets, shoes, old hats, coconut shells, plastic buckets, pots and pans, garbage cans, bird feeders, cups and coffee mugs all work, and that's only the beginning. After selecting the appropriate, or in some cases inappropriate container there is unlimited opportunity to trim, paint, decorate, customize and make this a truly uniquely your own work of art. Raid the junk drawer and button box, rummage through stored Christmas decorations, yesterday's collections, and whatever else can be found for stuff that makes a statement. Set the imagination free and see what happens.

It is best to use a container that permits some drainage, but, with careful watering, coffee mugs, ceramic planters, glass containers, etc will work well. As an example carrots, radishes, beets and peanuts growing against the edge of a clear glass or plastic container filled with a quality potting soil can provide a window on the world of roots.

A large plastic tote or laundry basket makes an inexpensive and efficient container for really big plants. Suggestion, rather than drilling holes in the bottom of these plastic containers, drill a series of 1/4" holes around the sides about 2" from the bottom. Fill the bottom of the container with stone chips or gravel and you have a built in water reservoir.

Closets, attics, thrift shops and yard sales are all sources of non-traditional containers that can be used in windowsill gardening. This can be a true exercise in creativity, as well as a source of memory stimulation.

Materials needed:
A container selected for its uniqueness
Uniquely yours decorations
Waterproof craft glue
aquarium gravel
crushed charcoal (untreated with any kind of fire-starter)
High quality potting mix
A warped sense of humor, the more off the wall the better
Seeds or cuttings that are appropriate for the container
A saucer, tray or other shallow container that will protect the windowsill from water stains

Putting it all together:
Where space is limited to the windowsill, a whimsy container can add much to the project. It's one of the ways we can empower the gardener as we brighten the garden. Each participant can chose the container that they find to be either fun or fitting.
1. Select the container appropriate for the plants being used. As an example miniature African violets will grow quite well in a coffee mug, as long as they aren't over watered.
2. Decorate, customize, be artistic with paint, junk, clippings, whatever you choose.
2. If there are no holes in the bottom for drainage and it is a container that is difficult to drill a hole into, place about ½" of aquarium gravel in the bottom of this makeshift container.
3. A small amount of crushed aquarium charcoal can be sprinkled on the gravel. This will help to prevent sour soil and the growth of soil borne organisms in the event over watering occurs.
4. Fill the container with potting soil.
5. Plant seeds or strike cuttings and water lightly.
6. Colorful gravel, plastic figures, silk flowers or any whimsical item can be added as the final touch.

Variations on a theme:
- These Thrift Store Gardens can be used as a fund raiser and the money donated to a charity or to fund a field trip for the participants
- They can be used as table decorations for a special event in the cafeteria or dining room.
- Participants can experiment with different plants, different soils
- Participants can have a "Pot Party" and show off their personally selected or created planters and pots.
- Participants can paint, decorate and customize their containers.

- Participants can share stories about the containers they are using.
- Memories can be triggered and moments shared.
- These containers can be reused if they outlive the plants.

This can be a great intergenerational project

Kyle, a shy young fellow of nine, chose a plastic model of a vintage 30's pickup truck he had assembled some time ago to bring to an intergenerational program at a nearby assisted living center. This gave Denny, his 83 year old "grandfriend," an opportunity to discuss his childhood during the great depression. Together they decided to fill the bed of this model truck with soil, plant lettuce seeds and see if they would grow. The seeds sprouted and they laughingly referred to this as "our truck garden."

Bernice had been a quilter all her life. When the two eight year old girls adopted her as an honorary Grandma they went to her box of scraps. They rummaged through , swapped stories, snipped and glued their way into a unique line of *"quilted flower pots"* that they actually sold to local gift shops.

Remember that this is supposed to be a fun project and the plants may only last a couple months. The creative container decor may also last only a short time, but we aren't creating art for the ages, we are making moments of joy. This is an opportunity to try something else when that time comes.

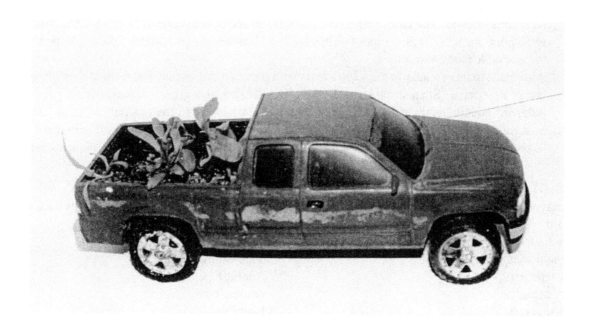

Aloe vera

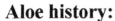

Aloe, *Aloe vera (and many other varieties)*
Lily family, *Liliaceae*
Native to Africa, now global
All parts safe
Rating: Very easy
Time frame: approximately 1 hour to initiate the project
Life span: Aloe will continue to grow for years
Size: Small scale project

Aloe history:

The ALOE holds a special place in the history of the people-plant connection. It may well have been the first plant humans used as a medicinal herb. It was growing in the Olduvai and the Great Rift Valley of Africa over a million years ago. The inside of the leaves contains a gel that has soothing and anti-bacterial properties. This makes it valuable as a treatment for sunburn, insect bites, rashes, burns and wounds.

- ✔ Because of this anti-bacterial quality it was a part of the embalmer's art in ancient Egypt. There are records of its use over 4000 years ago. Aloe plants lined the paths to temples and tombs because they symbolized everlasting life.
- ✔ Both Egypt's Cleopatra and France's Josephine used aloe gel as an anti-aging cream.
- ✔ It is mentioned several times in the Bible. In John 19, verses 39 & 40 Nicodemus brought a mixture of myrrh and aloes to wrap the body of Jesus.
- ✔ Aloe caused a war. Alexander the Great invaded and seized the island of Socotra in the Indian Ocean to obtain control of the aloe supply. Thus he could heal his troops and deny the opposition access to this valuable medical resource.
- ✔ Aloe came to this country in the 1700's and was a part of many herbal and medicinal gardens. It was one of the twelve "Spanish Mission Herbs." The Shakers also grew it extensively.
- ✔ After the atomic bombs were dropped on Japan aloe was used to treat radiation burns. Americans brought this plant back to the United States and it became a popular windowsill herb again.
- ✔ Today research is progressing in the use of aloe in the control of some cancers, diabetes and AIDS.

Uses of aloe:

This may well be the third most versatile herb known (after garlic and the chile pepper). It has been used for:

sunburn	Burns and scalds
stomach ulcers	Jellyfish stings
stinging nettles, poison ivy	Tree wound dressing
insect repellent	Rabbit repellent
beauty cream	Athlete's foot
dish-pan hands	Hair loss
animal wounds and injuries	Mosquito, fire ant, flea & tick bites

In many parts of the world the aloe leaves are used as lunch or dinner. It should be noted that some are allergic to aloe when taken internally, but usually not when used on the skin.

Materials needed:

An empty plastic 4 oz or larger plastic aloe cream jar, or container of your choosing or design.
Sufficient quality potting mix to fill the jar. You can add some play sand to the soil for a happier aloe.
1 to 3 aloe pups
Drill or punch to make drainage hole in the bottom of the jar
A sunny windowsill
A saucer or tray to put the container on to protect the windowsill

Putting it all together:

✿   Wash the jar and drill or punch a hole in the bottom for drainage, or water very carefully.
✿   Fill your chosen container with soil.
✿   Place the "pups" in the soil so that they are stable but not too deep or they may suffer crown rot.
✿   Water only when dry until well rooted and new leaves are forming.

Care & Feeding of Your Aloe

There are several hundred varieties of aloe, some grow into tree like plants over 5 feet tall, some are minute, some form vast mats or clumps. They are a succulent plant requiring little water and they are able to stand lots of abuse. They will blossom and the flower spikes can be several feet tall in colors ranging from yellow to orange or red.

Light: Aloes can grow in full sun, but they do quite well in filtered light or light shade. In full sun the leaves will show protective colorations and sometimes sunburn. Indoor they need to be in a sunny window for best results.

Soil: This is an adaptable plant that will take sandy soil, poor soil or a high quality potting soil. The important thing to remember is that it must be loose and well drained.

Water: This is a desert plant, but it is adaptable. It can accept evenly moist soil, but will rot out if kept soggy. The soil can become completely dry between watering with no ill effects.

Cold: Every plant has its weakness. The aloe doesn't like freezing weather. It will also rot out if there is a combination of cool temperatures and wet, soggy soil. A light frost will do minimal damage if the soil is dry. The key is to not over water.

Containers: Aloes work well in almost any container where there is good drainage. We have seen them growing in coffee cups and ceramic bowls, but watering has to be done carefully if this is the case. Note that aloes can be combined with other succulents and cacti to make a desert garden in a large pot or tray.

Feeding: They do best on a limited diet. Overfeeding can lead to weak growth prone to fungus disease. A weak solution of Miracle-Gro once every couple months is usually sufficient.

Problems: Very few insects think of the aloe as dinner. The biggest problems are from overwatering.

Propagation: Aloes form clumps or mounds by producing plantlets called pups at the soil line. Remove these pups from a mound and plant with the stem end in contact with soil.

African Violets in a Deli Tray

African Violets, *Saintpaulia ionantha*
African violet family, *Gesneriaceae*
Native to East African tropical forests
All parts safe
Rating: Easy
Time factor: less that 1 hour to set up. Four to six weeks for first results. Started plants will grow for years.
Size: Small to medium scale. Great group project.

History:

The African violet isn't a true violet but it is from Africa. It's a member of the *Gesneriaceae* family that includes lipstick vine, gloxinia and many other plants with interesting flowers and foliage. It was discovered in Africa by Baron Von Saint Paul-Illaire in the late 1800's and first introduced to Europe in 1894. This was the typical dark purple "old fashioned" violet that sat on Grandma's kitchen windowsill. This plant had a short blooming season that lasted only about two months per year. The plant breeders have now developed a wide variety of colors, leaf patterns, double and pinwheel flowers. There are miniature African violets and trailing varieties as well. The African violet has become one of the most popular house plants because it is easy to grow and the newer varieties will bloom almost all year long. They are adaptable and will tolerate some neglect, but, like people, the better the care the better they will bloom.

Starting new plants:

We all remember Grandma starting African violets from a leaf in a glass of water, or perhaps she struck that leaf in a pot of soil on the windowsill. Oscar Donovan, one of our participants in a horticultural therapy program in an assisted care facility had been a member in good standing of the American African Violet Association for decades. He also grew them commercially in his greenhouse complex. The fact that Oscar had spent most of his adult life in a wheelchair due to a motorcycle accident didn't slow him down one bit. He taught the group a "success guaranteed" method of starting African violets and shared some leaves from several plants he had thriving in his private collection. This is the way he taught us to do it.

Materials needed:

❀ A clear plastic deli or bakery department container, preferably containing cookies or donuts
❀ Sufficient African violet soil to cover the bottom to a depth of about 1 inch
❀ 3 to 12 African violet leaves, each participant can bring some to share.
❀ Sunlight from a north or east facing window, or Filtered light
❀ A dash of optimism
❀ A pinch of hope
❀ A smidgin of confidence

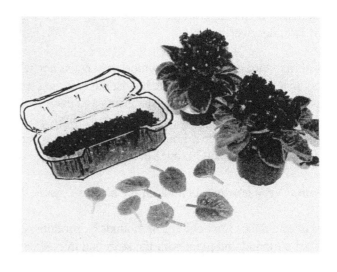

Putting it all together

1. The container needs to be empty. If it's still filled with donuts, cookies, potato salad or any other fresh food, share this with the rest of the group.

2. Wash the container and dry.

3. Fill with moist African violet or high quality potting soil until container is about half full.

4. Trade leaves back and forth within the group so that everyone has a good assortment.

5. Trim the leaf so that there is about 1 inch of stem.

6. Insert into the soil until the soil reaches the point where the stem becomes the leaf.

7. Take a deep breath and blow on the leaves for good luck.

8. Put the lid on the container and mark it with the date, and your name if this is a group project.

9. Place the container on the windowsill.

10. Wait until you see little leaves forming at the soil surface. This means you have roots, shoots and a new plant. The first member of the group to have baby plants gets to supply lemonade for everyone.

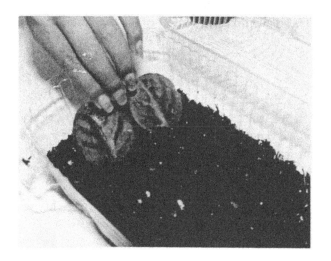

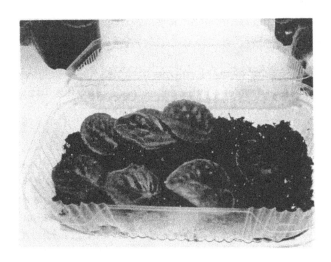

Now the fun begins as each baby plant is in turn plucked from the "Nursery" and potted up in its own planter. As they grow into real little plants they become great gift items. They may start blooming in about three to four months.

What to do while waiting for the roots to grow:

★ Paint clay pots in colorful designs, ready for the new plants.
★ Visit a local thrift store and discover some found containers.
★ Make gift cards.
★ Keep a Garden Journal complete with progress reports, photos, drawings, poetry.
★ Join, or start, an African violet club.

Variations on a theme:

Experiment with different kinds of soils, try rooting hormones on some while other leaves root au naturale.
Try rooting some of the leaves in water and see which method works best.
Try different plant foods, organic versus chemical, and note which performs best.
Have a contest and prize for grower of the first baby plant to burst into bloom.

The Care and Feeding of an African Violet

Light: African violets are at their best in a northern or eastern window. Bright afternoon sun can cause sunburn and a general decline in the plant's vigor. If you only have a southern or western window available a sheer curtain will help to filter the sunlight. African violets do very well under Gro-Lights if no windowsill is available.

Soil: These plants need an African violet soil or a quality potting mix. A cheap or heavy soil can create root problems and diminish bloom.

Water: African violets do best if kept evenly moist but not soggy. Most experts tell you to water them from the bottom by placing the pot in a saucer of water. This works well because the soil does become evenly moist, but they should not be left sitting in a saucer of water for more than an hour or two. Otherwise the soil becomes soggy and the plant's roots may begin to rot. Getting water on the leaves can cause brown spots or the loss of the leaves.

Feeding: There are special fertilizers designed for African violets. Some are time release pellets that feed for months, others are water soluble snack foods. It is best to avoid overfeeding, because this can lead to fungus problems, lanky growth and a decline in bloom.

Containers: Many claim that only clay pots should be used, some insist on using the "double boiler" method with an unglazed pot sitting inside a second container. Others prefer pots with a water wick. Most commercial growers use plastic pots because they are cheaper and lighter weight for shipping. You can use a yarn or cord wick run through one of the holes in the pot and placed in a tray of stones. By keeping the stones moist water is drawn into the pot and the optimum humidity level is maintained. We have seen African violets growing quite well in tea cups, Easter baskets, old sneakers, half a coconut shell and bamboo sections. Use your imagination.

Conversations

Everyone has a favorite African violet. What's yours? Why?
What memories do you have of a African violets from your childhood?
Did you have your own special house plants? What were they?
Do children today grow plants, either indoors or out?
How could we encourage our grandchildren to grow African violets or other plants on the windowsill?

Easter Basket Garden
From Hens & Chicks to Donkey Tails and Rabbit's Feet

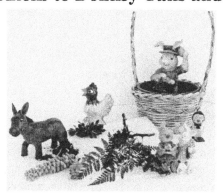

Objective: this is a just for fun project that begins with an old Easter basket, three plants and a healthy sense of humor. The plants were selected for their easy propagation and because one small plant will provide the startings needed for a group. We list three different plants but you can use your collective imaginations and available resources to customize this project as the participants wish.

Hens & Chicks

Hens & Chicks, *Sempervivum,* many varieties
Sedum family, *Crassulaceae*
Native to Europe, varieties found in Africa, Asia and the Americas
All parts safe
Rating: Very easy to grow
Size: 2 to 4 inches, mature plant size

Description:
In Europe this familiar plant is often referred to as house leeks, and it was marketed as artichoke cactus in the early 20th century. The varieties we commonly see are from Europe and are often classified as Alpine plants. There are other related plants found throughout the world. Plant breeders have developed dozens of hybrids with colorful foliage, variegated leaves or bigger and brighter flowers. There is one type of this popular plant that will reach twelve inches or more in diameter, but most are only two or three inches across. They all form perfect rosettes of fleshy leaves, with a whole flock of "chicks" surrounding the "hens."

They produce a flower spike with small almost daisy-like blossoms that can be white, pink, purple or orange. Sempervivums are *monocarpic.* This means that the plant matures, flowers once, then becomes mulch. Don't despair though. By the time they bloom there will be dozens of chicks to take over the growing space. It may take from 1 to 5 years to bloom, depending on growing conditions and variety. One of our favorites is called "Spider web" or "Bird's Nest" (*Sempervivum arachnoideum*). This small hen & chick is covered with fine white hairs that, in the high mountains where it lives, serve as a sun screen. Another variety with dark purple leaves is often seen during the Easter season. It is sometimes sold as "Chocolate Chickens."

In some parts of the world this is considered a "kid's plant," and is given to children to grow on their windowsill. It was a popular parlor and rock garden plant in Victorian England where varieties were traded and shared with house guests as a token of friendship.

Donkey Tail Sedum

Donkey tails, *Sedum morganianum, S. Burrito*
Sedum family, *Crassulaceae*
Native to Mexico & Central America
All parts safe
Rating: Very easy to grow
Size: 4 to 12 inches, mature plant size, sometimes longer

A brief note about donkey tails:

This rugged succulent is also known as Burro's Tail. It's known for its odd fleshy leaves clustered tightly along the pendant stems. The donkey tail is a popular succulent. There are several varieties that vary in coloration or size of leaf. Some will form stems three feet or more in length. This has been popular for several centuries as a rugged and adaptable curiosity. The Burro's tail is a completely safe plant for people and pets. Propagation is from individual leaves or stem cuttings. It has been used in window boxes, as a draping groundcover in large planters and pots and in hanging baskets. This plant is easily started from a fallen leaf or stem section.

Rabbit's Foot Fern

Rabbit's foot fern, *Davalia fejeensis,* and other species
Fern family, *Polypodiaceae*
Native to Pacific Islands and Southeast Asia, some relatives found throughout the tropics
Safe, but some have experienced a skin rash from handling the leaves
Rating: easy

About Rabbit's Foot Ferns:

This fuzzy little plant is also known as Hare's-foot fern or lacy bears-paw. There are varieties with white, brown or black fur on the creeping rhizomes. Close relatives that get somewhat larger are called squirrel's-paw and bear's-paw ferns. Relatives of this plant are found in Africa, the jungles of India and Australia.

The fuzzy rhizomes need to be on the surface so that they can breathe. They are adventurous plants and will even creep out over the edge of the pot. New leaves (fronds) will grow from these fuzzy fingers. This variety will produce leaves between 6 and 12 inches long and the fuzzy rhizomes.

Many varieties of Rabbit's Foot Ferns are deciduous and will gradually drop all their leaves for the winter. Never fear, they will grow new bright shiny green leaves in early spring.

These ferns make friends easily and grow well with the Hens & Chicks and Donkey Tails. They even enjoy the company of African violets, rex begonias, caladiums, carnivorous plants, ti plants and other popular indoor/patio plants. They even make a great ground cover for large indoor planters.

Rabbit's Foot Ferns are easily started from a section of the rhizome with a leaf or two attached. Simply place it on top of the soil and hold it in place with a hairpin, (or you can open a paperclip to make a "U" shaped pin).

Materials needed to plant an Easter Basket Garden:

1 to 3 small "chicks"
1 to 3 stems from the Donkey's Tail
1 starting of a Rabbit's Foot Fern
2 or 3 large pieces of shell from a dyed Easter egg, or any egg shell
1 Easter basket, used, yard sale or thrift store rescue
sufficient aluminum foil to line the inside of the basket
sufficient quality potting soil to fill the basket You can add play sand at the rate of 1 part sand to 4 parts soil
2 TBS aquarium charcoal, or crushed charcoal from the grill that doesn't have starter in it
2 to 6 TBS colored sand or aquarium gravel, at least two different colors
Silk flowers to provide some spring color
An Easter bunny figurine and any other animals you wish to use, including donkeys and chickens
Decor items of your choice; egg shells, plastic eggs, colored stones or small silk flowers
A good imagination
A good sense of humor is helpful

Putting it all together:

1. Line the basket of your choice, with the foil to protect it from moist soil.
2. Place a layer of fine charcoal in the bottom of the bonnet.
3. Add lightly moist soil until it is about 1/4 inch below brim.
4. Using your index finger, three holes near the center of the basket for the array of Easter plants.
5. Place the "Chick" in one of the holes and pack the soil firmly around it.
6. Next place the Donkey's tail and Bunny's foot in the other two holes and press the soil firmly around them.
7. Carefully place egg shells as a part of the whimsy decor.
8. Spread the sand or gravel around with the spoon.
9. Place the decor items and animal figurines around the plants.
10. Set your imagination free and make your Easter basket Garden as whimsical, absurd, outlandish, preposterous or beautiful as you choose.

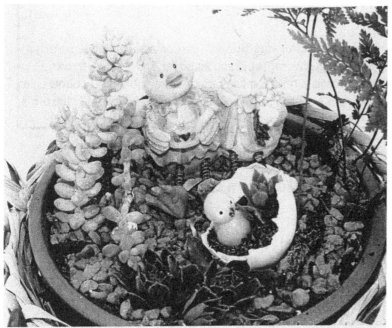
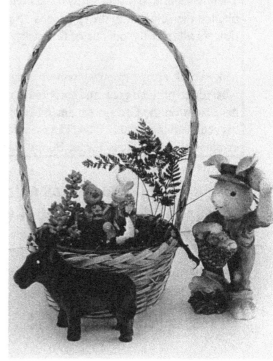

Care & Feeding Your Easter Basket Garden

Light: These plants are at their best when growing on a windowsill where they get at least four hours of direct sunlight. They may get a sunburn with exposure to too much sun.

Soil: A well drained soil like a quality cactus blend is ideal. You can make your own cactus mix by adding I part sand (use coarse builders sand or play sand) to 3 parts potting mix.

Water: These are all tough plants, but they are at their best with lightly moist soil. Soggy soil can cause problems.

Cold: Most varieties of Hens & Chicks are hardy to near zero. But Donkey Tails and Rabbit's foot ferns don't like temperatures below 40 degrees F.

Feeding: They do best on a limited diet. Overfeeding can cause weak growth. If you are using a good soil, you don't need to feed them more than every two months with a weak solution of Miracle-Gro.

Problems: No major insect problems, with these rugged and hardy plants. Most problems arise from over-fussing. The easiest way to kill these "barnyard plants" is by over watering or over feeding.

Notes from the field:

Nolen, a baseball fanatic, used a Braves Baseball cap with miniature baseballs and bats instead of Easter eggs. He used the sand to mark out a baseball diamond and planted a plant at each position.

Stella used craft ribbon to make the handle of her basket a rainbow of spring colors and decorated with sprigs of silk forsythia and brightly colored tulips.

Thelma decorated an old straw basket with pastel silk apple blossom twigs stuck in the soil as trees. She then planted the "chicks" in the egg shells. She chose not to use the ferns and donkey tails. But, she did glue silk flowers all over the outside of the basket.

Mike stuck sprigs of pussy willow around his plastic "Easter Egg Bucket" garden and was quite surprised when three of them grew and sprouted leaves. He used green craft sand and some little toy golfers to complete his Easter on the Green. An annual Easter egg hunt was a tradition he started at the public golf course near his senior living center. The elders would scatter plastic eggs around the course. Then they would take turns dressing in a ridiculous Easter Bunny costume when the children arrived.

Questions a group of young gardeners asked, most of which we couldn't answer.

Where does the Easter Bunny get the eggs?
Santa has reindeer, but how does the Easter Bunny get around?
What is the Easter Bunny's name?
Is the Easter Bunny a boy or a girl?
Do we really have to eat all those Easter eggs?

Bashful's Plant, Snow White and the Other Dwarfs

Also known as Sensitive Plant, Action Plant, Shame Me, Live & Die, Humble Plant & Touch-Me-Not
Sensitive plant, *Mimosa pudica*
Bean family, *Fabaceae*
Native to South & Central America
All parts safe, except for the small spines at the leaf nodes
Rating: Easy
Time frame: from seed to sprout 14 to 21 days, first touch response about 6 to 8 weeks
Life span: considered an annual, but have had it thrive on the windowsill for 2 - 3 years.
Size: Small to medium scale

A Discovery in Disney World:

The elderly gentleman in the wheelchair had been parked at the corner of the raised bed sensory garden. This was at the Opportunity Garden, the American Horticultural Therapy Association's showcase for EPCOT's International Flower & Garden Festival. The family had brought him to this paradise in central Florida, then left him in the shade of the Erythrina trees and the beauty of the flowers while they went off to experience one of this theme park's great attractions.

He looked so sad, sitting there by himself, so frail as he struggled to wipe the drops of perspiration from his brow. As he lowered his hand it brushed against the outstretched leaf of a plant growing in a container at the corner of the raised bed. It folded its leaflets and then the leaf stalk drooped against the stem. With great effort and a good deal of curiosity he reached out with a single aged and arthritic finger. Cautiously he touched another leaf. It too promptly folded itself into little more than a drooping stem. Again, with a blend of curiosity and caution he touched another leaf, then another, and still another. In a matter of minutes he had touched every leaf on the plant, and every leaf was folded so that the plant looked dead. He had a broad smile on his face as he studied the plant and watched the leaves slowly unfold and regain their rightful place in the sun. A small child wandered by. The elderly gentleman waved to him and touched one of the leaves. The child joined this gentleman and together they touched each leaf again, this time there was laughter as the joy of discovery was shared.

The child's mother appeared at the walkway and scolded the child for talking to strangers. She gave the old gentleman an angry look and quickly lead the youngster away. Soon the family returned from the technological marvel of a Disney attraction. The old man pointed to the plant, spoke to his family and touched a leaf. They ignored his comments, failed to share his curiosity and refused to take the time to experience this discovery themselves. They turned the wheelchair around and headed through the crowds toward the next attraction. The smile left the elderly gentleman's face, his eyes half closed and he slumped back into his wheelchair, surrendering to his mobile prison. Perhaps he was able to carry the memory of his discovery of this bashful plant with him. Perhaps he could not. Regardless he knew the joy of hands-on discovery, the thrill of the moment, the opportunity to be engaged, the simple pleasure of play.

More than you ever wanted to know about the sensitive plant:

This botanical plaything is a Sensitive Plant, the popular weed that folds its leaflets when touched lightly, and when tapped vigorously collapses the leaf stalk against the plant's stem. We marvel at this defensive mechanism. The folding of the leaf at the slightest touch protects it from grazing animals. The folded leaf reveals the small spines that are a not to gentle warning that this isn't a great snack.

If you want to get technical this botanical response to touch is called *thigmonasty*. This is not a common part of a typical plant's activity, but it is what makes a gourd's tendrils grasp and wrap around something that it touches. The Venus Flytrap has a more rapid response to being touched but, unlike a defense against being eaten, the Flytrap's movement is designed to catch lunch.

Because the leaves seem to turn away in shame when approached it is called "Shame Me" or "Shame Plant" in the Caribbean Islands. In fact its botanical name, *pudica*, can be loosely translated as ashamed. In other places it's called "Humble plant," "Shy Plant," and more commonly, "Touch-Me-Not." At Disney World it was referred to as the "Bashful Plant" in honor of one of the most popular dwarfs of Snow White fame.

All over the world it's regarded as a medicinal plant. It's most popular as a soporific, calming frayed nerves or inducing sleep. It is sometimes called "Sleeping Grass." It is said to have antibacterial properties and both crushed leaves and a tea from the leaves and roots are used to cleanse minor wounds. In Panama a rinse with tea made from the leaves is said to prevent baldness. In India this plant has been used in conjunction with several other herbs to treat diabetes.

We were told a story about a bar in Hawaii that kept one of these plants for a very interesting purpose. When it appears that a patron might have consumed too much alcohol and might not be safe driving on the city streets, he is given a sobriety test. The Sensitive plant, called the "alco-meter plant" is placed in front of the patron and he is instructed to touch a leaf. If the leaf folds up it's time to call a cab.

Materials needed:
Seeds for *Mimosa pudica*
A suitable container for a Bashful Plant, equivalent to a four or six inch pot
Snow White and the Seven Dwarfs figurines
Plastic gem stones for the mine
Sufficient quality potting mix to fill the container
A sunny windowsill
A copy of the book, a video or DVD of the Disney film Classic, *Snow White and the Seven Dwarfs*

Putting it all together:
1. Watch the movie, then do the fill-in-the-blanks questionnaire above.
2. Paint, decorate or in some way make the planter distinctly yours and a celebration of great literature and a classic movie for all who are children at heart.
3. Fill the container with your choice of potting mix.
4. Carefully place 6 to 8 seeds on the surface and firm the soil until it is about a ½" below the rim. Then cover with about a 1/4" of soil.
5. Water thoroughly and place in a sunny windowsill.
6. Read the book to a child and have him or her help you locate some whimsy for your chosen container.
7. When the seeds sprout, thin to 2 or 3 plants and keep soil evenly moist but not soggy. It is very important that these baby plants be given the sunniest spot on the windowsill or they will get spindly and die.
8. As this Bashful Plant grows you can place the Bashful dwarf figurine on the soil surface and begin to plant and grow the rest of the cast.

Notes from the field:

One of our Green Thumb Club members planted nine different plants in 4" pots decorated with stickers of each character. She then placed these on a Snow White Tray and placed the figurines around the pots. For the witch she used a puddle of green candle wax and a small witch's hat. We think she was mixing two different stories and that this witch was from the Wizard of Oz. She dismissed this observation with, "A witch is a witch is a witch. It's my garden and I'm doing it my way." She was, of course, right. It is her garden, but we still think her witch was from Oz.

Care & Feeding of Bashful

Light: The more sunlight the better. Bashful enjoys a southern or western windowsill.

Soil: Any reasonably good, well drained potting mix will work.

Water: Bashful enjoys wet feet. You will need to keep the soil evenly moist. When the soil is allowed to go dry Bashful will drop his leaves for good.

Cold: This isn't a freeze tolerant plant and outdoors is considered an annual in temperate climates. On the windowsill it may grow and bloom for several years.

Feeding: A weak solution of Miracle Gro monthly or two feedings of Osmocote annually is sufficient to keep it healthy and blooming.

Problems: The sensitive plant has very few insects and fungus problems. The greatest stress occurs when the soil is allowed to dry out.

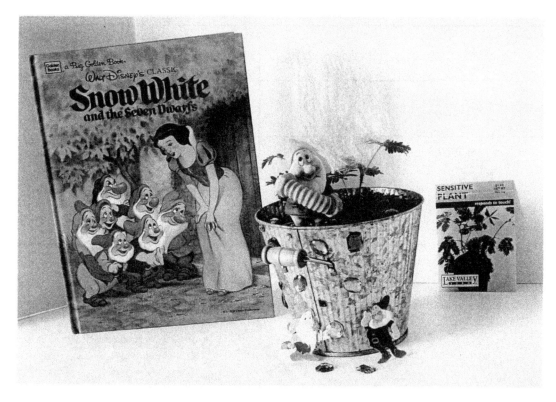

Snow White's Friends, a brief diversion

We are all familiar with the genius of Walt Disney and the story about how he created an whole new art form with the animated movie, Snow White. This sensitive plant is called Bashful's Plant. Let's see if we can come up with a plant for the rest of the cast. First you have to list all seven of the dwarfs. Then select a plant that seems to best symbolize the appearance or character of that individual . Let us know what you come up with.

Snow White Cast Member	Plant that symbolizes that character
Snow White	
Evil Queen, Witch	
Prince Charming	
1. Bashful	*sensitive plant*
2.	
3.	
4.	
5.	
6.	
7.	

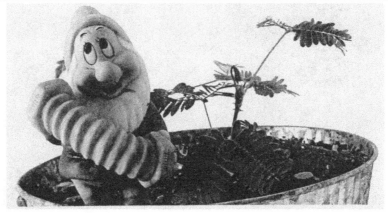

Making a Peace Card

A native American boy was talking with his grandfather.
"What do you think of the world situation?" he asked.
The grandfather replied,
"I feel like two wolves are fighting within my heart.
One is full of anger and hatred.
The other is full of love, forgiveness and peace."
"Which one will win?" asked the boy.
The Grandfather replied, "The one I feed."

Common Olive, *Olea Europa*
Native to the Holy Land and Mediterranean Basin
All parts safe
Rating: easy
Time: approximately 1 hour
Project category: Arts & crafts

As each of us makes our journey through life we encounter others with whom we might have disagreements, form resentments or exchange harsh words. Sometimes we are wronged, sometimes we commit the wrong. Regardless, the time comes to either say, "I'm sorry," or "I forgive." It was once said by one of our horticultural therapy clients in a hospice program, "We should count our success at living by the number of friends we've found, not the enemies we've made."

The following is a little project that can help to promote peace for each of us personally, for communities and perhaps, if enough of us take part, the entire world.

Materials needed:

☺ Paper, your choice of type and color. Handmade paper created by the participant is the best. 8½ x11" is best to work with, but you can use other sizes as well.
☺ Paint, colored markers, even crayons
☺ An olive leaf
☺ An envelope rescued, or borrowed, from a box of cards
☺ One great big loving heart
☺ A compassionate attitude
☺ A vivid imagination
☺ A big smile you are willing to share

Putting it all together:

1. Cut your sheet of paper in half, to produce two pieces 5½ x 8½".
2. Fold one half in half again to form a blank "Peace Card."
3. On the front draw a picture of what you think peace looks like, what symbolizes peace to you.
4. Color, paint, paste, create a collage of pictures from a magazine, use any form of artistic expression with which you are comfortable.

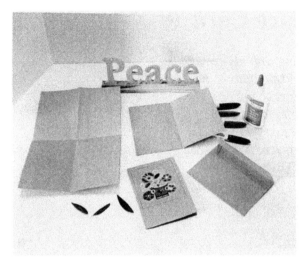
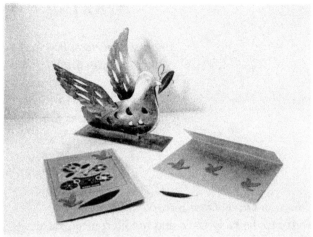

5. On the inside of the first fold of this "Peace Card" write lines of poetry, a quote from a prominent individual or personal thought of your own, verses from your favorite sacred text or other images that come to mind.

6. On the other half of this sheet of paper write a letter to someone that you can apologize to, forgive, accept or in some other way declare peace with.

7. Glue a single olive leaf onto this letter.

8. Be creative with the envelope for your Peace Card and letter. You are making a special, one of a kind, envelope.

9. Feel free to decorate it in any way your wish, then address it to the object of your peaceful sentiments.

10. Mail it with a smile, because you know that you have made a first step toward peace and sent off thoughts of hope.

11. Don't expect a response. You didn't create this Peace Card with the expectation of gain. If there is a response rejoice. If there isn't, know that your heart has been lifted, and your mind filled with peace.

12. Smile, you've done good, and you've done it well.

This is a project that can have a healing affect as a part of an alcohol or drug abuse program, programs for victims of violence and abuse, hospice programs and many others. Variations include the creation of buttons with an olive leaf, a group can create a tree with each olive leaf representing a prayer for peace or an act of kindness. It is empowering to have the participants determine the details of their project.

Olive leaves can be obtained from an olive grove if you live in an area where they are grown, otherwise contact the authors at petals_pages@msn.com for sources.

Conversations:
The following are some questions that came up in several groups doing this project.
1. How does faith affect our concept of peace?
2. How can we start making peace with someone who has wronged us?
3. What do we really mean when we say peace?
4. What are some of the symbols of peace around the world?
5. What would happen in world peace broke out?

Rainbow in a Bottle

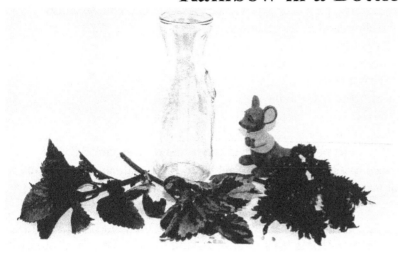

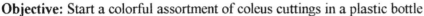

Objective: Start a colorful assortment of coleus cuttings in a plastic bottle

Coleus, *Coleus blumei*
Mint family, *Lamiaceae*
Native to much of the tropics
All parts are safe
Rating: Very easy
Time: 1 hour to initiate project, 3 to 4 weeks until cuttings are ready for potting.
Life span: Coleus are effective for about a season
Size: Small to medium scale project.

Coleus facts:

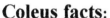

There are over 150 species, and over 500 hybrid varieties of coleus. Some varieties will grow into 3 or 4 ft. mounds of colorful foliage. Coleus leaves can range from green to pink, red, purple and white in dramatic combinations. Some have large leaves exceeding six inches in length while others have leaves less than one inch long. Some have smooth leaves, others are crinkled, some are "duckfoot" shaped and some are thick and fleshy. Coleus can be pinched back (pruned) to keep them from getting leggy. Most varieties are grown for their leaves so the flower spikes are pinched off, but this isn't necessary for the health of the plant. Other varieties are grown for the flower spikes. Some coleus relatives produce a fleshy tuber that can be eaten. One, Hausa Potato, was popular in Africa as a food source. Other close relatives have edible leaves. Do not eat coleus leaves however. They are bitter and the texture is unpleasant in the throat.

Materials needed:

At least three varieties of coleus with varying colors & leaf forms. Cuttings should be 6 to 9 inches in length. A bottle, vase, antique milk bottle or anything else that will hold water. A plastic water, juice or soft drink bottle also works well.
A handful of small stones, (You can use decorative aquarium gravel or sand as well).
Water
A sunny windowsill
A strong appreciation for all the colors of the rainbow

Putting it all together:

1. Clean bottle or container with soap & water, rinse well.   If it has a label you can remove, do so.
2. Carefully place ½ cup of stones, gravel or sand in the container.
3. Fill almost to the top with water.
4. Select three cuttings. These can be assorted for the rainbow affect.
5. Trim leaves from the bottom 3-4 inches of stem.
6. Make a fresh cut on the base of the stem and place in the water.
7. Print your name on a label and put on the side of the container, if this is a group project.
8. Place on a sunny windowsill and excise moderate patience.
9. After roots are well formed the plants can be potted up, three in one 6" pot or in separate 4" pots.
10. As they grow the tops can be trimmed to make the plant full and bushy. The cuttings can be shared with friends, or you can start the process all over again. Tie a ribbon around the bottle of started plants and use as a gift.

Note: While waiting for the cuttings to grow roots be imaginative and design a rainbow decorated container for your coleus' new home. Zelda, one of our Green Thumb Club Members, used metallic glitter paint on a coffee can to make a beautiful "Rainbow planter." Leroy was so intrigued by coleus that he rooted dozens of cuttings and gift planters for each member of the staff at Weldon's Adult Day Camp.

Care & Feeding of Coleus:

Watering: Keep your coleus plants lightly moist. They will do best if they don't go completely dry between waterings. Be certain to water when it starts to wilt. Note: They don't do well in soggy soil either.

Light: Indoors coleus need a sunny windowsill. Outdoors they will thrive in light shade, but there are varieties that enjoy full sun.

Soil: While coleus are adaptable and will grow in almost any soil, they are happiest in a quality potting soil.

Containers: Coleus will suffer from over crowding or being rootbound. To be at their best they will need room to grow a healthy root system. Most varieties will do well in a 6" or 8" (1 gallon) pot. You can also use a decorative planter, bucket, basket or other imaginative container. Some of the trailing types are attractive in hanging baskets.

Feeding: Often we tend to overfeed plants that we are growing in planters. One feeding a month with Miracle-Gro is usually all they need to keep them healthy. Overfeeding can cause a loss of color, weak, spindly growth and increased attack from insects.

Cold weather: They are frost sensitive, but if kept from freezing will last for years.

Pests & Problems: Indoors where the air is very dry coleus will often be attacked by spider mites. You will see the fine webs and the leaves will begin to loose their vivid color and look dull with a salt and pepper dotting of yellow spots. Outdoors the biggest problem is mealy bugs. These appear as cotton-like dots on the underside of the leaf or where the leaf joins onto the stem. These pests can be removed with a moist Q-Tip.

Cactus Spines

Cactus fascinate us. First of all because, they often look weird, but beyond that, we are intrigued by their defensive armor and their incredibly beautiful flowers. They are called succulents, a term that means the plant has adapted to a dry climate by devising ways to store moisture or control moisture loss through its leaves. Many cacti have done this by discarding leaves altogether in favor of a swollen stem. They also produce a waxy protective coating that slows the loss of water through these stems. For some cacti the spines are so dense they help to generate some shade from a sun that can be intense. These are relatively easy plants to grow if we are willing to satisfy a few of their basic needs: light, moisture, proper soil mix, appropriate temperate and a feeding schedule that matches their growth cycle.

Let's see how well you can do with this prickly little cactus quiz

1. TRUE or FALSE. All cactus are desert plants.

2. TRUE or FALSE. Most cactus come from the deserts of Africa.

3. TRUE or FALSE. All cactus have spines.

4. TRUE or FALSE. Nothing eats a cactus.

5. TRUE or FALSE. The "Yellow Rose of Texas" is a cactus flower, not a patented rose recognized by the American Rose Society.

6. TRUE or FALSE. The "jumping cactus" of the Arizona deserts is capable of shooting its spines into anyone who gets within four to six inches of the plant.

7. TRUE or FALSE. The desert "Loco weed" is a poisonous cactus whose spines are hollow and work like rattlesnake's fangs when anyone touches against them.

8. TRUE or FALSE. The pads of prickly pear cactus are both edible and nutritious.

9. TRUE or FALSE. The Christmas cactus isn't a true cactus and is actually closely related to the poinsettia.

10. TRUE or FALSE. The hallucinogenic plant called peyote cactus is really a mushroom.

Answers to the quiz: *1- F, some cacti are native to tropical jungles,   2 - F, all cacti are from the New World,   3- F, some have soft hairlike spines, others have no spines at all,   4- F, turtles, some insects and even cattle, sheep and goats will dine on young cacti,   5- T or F(Legend says it referred to a mistress who distracted Santa Anna during the Battle of San Juacinto in the Texas War for Independence. Many experts insist that it refers to a cactus flower. There is now a patented Yellow Rose of Texas). 6-F, no cactus is capable of "shooting" its spines, although it sometimes feels like it. 7-F, the locoweed is a member of the legume or bean family. 8-T, the "nopalitos" also seem to be beneficial for diabetics, and they taste good too. 9-F, the Christmas cactus is a true cactus and calls the jungles of Mexico, Central and South America home. It's not even a distant cousin to the Poinsettia. 10-F, peyote is a true cactus.*

Olé, a Fiesta Garden

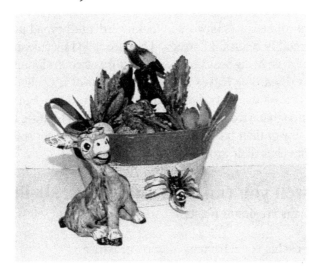

Assorted succulent plants from several plant families
Native to the arid lands of planet Earth
Most are safe, some have spines, some *euphorbias* may cause skin irritation
Rating: Moderately easy
Time factor: two 1 hour session on two different days; one to prepare the garden and one to plant it
Size: Medium size project

Most cacti have spines and this can be a hazzard, or at least uncomfortable. We suggest that great care be taken when handling these plants, but roses also have thorns and we take the necessary precautions and enjoy them. There are many other succulents that don't have spines. See the suggestions below.

Materials needed:

1 six or eight inch terra cotta saucer, or cereal bowl (some have used old cookie tins)
Sufficient cactus soil to fill this saucer
1 cup of Fine gravel or coarse sand (Can use play sand, but not beach sand)
"Uniquely yours" desert decor such as:
      Unusual rocks, stones, crystals, or other symbols of the desert
      A small piece of driftwood or weathered root from a tree or shrub
      Pieces of broken pottery or perhaps an arrowhead
      Miniature birds, animals, toy snakes & lizards, a burro, wagon wheels, etc.
Craft paint textured with sand. You can add the sand or use the ready-mixed paints.
3 to 5 desert cactus or other succulent plants
Dwarf Marigold seeds
Tongs to handle the spiny cactus
A CD of Flamenco music
Mild salsa and some nachos
A sunny windowsill
A vivid imagination and a memory of the great western movies, The Cisco Kid or Carmen Miranda.

Suggested "finger friendly" cacti and succulents for your desert garden:

Hens & Chicks, use the chicks for your garden
Kalanchoes, many varieties, most start easily from cuttings
Jade Plants, several varieties to chose from, all start easily from cuttings
Burro's Tails, start from cuttings
Panda Plant, has soft fuzzy leaves, start from cuttings
Christmas Cactus, start from cuttings
Old Man Cactus, use a young plant
Elephant Bush, a portulaca shrub from Africa, easily started from cuttings
Bishop's Cap, use a baby plant
Living Stones, use baby plants, lots of light and very little water
Aloe Vera, plant the pups (offsets)
Ice Plant, many varieties, can be started from cuttings, needs lots of light
Portulaca (Moss Rose) a rainbow of colors, easily started form seeds or cuttings. Needs lots of light

Putting it all together:

1. Play the Flamenco music CD and dine on some salsa and nachos, preferably sharing this experience with friends.
2. Paint the outside of the clay saucer, cereal bowl, or more unique container with the sand textured paint. Several colors can be used to create a "Painted Desert" effect. Now let it dry well.
3. While the paint is drying gardeners can share more salsa and chips.
4. They can also be collecting or selecting their own unique "desert decor."
5. Fill the saucer with the cactus soil (or good potting soil with coarse sand added) to about ½" from the rim.
6. Place the plants or cuttings you have chosen for your mini-desert landscape. If you are using cacti with sharp spines, use the tongs to position them. It is best to limit the garden to 3 to 5 plants. Too many plants in this small space will crowd out each other, and the garden looks more like a jungle than a desert.
7. Cover the surface of the soil with coarse sand or colorful aquarium gravel to help create the desert image.
8. Place your rocks, crystals and other specially chosen desert decor where you want it.
9. Optional: In a paint cup dilute some white glue with water (equal parts) and spread over the sand or gravel, gluing your decor in place. This helps to hold every-thing in place and keep the garden looking fresh.
10. While you are waiting for the glue to dry, try to remember the name of the Cisco Kid's sidekick

Why the Marigolds?

In the early 1500's a Spanish priest/botanist accompanied the conquistadores on their exploration of Mexico. He gathered the seeds of many plants including a medicinal plant that he called "Mary's Gold" in honor of the Virgin Mary. As the Catholic religion took hold in the new world this flower was adopted for the celebration of "Dia de los Muertos" the day of the dead celebrated on Nov. 1st.

The original inhabitants decorated their homes with flowers of all kinds and colors during the "festival of flowers." One of their favorites was the marigold, which was called *zempasuchil*. The role of the marigold in the celebration of the Dia de los Muertos continues today. It is a tradition throughout Latin America. We can plant these marigold seeds in September and have them in bloom by the end of October.

On a sunny windowsill the marigold will provide color for your cactus garden for a two or three months. This is a short lived annual plant and will produce seeds then fade away. You can dine on the bright colored petals of this flower and the leaves have ben used as a seasoning in soups and stews by both the Native Americans and the Hispanic settlers.

A few creative examples of Fiesta Gardens:

We have seen some truly imaginative deserts created by some of our Green Thumb Club members. Johnny found a little bird's nest in a box of craft stuff and several plastic turtles and lizards. The nest was placed in the Jade plant and the lizards and turtle was placed under and beside the other plants.

Lisa scattered chia seeds (from an abandoned Chia Pet) in a cluster of stones on about half of her desert and grew a mini-forest of this blue flowering sage.

Maria Rosera, with her youth group, created a landscape in a large baking dish complete with wall built from hand formed miniature adobe bricks, and a plastic burro that had once been a part of a Nativity set.

Jose, a student in a drug abuse center, carved a Sphinx and a pyramid from soap and planted areca palm seedlings around his mini-oasis.

One intergenerational program had the elders and youths create desert scenes then held a "flower show" open to the public. The gardens were sold as a fund raiser and the ribbons were awarded to the best entries. We were told that every participant took part in the pizza party.

One group of elders chose a plastic chip & dip tray shaped like a sombrero as their planter. They did such a great job that they were asked to create several more to serve as centerpieces in the dining room.

The potential is limited only by the creative mind and the time & materials available. Have fun. Remember, the choice of plant material, decor and whimsy is up to you. Play, experiment, set your mind and hands free.

The Care and Feeding of Fiesta Garden

Handling plants with spines

The best way to handle small cacti is with a small pair of kitchen tongs.

Using folded newspaper is another way. Many use gloves. Tough gardeners use their bare hands, but usually only the first time.

Keep a roll of masking tape handy. If you get spines in your fingers or hands gently place a piece over the area where the spines are and peel off. If this doesn't work you can gently apply hand lotion, Crisco or liquid soap. Don't rub, let the lubricant work the spines out.

It is advisable to replant most cactus every two or three years. Many texts say annually, but this isn't essential.

Turning the planter monthly will help to keep growth symmetrical.

Light: Not all cacti and succulents were designed by Mamma Nature to grow in full sun. It's our responsibility to learn as much as possible about the plants in our care. Too much direct sun can cause sunburn. Insufficient light can cause *etiolation* (the thin weak growth desperately seeking light). Indoors a southern or western window is good, but a northern or eastern one also works for many succulents.

Soil: The ideal potting soil for cacti and most other succulents is one or two parts highest quality potting soil and one part coarse builder's sand. Don't use beach sand. One of our Green Thumb Club members insists that she can grow cactus best when she adds crushed egg shells to the soil.

Watering: This is the single most critical consideration. You have to decide whether the goal is to have the plant survive or thrive. Because these plants are rugged they will take months of neglect but the following schedule will encourage more bloom, better growth and a longer life. Most cacti and succulents are at their best when the soil is almost dry between waterings. A dormant period from November through December helps to harden the summer's growth. Water the first of Nov. Water again the first of Dec. If you are growing marigolds you can keep the soil moist but not soggy for best results.

Feeding your desert: Many growers use a liquid balanced fertilizer like Peters 8-8-8 or Miracle-Gro every six to eight weeks. Slow release fertilizers can also be used and should be applied once a year.

Pests: There are only a few pests that attack these plants, and they are easy to control. Scale and mealy bugs on cacti and most succulents can be controlled with mist Q-Tips or alcohol swabs. Note that extensive use of alcohol can destroy the natural protective coating on the leaves and stems.

Cactus precautions:

While some cactus contain hallucinogenic drugs called *mescalins* (Peyote as an example) few cactus are considered poisonous. But bacteria can cling to the spines and cause an infection if puncture wounds aren't washed well. Many succulents in the Euphorbia family, like the pencil cactus, do contain a milky sap that is toxic. Some can cause a skin rash from contact, other are a problem only if ingested.

Cactus resources

http://www.aridlands.com/ **Lots of information on a wide variety of cacti and succulents**
http://www.shoalcreeksucculents.com/ **These people grow and sell some very rare and unusual plants. They also provide a good deal of information**
http://www.cssainc.org/ **The Cacti and Succulent Society of America is a treasure trove of information**
http://www.succulent-plant.com/ **A wealth of information on succulent plants form all over the world**

Cactus for dinner:

You might not expect to find a cactus on your dinner plate, but South of the Border it's not uncommon fare. There are both cactus pads and fruit for your dining pleasure. If there are folks in your group or Green Thumb Club with a Hispanic heritage they may be able to share some recipes for these delightful and nutritious fruits.

Tunas, that's what we call the fruit of the Opuntia (prickly pear cactus). Try sampling the cactus fruit called tunas, available at most produce counters. These *tunas* or *pears* can be eaten raw, used in cooking or made into a delightful jelly. Native Americans dried them for use during the winter and some people living in the deserts make a delicious drink from the juice of this fruit. The fruit of the many other cacti are also edible, some are fleshy, some bitter, others mealy.

Nopales or **nopalitos** are another nutritious cactus treat. These cactus pads can be found in the produce department of many grocery stores. These take some preparation before eating. You have to remove the spines then they can be eaten raw, roasted, baked, fried or added to a variety of dishes. You can also find these

Nopales in jars in the Hispanic foods section of your favorite supermarket. They are quite tasty and can be eaten in a salad, added to pasta dishes, diced and used to top baked potatoes and the potential is unlimited. Don't hesitate to sample this delightful and uncommon food.

Tequila, may not be considered a health food but it is a part of many fiestas. Agave is the source of tequila, a good topic of discussion, with or without samples.

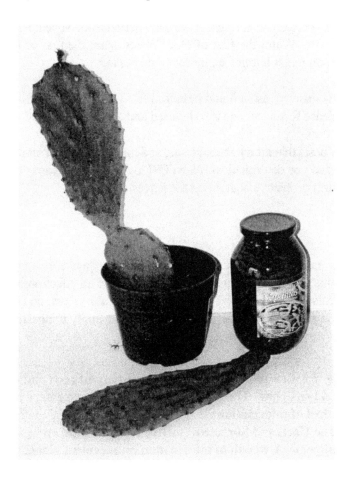

Digging deeper:
Compile a list of Mexican flowers: include marigolds, dahlias, Poinsettias and Christmas cactus
Make some of the colorful tissue paper flowers that brighten so many Hispanic homes
www.michaels.com/art/online/ProjectPrint?width-80&pid-e02913

The Legend of the Creator's Smile

Many years ago, in a small village along the Amazon River, a little girl lived with her grandmother and grandfather. In this village there was much fighting, yelling, anger and sadness. Few of the people in this village ever smiled. Even fewer were willing to help each other. This little girl was sad herself because of all the unhappiness that everyone else carried with them.

Her name was Florita. She would walk the jungle trails with her grandparents to gather avocados, herbs, and the roots of yams and sweet potatoes. She would help Grandfather gather firewood and tie the palm fronds on the roof to keep the rain out. She would help cook the meals and sew the clothes and weave the baskets. As Grandmother grew older and her arthritic hands hurt more and more, Florita would do more and more of the cooking. As Grandfather grew older his eyes grew cloudy and he could no longer weave the stories into the baskets, so Florita became a very good basket maker. Even with all the unhappiness in the village these three were happy together and in the evening Grandmother would tell stories around the fire, and Grandfather would play his bamboo flute and they would all sing the songs about beauty and harmony.

One of the songs Florita learned was about a bright red flower that bloomed in the trees. Grandmother told her this was a gift from the Creator, a message to the people about what was truly of value. The song told about a plant that healed no illness, nor was it good to eat. But it had great value because it celebrated beauty. In this song the Creator told the people that this flower would only be found high in the trees, and only those seeking peace and happiness could see it. The beauty of these flowers would heal an unhappy heart, replace anger with joy and turn enemies into friends. It was said that when peace came to live in everyone's heart all would then share the beauty.

"The beauty of the flowers is said to be the smile of the Creator," Grandfather said.

Florita asked, "What does this beautiful flower look like?"

Grandmother shook her head, the sparkle gone from her eyes. "I have never seen one. I guess the Creator has never smiled on me." She was wringing her arthritic hands as she spoke, and her smile disappeared.

Florita turned to Grandfather, "Have you ever seen this flower?"

Grandfather looked down, his clouded eyes gazing into the flames. "No, and with these eyes, I never will." and his smile was gone as well.

Their sadness troubled Florita. She left the fire and went to the home of the medicine man. "Have you ever seen the flower in this song, *The Smile of the Creator*?" She asked the old man who was hanging bundles of herbs from the beams that supported the roof of his home.

"Once when I was a child," he answered as he smiled down at Florita. "I was angry with my brother and had run into the jungle to hunt. Soon I felt sorry for what I had said, but didn't know how to put the words back into my mouth. A bright green parrot flew in front of me and led my eyes high into the trees. There I saw it."

"What did it look like?" she asked.

"It was too high for me to see it well, but a strange thing happened. The parrot flew into this huge plant growing high in the tree and broke loose a piece of the stem, a piece covered with bright red flowers, and dropped it down to me. I couldn't help but smile as I saw it falling closer and closer to me. I ran to stand under it and catch it before it hit the ground. I studied the flat stems and the strange, most beautiful flower I had ever seen. My first thought was, 'I must show this to my brother.' I forgot that I was angry with him. I clutched the flowers to my heart and ran all the way back to the village. We both smiled and all anger was gone. That evening we sang the song of the flower for all the people. Many others demanded to see where it grew. We went out day after day, but never saw it again."

"Then you can't tell me where I can get the flower for Grandmother and Grandfather?" she asked.

"No Child, I wish I could, but it is very rare."

She returned to her grandparents home, retired to her sleeping mat and tried to sleep, but through all the darkness of night she saw many kinds of flowers, all colors and all shapes dancing in her head. Finally, just before sunrise, before Grandfather fed the wood to the fire, she was outside the doorway selecting just the right basket to take with her into the jungle. She had an idea, but even as she took the first steps toward the trail and away from the village, she was afraid. She feared the night jungle and she feared that she would fail.

She started down the trail leading east. She was far from the village when the sun rose to greet her. She said her prayer to the rising sun and just as the last words of thanks for a new day were released a brightly colored parrot flew from the trees toward the sun. "Follow me," it said, and she ran as fast as she could. The parrot led her deeper and deeper into the jungle, deeper than she had ever been before.

Finally, the parrot disappeared into an enormous, ancient tree covered in moss and vines. High up in this tree she could see a mass of red and green. In her heart she knew this was the flower she was seeking. She could see the parrot sitting in the cluster of color, adding her beauty to the flowers. Then she began to tear stems from the massive plant and drop them down to Florita. One by one they fell gently into her arms. She carefully placed each one into the basket. Then she would run to catch the next piece of pure beauty released by the parrot. Soon the basket was full and she was exhausted. Clutching the last stem to her heart she fell asleep, with her head on the basket, and a smile on her lips.

The voice in her head began to speak to her. The voice sounded like the parrot, and this is what it spoke, "Take these flowers back to your village and plant one branch at the door to each home there. Your neighbors will begin to work together and they will build a big fire. Everyone will bring food to share and it will be a grand feast, The Feast of the Creator's Smile. Your Grandmother and Grandfather will sing the song and you will teach everyone how to care for this beautiful plant, but it will only grow if each person cares for the plant of another, not their own."

"Why?" Florita asked the parrot.

"Because, you are tending the Creator's Smile, and this is a great gift. A smile is only of value if it is given away. Smiles are also like infants. They need to be nurtured and cared for. If this is done then everyone will have many smiles growing at their doorways. These flowers, these smiles, will be a greeting to all who pass, and an invitation to enter and visit."

Florita awoke, smiled at the flower in her hand and placed the headband of the basket on her forehead. For an instant she was afraid she was lost, but there was the parrot sitting on a stump waiting for her, waiting to lead her home.

It was late in the afternoon when she returned with her basket filled with the flowers called the Creator's Smile. All the arguing stopped as she knelt by the doorway of Grandmother and Grandfather. She planted the first stem of flowers there, just as the parrot had instructed her to do. Grandmother knelt down and with hands no longer pained by the arthritis of age helped her granddaughter plant. She gave a beautiful smile to her granddaughter.

Grandfather held the flower close to his clouded eyes and the clouds cleared and he could see the beauty, and he also gave a beautiful smile to his granddaughter.

As Florita, Grandmother and Grandfather went from home to home, doorway to doorway planting, others in the village began to help. Soon there was laughter and happiness where once there had been anger, fear and fighting. The entire village was filled with smiles, all a reflection of the Creator's Smile that had before the sun set that day turned every home into a warm and inviting place filled with happiness, and a sense of peace they had not known for many years. Now everyone could see these beautiful flowers and share the peace and happiness. The feast was good, there was much singing and dancing, and more smiles than stars in the heavens were shared that night. And ever after each person cared for their neighbors flower and nurtured their neighbors' smiles.

And, that is the story of the flower we know as the Christmas cactus, known to the people of this village from another place and time as the Creator's Smile as it was shared with me. May your Christmas cactus also be the Creator's Smile and may it be the gift of peace to you this season and forever.

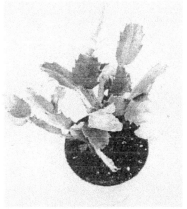

Christmas Cactus, Growing Fond Memories

Christmas cactus, *Schlumbergera Bridgesii* & others
Family, *Cactaceae*
Native to Mexico, Central and South America
All parts safe
Rating: easy
Time frame: Start cuttings in June for bloom by Christmas
Life span: Christmas cactus can be a part of the family for generations
Size: Small size project for the first year or two, plant will eventually mound to 8 to 12 inches.

History of the Christmas Cactus:

These are true cacti and they can be found growing in the trees of the tropical jungles of Central and South America as semi-epiphytic plants much like many orchids and bromeliads. This family of plants is rugged, with cousins that bloom at various times of the year. Often this bloom cycle matches a popular holiday, such as Christmas (of course), and Thanksgiving, Easter or Mother's Day.

This was a favored Christmas plant long before it was cool to have Poinsettias. Your Christmas cactus is absolutely safe, has no spines, is non-toxic and not harmful to pets and small children. It will continue to grow and live for years, often being handed down from generation to generation. They will spread to six feet or more in diameter and develop stems like tree trunks with bark on them as they age. Many of us have memories of Grandma's Christmas cactus, and wonderful stories to tell as well.

It propagates easily from cuttings, even when in bud, inserted into slightly moist soil. This is a plant that is easy to hybridize and many new varieties have been developed in the past 30 years. We now have a wide range of colors, blooming periods, and forms to choose from. Many of these newer varieties will grow and flower without all the fussing that was necessary with some of the originals.

Care instructions once included precise temperature controls, limiting the light by locking the plant in a closet, withholding water, special feeding, and a host of activities to trick the poor thing into blooming. Not so today. They are easy to encourage into bloom, are fun to grow and are quite durable. They willingly tolerate a good deal of neglect. In fact most Christmas cactus that don't survive are "fussed to death."

Materials needed:

3 to 5 cuttings (about 3 to 6 inches long) from different plants that have been in the family or belonged to friends. If there are no traditional plants available for cuttings, start a new tradition with a newly acquired Christmas cactus. Cuttings can be shared if this is a group project.
A Christmas cookie tin or coffee can with paper label removed
Sufficient potting mix to fill the container
Photos of family members, and yourself
Clip art from last year's Christmas cards
Craft paint
Craft sealer, waterproof, like Mod-Podge

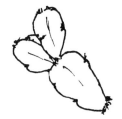

Putting it all together:

1. Take cuttings that look like a letter "Y." Let the cuttings dry for 1 to 3 days.
2. Punch or drill several drainage holes in the bottom of your chosen container.
3. While the cuttings are curing you can decorate the container by painting and/or gluing the photos or clippings onto it.
4. Waterproof it with the sealer and let dry.
5. Fill your chosen container with the soil mix. A mixture of 3 parts quality potting soil and 1 part coarse sand works very well.
6. Insert cuttings in the soil mix so that at least half of the bottom joint is in the soil.
7. Let soil mix go almost dry between waterings.

You will know that the new plants have roots when new sections of stem begin to grow at the ends of the original joints.

The Care and Feeding of a Christmas Cactus

Light - Outdoors it thrives in medium shade, indoors it's at its best in a sunny window. Too much bright sun can cause bleaching or sunburn.

Water - This is a tropical plant, not a desert plant. It likes to be kept lightly moist, but not saturated. Don't keep it sitting in a saucer of water, and avoid subjecting it to prolonged periods of drought. They can be outdoors under a tree for most of the year without any special care. It can be drier during the winter months.

Cold weather - These plants call the tropics home and shudder at the thought of a frost, or even temperatures below 40° F.

Humidity - Christmas cactus enjoy the same relative humidity people do, about 30%-40%, but can handle much higher humidity levels in warm weather.

Soil mix - A high quality potting soil is best. Some experts add some sand, and this can help prevent root rot. We have seen some great results with prepared African violet soil and cactus mixes.

Containers - The important factor in a container is that there be provision for good drainage. Some prefer clay pots, but Christmas cactus thrive in plastic containers and hanging baskets, even metal buckets will work well. Be creative and use found containers, just for the whimsy.

Feeding - You can use a ½ strength solution of Miracle-gro once a month during the active growing season or apply Osmocote for flowering plants twice a year. The important thing is to not over feed.

Problems - Over watering is the biggest problem. There are few insect pests.

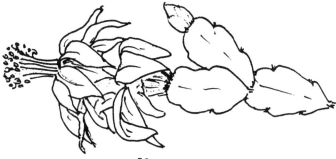

Botanical Big Game Hunters

It may sound like science fiction, but it's a fact, there really are plants that hunt, kill and eat animals. In fact there are over 500 species if insect-eating (carnivorous) plants that employ the most ingenious and diabolical methods of trapping their prey. Let's see how well you can separate the science fact from the science fiction about these fascinating plants. Simply circle FACT or FICTION for each of the statements below.

1. **FACT or FICTION**   A tiny, rootless, carnivorous plant floats about in the water and captures microscopic aquatic animals.

2. **FACT or FICTION**   Almost all carnivorous plants, the most highly developed of all plants, are members of the orchid family.

3. **FACT or FICTION**   In Australia a gigantic species of Venus flytrap has been known to catch and seriously injure small children, although no deaths have been documented.

4. **FACT or FICTION**   The exotic pitcher plant produces hollow leaves that contain acids similar to the gastric juices produced by the human body.

5. **FACT or FICTION**   Each leaf of the Venus flytrap is equipped with a set of triggering hairs. The leaf will spring shut only if these hairs are touched in a certain way.

6. **FACT or FICTION**   One type of sundew grows so large that people hang the leaves in windows to serve as organic fly paper.

7. **FACT or FICTION**   Many carnivorous plants produce fragrances, perfumes and scents to lure insects. The poor insect is expecting a romantic dinner and finds out that he is the main course.

8. **FACT or FICTION**   In Malaysia there are several species of unusual insect-eating plants that are not rooted to one place. They are capable of slithering through muck, mud or moss to locate nests of ants or termites.

9. **FACT or FICTION**   Lizards, frogs and praying mantis use carnivorous plants as restaurants. The plant traps lunch and these critters enjoy the meal.

10. **FACT or FICTION**   A carnivorous plant exists that never produces a leaf and rarely sees the light of day. It literally lassoes, then poisons and devours its prey.

Answers to Botanical Big Game Hunters:

1. **FACT**, The rootless bladderwort serenely floats about near the surface of its swamp water home. Its stems are covered with minute bladders that trap minute water animals for lunch.

2. **FICTION**, There are no flesh-eating orchids.

3. **FICTION**, If you missed this one you have been watching too many bad sci-fi movies.

4. **FACT**, Some pitcher plants are patient and wait for their victims to decay; others actually digest them.

5. **FACT**, There must be at least two contacts made; either two different hairs or the same hair twice. These contacts must be made within moments of each other.

6. **FACT**, The peasants in certain areas of Portugal do hang the 6 to 12 inch leaves in the windows to capture flies, mosquitoes and other insects.

7. **FACT**, Most carnivorous plants still depend on insects to pollinate their flowers, thus they use a floral perfume. There is also a fragrance produced in the leafy traps that is inviting to the bugs.

8. **FICTION**, Some bladderworts float about in the water, but no carnivorous plants go hunting for their game.

9. **FACT**, They hide and wait for bugs to come to the plant, then steal the hungry plant's dinner. Sometimes they slip and fall into the pitchers of pitcher plants, becoming a big meal themselves.

10. **FACT**, There are at least fifty species of fungi that trap microscopic nematodes by snaring them with their mycelium.

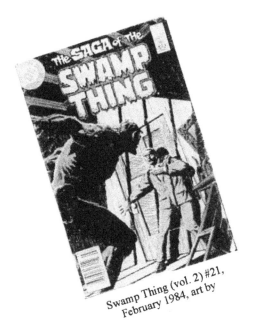

Swamp Thing (vol. 2) #21, February 1984, art by

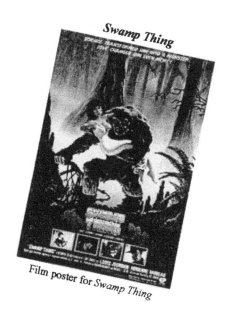

Film poster for *Swamp Thing*

A Flesh Eating Garden of Horrors?

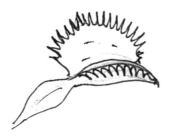

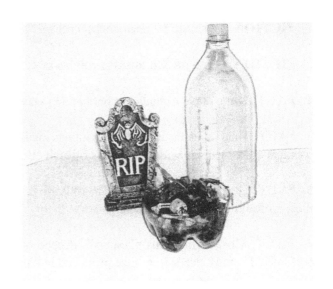

Venus flytrap, *Dionaea muscipula*
Venus flytrap family, *Droseraceae*
Safety factor: All are safe, there are no carnivorous
plants known to dine on people or pets
Rating: Difficult
Time frame: 1 hour to initiate project,
will need to be transplanted in 12 to 18 months
Size: small scale project

Venus flytrap, *Dionaea muscipula*
This native of the Carolina swamps is the most popular of the meat-eating plants. The leaf is composed of two parts that spring shut when two of the three trigger hairs are touched. It doesn't shut tight at first, this allows an insect that is too small, or too large, to escape. After a few seconds the trap is firmly closed and there is no escape. It will open again in 10 or 12 hours if the prey is a stone, twig or other indigestible item. The leaf secretes digestive juices much like your stomach does and the insect is dissolved, except for the skeleton. In a few days the digestive juices are absorbed by the leaf and it opens. When skeleton of the bug dries and blows away the leaf is ready for another meal.

Each plant develops only seven leaves. If you plant grows more than this number then it is multiplying and you now have two plants. They will bloom if they are happy with the care you are providing. The stalk of white or pink flowers may be followed by seeds that will readily sprout if deposited on the moist soil. This is one of those plants that it is impossible to over water. Venus flytraps may go dormant if they are exposed to cool temperatures, or go dry. Often we think they have died and discard them when they are only taking a vacation.

Other hungry plants:
The Venus flytrap isn't the only plant with an appetite for flesh. There are some plants that actually invite insects over for dinner. Of course the insect is the main course. These are known as carnivorous plants and in some places they are so large that they can capture and devour small mammals and birds. The ones we commonly see in the garden center aren't quite that vicious however.

Carnivorous plants belong to a number of plant families and the ability to eat insects and other creatures was learned through eons of evolutionary education. These plants usually grow where the soil is seriously lacking in nutrients, or too acid to be usable. They had to find another way to sustain life. Most of the carnivorous plants are native to bogs and wetlands where usable nitrogen is almost non-existent. These plants are the "Horror of the Dismal Swamp" to the bugs. They include Pitcher Plants, Sundews and many others.

Carnivorous plants aren't easy to grow, but if we can satisfy their basic needs it is possible to keep them quite happy. We can even coax some of them into bloom. You can cut the bottom from a 2 liter plastic bottle and place the bottle over the potted plant to make a mini terrarium for your "Little Shop of Horrors."

They will thrive if you give them:	They will die if:
☺ Lots of humidity	☹ They dry out
☺ Soil that is constantly soggy	☹ They are fed MacDonald's hamburgers
☺ Lots of sunlight	☹ They are handled too much
☺ An even temperature above 45 degrees	☹ They don't get enough light
	☹ They overdose on plant food

Keeping bug eating plants growing:

The best way to grow bug eating plants is in a terrarium sitting on a windowsill. You can make a mini terrarium from a bottle. If you are growing them in a pot it should be kept in a saucer of water so that the soil is always soggy. If they are in a tray filled with stones and water the immediate atmosphere will also be humid enough. Remember, air conditioning dries the air. Don't worry about finding insects for them to eat. There are sufficient nutrients in the soil to maintain the plants.

Materials needed for a flesh eating garden:

Your choice of two or three different carnivorous plants
A clear two litre soft drink bottle
2 or 3 cups of coarse sphagnum moss, or orchid moss (African violet soil also works well)
Skeleton, dried chicken bones or a warning sign for the bugs (you can make the sign yourself)
An old *Swamp Thing* comic book or the *Little Shop of Horrors* movie
A couple small flies or moths, alive

Putting it all together:

1. Read the *Swamp Thing* comic book or watch the *Little Shop of Horrors* movie with friends.
2. While reading or viewing, enjoy a juice or soft drink in a learn plastic bottle.
3. After the movie, wash the bottle well and gather the rest of the materials.
4. Measure up from the bottom on the clear plastic bottle about four inches and cut all the way around.
5. Do not punch drainage holes in the bottom, but do make two one inch slits on the bottom edge of the top section. This makes it easier to place the two sections together.
6. Put about two or three inches of the sphagnum moss in the bottom and moisten well.
7. Position the plants in the moss and place the skeleton, bones or sign near the plants as a warning to the bugs.
8. Place the top over the bottom half to make a mini-terrarium, the ideal home for your flesh eating garden.
9. Chose a good name for your new "Monster Plant."
10. After a week for the plant to feel at home, set the captured insects free in the bottle and replace the cap.

Care & Feeding of your Little Shop of Horrors

Light: Most carnivorous plants do best with a sunny windowsill. A Northern or Eastern exposure works well.

Soil: The coarse sphagnum or orchid moss is generally the best to use for most carnivorous plants, but any porous, soil rich in organic matter will work, including African violet soil.

Water: Your flytrap is a bog plant and cannot be overwatered. They also enjoy high humidity. This is why they are at their best in a terrarium. They can actually survive for over a month underwater.

Temperature: These plants will go dormant if exposed to cool temperatures. Some will go dormant even if they don't get a chill, but be patient.

Feeding: No fertilizers please. Small insects occasionally but nothing too large, and no ants either.

Problems: Unlike most plants, they are quite capable of defending themselves against most insects, except ants. The biggest problems involve dry air, dry soil and feeding with chemical plant foods.

Digging deeper:

Gracie, a green thumb club member, painted window frames on her plastic bottle and glued a sign proclaiming "Little Shop of Horrors" above the door.

Cal downloaded some pictures of monsters from the internet and glued them around the outside of an old 10 gallon aquarium containing an ever increasing variety of botanical big game hunters. His mosters included Dracula, Frankenstein, Godzilla, Hitler and Osuma Bin Laden. This became quite a center of conversation in the lobby of the senior care facility he called home.

Marita glued plastic flies and mosquitoes on the outside of her 2 litre terrarium. She also experimented with sphagnum moss as the growing medium and was quite surprised to fine that it grew and soon she had a carpet of fine green moss surrounding her Venus flytrap.

Landis, a retired science teacher used his pet flytrap, named Audrey, as a prop when he entertained the children that were a weekly part of the intergenerational science club he started at his assisted living center.

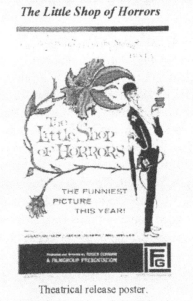

The Little Shop of Horrors

THE FUNNIEST
PICTURE
THIS YEAR!

Theatrical release poster.

A Literary Quiz for Gardeners of All Ages

1. Peter Rabbit was guilty of trespassing and theft when he stole _____ from Mr. MacGregor's garden.

2. Bre'r Rabbit escaped from Bre'r Fox when he said, "Please, Whatever you do, don't throw me in that there _____."

3. In the Dr. Seuss story "The Lorax" the Lorax is trying to save what unusual species of tree? _____

4. What did Jack trade the handful of beans for in Jack & The Beanstalk? _____

5. Charlie Brown waited for Who on Halloween?

_____

6. Little Jack Horner sat in a corner eating his Christmas pie.
   He stuck in his thumb and pulled out a _____,
   And said, "What a good boy am I."

7. Thumbellina went sailing in a _____

8. "Run, run, as fast as you can.
   You can't catch me,
   I'm the _____ _____

9. In Alice in Wonderland the Walrus told a tale of _____ and kings.

10. In the Disney version of the popular fairy tale, Cinderella rode to the ball in a coach the fairy godmother made from a _____

Answers:
1. Carrots,   2. Briar patch,   3. Truffella trees,   4. The family cow,   5. The Great Pumpkin,
6. Plum,   7. Pea pod,   8. Gingerbread man,   9. Cabbages,   10. Pumpkin

The Botanical Zoo

Many of the plants we know and love, and even some of those we aren't too fond of, have for one reason or another acquired animal names. Sometimes this is because of a similarity to a given animal such as soft and fuzzy textured Lambs Ears. Sometimes it is because the plant is considered a part of the animal's diet, such as the common Pigweed. Sometimes it's a matter of myth and legend such as the Snake plant, otherwise known as sansevieria. Let's see how well you can do on this little quiz about plants with animal names.

1. A flowering plant in the lily family common to the Rocky Mountains is known as _____ grass.

2. A medicinal herb, food source and sometimes ornamental shrub is known as the Chinese _____ berry.

3. A very popular flowering plant is called snap _____.

4. A plant that was thought to discourage a certain common pest is known as _____ bane.

5. Geraniums produce a distinctive seed pod that gives them another common name, the _____ bill.

6. A variety of tomato that produces a large irregularly shaped fruit is the _____.

7. Some crested varieties of the brightly colored celosia are called _____.

8. Many members of the Goosefoot (Chenopodium family) are nutritious and delicious, but some consider them weeds. You may know these easy to grow vegetables as _____ quarters.

9. A native wild flower of the forests is sometimes called Dog-Tooth Violet, but it is also known as the _____ lily.

10. A popular house plant for hanging baskets that produces numerous 'leggy' offspring is commonly known as the _____ plant.

11. A plant that produces cute and colorful flowers that some think look like tiny mischievous faces is Mimulus. It is sometimes called _____ flower.

12. A fern that produces fuzzy creeping rhizomes and fine, lacy leaves is commonly known as _____ _____ fern.

13. The Calathea produces large colorful leaves, giving it the common name _____ plant.

14. A member of the grape family grown as an indoor hanging basket plant is often called _____ ivy.

15. Aphelandra produces yellow flower spikes and green and white striped leaves, giving it the common name _____ plant.

Bonus: A foul smelling though edible swamp plant common throughout much of North America is known as _____ cabbage.

Answers: 1. Bear, 2. Wolf, 3. Dragon, 4. Flea, 5. Crane's, 6. Beefsteak, 7. Cockscomb, 8. Lambs 9. Trout, 10. Spider, 11. Monkey, 12. Rabbit's foot, 13. Peacock, 14. Kangeroo, 15. Zebra, Bonus, *Skunk*

Behold the Mighty Dandelion

You are invited, she said
to a party, to meet people, unfamiliar and new.
Will there be food? I asked.
Yes, was her reply. My specialty, my own, my original, dandelion stew.
I could not decline the invitation
to meet unknown friends and taste uncommon foods too. Anon

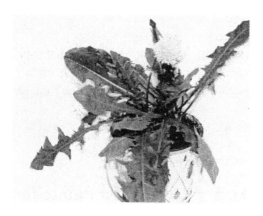

You can shock your friends by growing Dandelions on Your Windowsill.

Dandelion, Botanical, *Taraxacum officinale*

Daisy family, *Asteraceae*

Safety factor: All parts are safe, some even nutritious

Rating: Almost too easy

Time frame: 1 hour to initiate project, will need to be transplanted in 12 to 18 months

Size: Small size project

The dandelion is among the most hated of plants, yet it isn't poisonous and has no thorns. In fact, it's a healthy food source, and has been the universal toy of childhood for uncounted generations. Let's take a new look at this despised plant. Throughout history the dandelion has been there for the joy and amusement of children of all ages. It has been a traditional and versatile toy that has an A1 safety rating, is inexpensive and available almost everywhere. It provides nutritious spring greens and has been used as a medicinal herb to treat a wide range of ailments. It's such an effective diuretic that in the British Isles it's called "pissabed."

Materials needed:

A playful attitude and a sense of humor

A container of your choice equivalent to a four inch pot

Sufficient potting mix to fill the container

1 dandelion seedhead that you have collected from the wild, or seeds purchased from a mail order catalog

A magnifying glass

1 clear plastic sandwich bag

A sunny windowsill

Friends of all ages, must be willing to play, and a camera to make a photo record

Getting started:

1. On a beautiful morning set out on a quest for a dandelion seedhead, filled with parachutes ready to launch into the wind. Take a friend, the magnifying glass and sandwich bag with you on this backyard safari.
2. Observe the intricate structure of this seedhead and note the way the parachute is designed to carry the seed. This is great engineering and a work of art as well.
3. Carefully collect the seeds and place in the clear plastic bag.
4. Fill the container of your choice with the potting mix.
5. Carefully place between 10 and 15 dandelion seeds on the surface and press into the soil, then cover with about 1/4" of soil or decorative colored sand.
6. The seeds will sprout in about two weeks
7. As the plants are growing you can do research by asking friends what they used to do with dandelions. We have provided a starter list, but this is only the beginning. The rest is up to you.
8. As the tender new leaves begin to grow they can be harvested, one from each plant, and added to a salad or added to a pot of cooked greens.
9. In about two or three months from sprouting the dandelion plants will give you the first flower buds.

Care & Feeding of a dandelion

Light: The more light the better. Put this plant in the sunniest window, or move outdoors after seeds sprout.

Soil: For a dandelion almost any soil will do, but of course, the better the soil the better the plants will be.

Water: Keep evenly moist for best growth and tenderest leaves.

Feeding: Any plant food will work, but don't overdo it.

Problems: Insufficient light will produce spindly, weak leaves and no flowers. Just a note of interest, the popular Wooly Bear caterpillar does enjoy dining on dandelions. You can place your dandelion plant and a young Wooly Bear in a large pickle jar terrarium and watch them both grow.

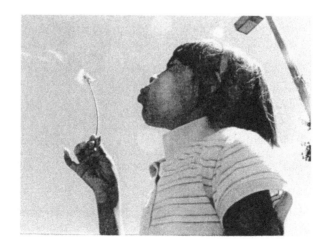

The Dandelion, Universal Toy of Childhood

When Melissa and Eddie were young they lived in a small house in the older part of town. The roof bowed under the weight of years and the white paint was flaking from the warped siding. Mama tended a garden in the back yard to put food on the table while Papa worked two jobs to keep the rent paid. This was a poor neighborhood, but the kids still had a lot of fun. It was in the early fifties, before color TV, and long before computers, video games and all the electronic entertainment we have today. Melissa and Eddie lived in a house without even a black & white TV, but they did enjoy the family radio. These two children didn't have much in the way of store bought toys, never saw the Sears & Roebuck Christmas catalog and only once had they set foot in the Gimbles Department in downtown Pittsburgh.

But they had fun, lots of fun. They played games, used their imaginations, invented their own entertainment, and they read books from the B. F. Jones Memorial Library. One Sunday afternoon in late May the lilac bushes were just opening the first of their tiny lavender flowers. The perfume from these first lilacs of spring spread over the entire yard. This was an event with special meaning because Mama had this rule, "When the first lilacs bloom you can go barefoot."

They had just finished helping their parents plant the seeds for beans, squash and cucumbers in the garden. Melissa picked a couple of the bright yellow dandelion flowers blooming against the fence. She noticed the yellow pollen on her fingers and playfully dabbed the flower against the back of Eddie's shirt. Soon they were both wearing yellow polka-dot clothing and even had yellow dots on their faces, arms and hands.

This is the way one of the best afternoons the whole family had ever enjoyed began. Mama gave the children a pan and sent them out to pick as many dandelion flowers as they could find. When they asked her what she was going to do with them she answered, "It's a surprise." and would tell them nothing more.

They soon returned with a pan overflowing with the bright yellow blossoms. Mama led them into the kitchen where they washed them while she gathered a lemon, some brown sugar, some corn starch, and milk. They wanted to know what she was making but she still wouldn't answer. She stirred the cornstarch and water on the stove until is was almost boiling. Then she added the sugar and as much juice as she could squeeze from the lemon. Soon she removed the pan from the burner and began picking the dandelion flowers from the towel where they had been placed after they had been washed. She pinched off the stem as close to the flower as she could then carefully dropped each one into the sauce. Melissa and Eddie took turns stirring until almost all of the dandelions were in the pan.

Melissa finally asked, "Are we making dandelion pudding?"

Mama smiled as she placed the pan in the fridge and put the last handful of flowers in a bowl of cold water. In about an hour they were all sitting on the back porch enjoying Mama's Dandelion Pudding. She explained that you can also make dandelion soup, dandelion ice cubes, dandelion blossom tea and candied dandelions.

After the last of the dandelion pudding was licked from the spoons Papa led them all into the backyard, just beyond the garden to the fence where they had picked the flowers. He carefully selected a bud with a long stem and plucked it from the plant. He then made a loop with the stem end, so that it looked much like a lasso. The bud was several inches from this loop. He aimed it at Eddie and pulled real fast. The bud popped off and flew through the air, hitting Eddie in the stomach. All four of them spent the next half hour firing their dandelion cannons at each other. Finally, there were no more buds to be found. But they did have a piles of stems all over the yard.

"Let's see how long a chain we can make," Mama said as she showed them how to make a loop out of a dandelion stem.

Within minutes they were taking turns adding links to their dandelion chain. Soon it reached from the rocking chair on the porch to the gate just beyond the garden and back again. Everyone agreed that this was the longest dandelion chain ever. The Guiness Book of World Record wasn't around then, but if it had been, they would have been in it.

Eddie picked up one of the largest stems and put it to his mouth. When he blew through it is made a whistling sound. He could coax a wide range of tones from this dandelion flute by pinching the end with his fingers.

Papa reached down and picked a leaf from one of the biggest dandelion plants and cupped his hands. When he blew across the leaf it made a strange rasping sound. Soon everyone was experimenting with different stem lengths, and large and small leaves. Before long they had a Dandelion Band. The neighbors came over to see what all the noise was, and they joined in too.

Old Mr. Janeki from the house on the other side came over and told them how he used to make coffee from dried and roasted dandelion roots. Mrs. Bernelli showed Mama how to boil the leaves twice to get rid of the bitter taste and then mix them with bacon and onions for a delicious meal. Soon other neighbors were dropping by and they all shared their favorite ways to eat, or play, with dandelions. It was agreed that they would all get together next Saturday afternoon and have a dandelion party.

It was so much fun. They shared dandelion blossom iced tea which they drank with dandelion straws. Two people made dandelion soup, Mr. Concelli brought his churn and the kids helped him make some home-made dandelion ice cream. Others brought batter fried dandelion flowers and leaves for salads and dandelions cooked with spinach. Dandelion fritters and several kinds of dandelion candy were also shared. The kids all invented new dandelion games, made all sorts of dandelion toys, made intricate dandelion braids and several kids worked together to create a giant portrait of a dandelion, made completely from dandelion flowers, stems and leaves.

It was so much fun that they made it an annual Dandelion Party. The entire neighborhood got together and shared special foods, games and dandelion toys. The children even made up a dandelion song.

Share the fun

Dandelions grow all over the country and we call them weeds, but they are delicious, nutritious and can be made into a multitude of toys. If you have a good dandelion story to share, or know of a use for the dandelion that might be of interest to others please send it to us at petals_pages@msn.com

A Little Coconut Quiz

The coconut is one of the most popular foods in the world and is the most widely grown palm. This symbol of the tropics provides a nutritious fruit and a flavorful liquid called coconut water (sometimes referred to as coconut milk). It's the source of a valuable oil used in food preparation, soaps, shampoo, cosmetics and even the manufacturing of paints.

1. TRUE or FALSE. The liquid inside an immature coconut is sterile and contains a natural sugar, making it a healthy, refreshing drink.

2. TRUE of FALSE. In some parts of Africa cutting down a coconut tree was once considered murder.

3. TRUE or FALSE. The smoke from burning coconut husks is considered a natural mosquito repellent.

4. TRUE or FALSE. Coconut husks have been used to make cigarette filters.

5. TRUE or FALSE. On the islands of Polynesia dried coconut fibers are shredded and used to stuff pillows and mattresses.

6. TRUE or FALSE. Sap from the fruiting stem of the coconut is used to produce an alcoholic beverage called *arrack*.

7. TRUE or FALSE. Coconut palm trunks have been hollowed out to make canoes.

8. The coconut, in various parts of the tropics is referred to as is:
(a) the tree of abundance,   (b) the tree of life, (c) The tree from heaven.

9. TRUE or FALSE. Copra, the dried flesh of the coconut is the source of cocaine ?

10. TRUE or FALSE. One of the rarest gemstones in the world is the famous "coconut pearl" which forms within the wall of a coconut shell.

Answers are on page 65

A Garden on the Half Shell, Coconut Shell, That Is

Coconut, *Cocos nucifera*
Palm family, *Arecacea*
Possibly originated in Africa or Western Pacific, now pan-tropical
All parts safe, fruit and sap are edible
Rating: easy, hand dexterity required, but no lifting or detail work is required.
Time: two sessions of an hour each to make this planter. It will last for about 3 years.
Size: Medium size project

Materials needed:

1 coconut with husk removed, available from the tree or your local supermarket
a drill to make a hole to drain the coconut water
1 glass to hold the water for tasting and sampling
a saw to cut the shell in half
sufficient potting soil to fill one half shell
water-proof wood glue, although some have used Super Glue
1 to 3 areca palm seedlings to plant in the planter, or you may substitute your favorite tropical plant

Putting it all together:

1. Select your coconut and wash with warm water.
2. Drill a 1/4" hole in one end of the coconut to drain the coconut water.
3. Drain the water into the glass, add ice cubes and sample. Share some with a friend.
4. Cut the coconut in half with the saw. Be careful with this part of the project.
5. Wash the two halves and scrape out the coconut to sample and share, or use in a cooking project.
6. Use the saw to cut the end off of one of the halves so that the other half will set in it.
7. Glue the planter half into the base half and let glue dry for at least 24 hrs.
8. Paint or trim the planter using craft items at hand.
9. Fill with soil.
10. Plant the areca palm seedlings, or plant of your choice.

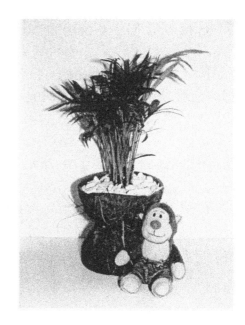

Variations on a theme:

1. Paint, decorate, be creative with the coconut planter. You can use beads, pearls, ribbon, macrame cord, twine or whatever else is available.
2. Make a hanging basket out of the half shell by drilling three holes around the edge and using twine or heavy string to make the hanger. You can also make a macrame hanger for it.
3. See the project on page 166 "Put the Lime in the Coconut and Call Me in the Morning"

Starting a coconut from seed

You can start a coconut palm from seed as a group or individual project. Yes, this is a big seed, but all it takes is a big pot and a whole lot of patience.

1. Start with a fresh coconut, preferably with the husk still intact and a three to five gallon nursery pot.

2. Fill pot about 2/3 full of good sandy topsoil.

3. Place coconut, husk and all on its side in the pot.

4. Fill with soil until only the top 1/3 of the coconut is above the soil surface.

5. Keep moist and wait. . . . It takes from 3 to 6 months for the coconut to sprout. But, its worth the wait.

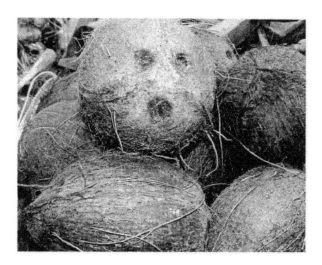

Answers to A Little Coconut Quiz:

1. TRUE In fact, this coconut water, or milk, was used by field surgeons during WWII as an intravenous glucose solution when the medical preparation wasn't available.

2. TRUE

3. TRUE, and yes, it does work. In the Phillippines people will "bathe" in the smoke before going where mosquitoes are prevalent.

4. TRUE, the husk is burned without oxygen to produce porous activated charcoal that is used in the production of some gas masks, cigarette filters, aquarium filters, and filters to remove radioactive particles in the air at nuclear power plants.

5. TRUE, When shredded the fiber has resilience and makes a good stuffing material for cushions, pillows, furniture and mattresses.

6. TRUE, this sweet sap is used to produce a coarse sugar, wine, vinegar and coconut beer. When fermented and distilled, the alcoholic beverage is called Arrack.

7. TRUE. The trunk is also cut into lumber for building, furniture and fence posts.

8. A, B & C. It is known by all three names plus many more.

9. FALSE, copra is the dried flesh of the coconut and is used as food, the source of coconut oil, and to manufacture cosmetics, medicines and many food items ranging from ice cream to cookies.

10. Maybe TRUE, maybe FALSE. There is no scientific proof of a coconut producing a pearl and there is nothing within the coconut that matches the chemical composition of a pearl. Yet, there are collectors of rare and exotic gem stones that claim to have the incredibly rare coconut pearl.

Coffee Plantation on the Windowsill

"Strong coffee, much strong coffee, is what awakens me." Napoleon Bonaparte

Coffee, *Coffea arabica*
Gardenia family, *Rubiaceae*
Native to East Africa and the Arabian peninsula
All parts safe, seeds contain caffeine (will keep you awake for the rest of the project)
Rating: easy project for everyone
Time: 1 hour to initiate, Will grow for years and bloom in 3 to 5 years, a long time to wait for a cup of coffee.
Life span: Coffee trees can thrive for years, but will need a larger container every 3 or 4 years.
Size: Small scale project in the beginning, but can eventually grow into a large scale project.

A Cup of Coffee Trivia

1. At one time, ground coffee was smoked in a special pipe to ease breathing difficulties.
2. Women in some parts of Europe were, in the 16th century, forbidden the pleasure of a good cup of coffee because it was believed to make them irritability or moody.
3. Approximately 450 million cups of coffee are consumed in the United States every day.
4. Coffee is in the same family as gardenias and the quinine tree.
5. Caffeine is on the International Olympic Committee's list of prohibited substances.

Coffee Culture:

The ripe beans were chewed by prehistoric African hunters to keep themselves alert during the hunt, and probably late night poker games around the campfire. To date there is little scientific evidence of this poker pastime, but we suspect that the Leakeys are working on it. They also made a tasty fermented drink from the coffee beans. The archaeologists claim this is a great way to relax after a hard day at the dig.

It was the beverage of choice in "Merry Ole England" years before tea found its way from the Orient to London's drawing rooms. By the 1650's, coffee houses were the favorite hangouts of the intellectual crowd. Ideas, lofty thoughts and creative inspiration flowed so freely that these drinking establishments were commonly referred to as "penny universities," the price of a cup of coffee then. This was obviously before the Starbucks era.

Coffee was forbidden by the Medieval church as the drink of the devil, but it remained popular with the philosophical and intellectual elite who enjoyed and respected the stimulating effect coffee has on the mind. It was even recommended medicinally for everything from allergies to depression. It's used today as an antidote for some poisons, to ease some breathing difficulties and enhance the effect on certain pain killers.

Growing Your Own Windowsill Coffee Plantation

The coffee plant is both attractive and easy to grow. In climates where frost warnings are never a part of the local weather forecast, it can be grown as a landscape plant reaching 8' to 15' in height. For those of us who shovel snow for winter time exercise, it is better treated as a magnificent house plant, pruned to a size that suits the space and decor. It's quite happy outdoors during warm months. Your pet coffee tree enjoys moderate shade outdoors or a sunny window indoors.

Materials needed:

4. 1 coffee mug filled with freshly brewed coffee
5. 1 empty coffee mug, carefully selected from a yard sale, thrift store or closet. Choose one that you find beautiful, humorous or cheap.
6. Sufficient moist potting soil to fill your coffee mug. Don't use the cheap soil found at you friendly neighborhood discount store. That stuff is an insult to weeds and hardens into adobe bricks.
7. 1 teaspoon of crushed charcoal, if using charcoal from the grill, make certain it doesn't have any fire starter or additives in it. These can kill your plants.
8. 1 to 3 coffee seedlings, or green, unroasted coffee beans.
9. A deep appreciation for a fine cup of coffee, decaf or regular

Putting it all together:

1. Take a sip from your cup filled with coffee, to put you in the mood for this project.
2. Mix the charcoal thoroughly into the soil.
3. Take another sip of your coffee. You have earned it by mixing the soil.
4. Fill the other coffee mug, the one without the coffee in it, with the soil you mixed so well.
5. Now take another sip of coffee and meditate for a moment to prepare yourself mentally for the next step.
6A. If you are using seeds, evenly space three seeds and press into the soil to a depth approximately twice the thickness of the seed. Cover the seeds well, wipe your hands on your shirt and have another sip of coffee to celebrate a job well done.
6B. If you are using seedlings it gets a lot more complicated so perhaps you had better have another sip before starting. Good, now you seem ready to proceed. Raise your right hand (can substitute the left if you insist) and hold up your thumb. Now rotate your hand so that the thumb is pointing down. Then press that thumb as deeply into the soil as you can. This makes a suitable hole for your seedling to occupy. If you are planting 2 or more seedlings you can either make the hole larger and plant them all together, or you can make separate holes. Then put the seedlings in the hole and pack the soil firmly around them.
7. Have another sip of coffee, then add about two tablespoons of water to the coffee mug containing the plants or seeds, not the one you are drinking from.
8. You have successfully completed this project. Sit back and enjoy whatever is left of the cup of coffee that you have been sipping throughout this process.
9. You can now show off your new coffee plantation, or at least the seedbed for the above mentioned plantation, to your friends, neighbors, family or total strangers.
10. Have another cup of the fine stuff you brewed and invite the acquaintance or acquaintances from step 9 to have a cup with you and share some conversation.

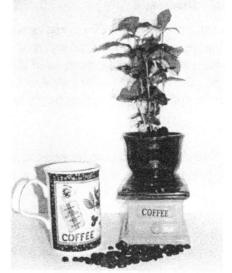

67

Coffee notes

Coffee plants do best in a coarse, compost rich soil that is kept evenly moist.

Frequent feedings with your favorite organic fertilizer during the warm months will keep your coffee plant happy and healthy. If you aren't an organic gardener, then feel free to use your favorite balanced chemical house plant food. After all, it seems only right that, when growing your drug of choice, you make that plant chemically dependent too.

Don't hesitate to prune, trim and shape the coffee plant as it's growing. This makes it fuller and encourages more flowers. If you look closely at the commercials on TV, you will notice that even Juan Valdez carries a pair of pruning shears as he roams his mountainside plantation.

The bright, shiny, dark green leaves make this an attractive and dramatic specimen indoors or on the patio. Having a coffee tree in your living room makes a great subject for after dinner conversation. Warning! You will be asked, "Can you really grow coffee beans on that thing?" The answer is, "You betcha." After years of care and nurturing through sickness and health; if you have led a good life and achieved harmony with the universe, you may find clusters of fragrant creamy-white flowers on your pet coffee tree some morning. Incidently, the highly fragrant flowers form all along the stems.

These flowers, if pollinated, are followed by "berries" or "cherries" that usually contain two seeds each. When ripe these berries are red, the pulpy husk can be removed and the beans dried. Then you need to roast them in the oven before you can reach for the coffee maker. Sure, it's easier to purchase a bag or coffee from the local supermarket, but there's a real thrill in sipping a cup of the stuff you grew yourself.

Digging Deeper:

Don Francisco Coffee has a great web site with some interesting facts about the history of coffee, coffee terms, coffee recipes and much more. **http://www.don-francisco.com** The following is from their web site and makes an interesting springboard for discussion. Sit back, enjoy a cup of your favorite coffee and some good conversation.

Alzheimer's Disease:

A recent study at a Dementia Clinic in Lisbon, Portugal concluded that Caffeine intake was associated with a significantly lower risk for Alzheimer's disease. **www.coffeescience.org/alzheimers**

Parkinson's Disease:

Recent studies from the Mayo Clinic, Harvard School of Public Health, U.S. Veterans Administration and other medical centers prove that drinking from 2 to 4 cups of coffee a day may lower the risk of colon cancer (25%), gallstones (45%), cirrhosis of the liver (80%), and Parkinson's disease (50-80%), among other diseases. It can even reduce the incidence of asthma (25%) due to the presence of the chemical *theophylline* in coffee. **www.coffeescience.org/parkinsons**

Diabetes:

A recent US study shows that people who drink several cups of coffee a day can greatly lower their risk of developing diabetes later in life, even if they are overweight. **www.coffeescience.org/diabetes**

Composting Your Problems

We are all familiar with the old line, "When life gives you lemons, make lemonade." Gardeners have a special advantage with life's little problems and annoyances. This simple activity has opened the door to healing for many people of all ages. It isn't a solution, but it is a starting point.

Many of us seem to collect problems. We set them on our mental book shelves, or store them in the closets of our minds, until they become uncontrollable clutter. This is the real monster in the closet. This is the demon that stands before us and tells us we are failures, that we needn't try again because of something that happened in the past. Or perhaps it's the ghost of the future warning us that if we try we might do something wrong, we might fail. It's the scolding finger waved in our faces telling us we can't do something as well as someone else or might not know something we should, so why bother. Perhaps you are troubled by hurt feelings, by the rude or ignorant behavior of someone you know, work with or love. This may be a wound called guilt that won't heal, an obstacle that you can't get past. These are the chains that bind us, hold us back, keep us from trying. We call these chains fear, anger and pain. They keep us from happiness, friendship, emotional freedom. They convince us we are worthless when the truth is we are all priceless.

This little project was first reported to us by a horticultural therapist friend working at a drug rehab center. It has been modified and adapted for numerous venues. We think that it has value in many horticultural therapy programs where clients and staff, family and friends, need to get beyond the conflict, problems, difficulties, hurt feelings, wounded psyches, emotional scars, anger, fear, inertia and all the other burdens that each of us carries with us every day.

Materials needed:
1. 1 or more 3" or 4" clay pots, or containers of your choice
2. a piece of recycled paper
3. a writing implement
4. sufficient quality potting soil to fill your selected container
5. a plant, cutting or seeds that symbolize beauty, peace, joy or forgiveness to you
6. Paint or waterproof markers to customize your clay pot

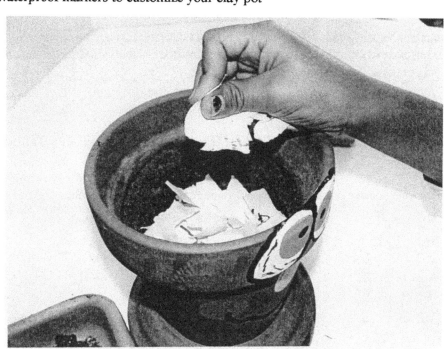

Putting it all together:

1. Place 2 or 3 tablespoons of soil in the pot.
2. Identify your problems, fears, emotional injuries, acts of unkindness, elements of regret, causes of hatred or anger.
3. Write them on the piece of paper, in as great a detail as you need to. Don't worry about spelling, grammar or choice of words. No one else will see this.
4. Tear the paper into small pieces and put them into the pot.
5. Fill the pot to the top with more soil.
6. Plant seeds or cuttings.
7. Water is cleansing and purifying. Add water.
8. Gently place the new plant in the sunlight, the source of energy and healing.
9. Discover patience as you watch the problems turn into compost and the seeds of peace and hope and joy and forgiveness grow. During this "patience period" you can use the markers to make the clay pot a thing of beauty.
10. Give it to a friend, an enemy or a total stranger. In some programs the gardener is encouraged to give the composted problems and the new plant to the source of the conflict or object of guilt.

You have transformed your problems into compost to nourish a new life. Then you have shared the end result of this project with someone else. Two lives, at a minimum, have been touched, two people, at a minimum, have smiled, and perhaps people you don't know and will probably never see have had their lives enriched because you made compost from your problems.

Variations on a theme

- A group can mix their problems together as they tear them into small pieces. When problems are shared they become much more manageable.

- Individuals can write down more than one problem. In fact, a "top ten" list can be compiled.

- The problems can be discussed, but only if the clients choose to. Having the opportunity to say "NO" is empowering, even when refusing to participate means that the individual passes up an opportunity to get second opinions, suggestions and understanding.

- The pots can be decorated by each individual.

- The problems can be ceremonially burned and the ashes mixed with the soil. Fire is also cleansing and purifying.

- Use more than one species of plant in each pot to increase chances of success.

Suggestions

✌ Select seeds, cuttings or plants that have significance for you as an individual, perhaps in some way relate to how you define the "best of yourself."

✌ Select seeds or cuttings that will grow with relative ease so that chances of failure are minimal.

✌ If this is being done with a group, as the horticultural therapist you can have a couple extras started to replace any failures that might occur.

✌ Clients can write a daily journal as they wait for the seeds to sprout or the cuttings to take. This can include feelings, expectations, daily thoughts, art work, poetry, any form of expression.

✌ Group discussion can be a part of the project as friendships form and individuals become more comfortable with each other. Often an unofficial support group grows along with the plants.

Digging deeper:

This is an project that works well with many age groups, ability levels and venues. Victims of abuse, individuals suffering from depression, PTSD, major illness, accident victims, individuals going through life traumas, such as a job loss, divorce, retirement, and those stressful times that confound every one's life on occasion.

One successful project was done by a group of pre-teens who had experienced bullying. This was a way for them to confront the fear, get beyond it and take positive action.

In one senior care facility there had been major changes in administration and a good deal of uncertainty within the staff and confusion among the residents. The tension created intense insecurity and anger bordering on hostility. The members of the staff and a number of the residents did this project together and in the process, began talking and discussing their concerns and problems. It ended in a pizza party the first evening and a patio garden about a month later.

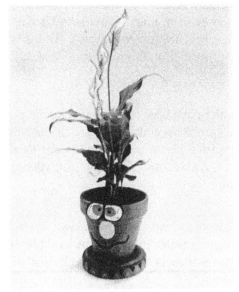

The Edible Bouquet, a Bloomin' Salad

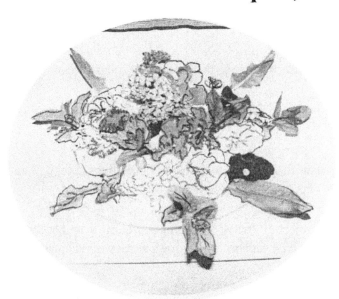

In this salad you could dine on:
Basil, Calendula, Carnation, Chives,
Dianthus, Geranium, Lilac, Mint,
Mustard, Nasturtium, Pansy, Radish,
Miniature rose & Snapdragons

This is a great group project

We enjoy the colors, fragrance and form of flowers, but we don't usually think of dining on them. Of course we eat our broccoli and cauliflower, and in the American Southwest we dine on squash blossoms, but aside from a table centerpiece or an occasional tea we don't see too many flowers on the dinner table. Yet there are many flowers that can add so much to a meal, a snack, a drink or a dessert.

This is a long term project that calls for group activity. It can be a fun gardening and dining effort that works well for a senior care facility, intergenerational program, classroom or community. Because there are opportunities for gardening, food preparation and social dining, this project has potential for almost everyone.

Caution:

Not all flowers are edible. In fact some can be guilty of anti-social behavior. Some don't taste good and some can cause allergenic reactions while others are downright toxic. This is why it is important to know positively what flowers you are putting on your plate. But, this is the same with leaves and seeds; some of them are very nutritious while others are poisonous.

There is also a great danger from the pesticides used in commercial plant production. The residue left on flowers and buds can cause serious problems and reactions. This is why it's important to grow your plants organically rather than use flowers from plants purchased at your local garden center that may have been sprayed with insecticides, fungicides, weed control chemicals, growth regulators or any of the other chemicals in the commercial grower's arsenal.

It is important that you grow your plants without any of these lawn & garden chemicals, whether you are going to eat the flowers or not. You can use a water soluble plant food like Miracle-Gro or Peters Plant foods in moderation, but even many of these fertilizers can cause you physical discomfort.

Materials needed for each participant:

1 to 3 six inch pots or decorative containers
Sufficient soils to fill the containers
A bright sunny windowsill. The more sunshine you can provide, the more flowers you will get in return.
Seeds selected from the list below
Access to a kitchen and a dining room
A sense of adventure
Courage sufficient to taste the floral dishes the group has prepared

Getting started:

1. Get your group together for a discussion and go through the list of edible plants that can be grown on the windowsill. Research edible flowers and recipes.
2. Decide who is going to grow what. Participants can grow their favorites or make a copy of the list below, clip apart and put in a flower pot. Each participant can then draw 1 to 3 plants to grow. One group placed seed packets in the pot to draw.
3. Have a ceremonial planting session complete with open discussion.
4. Plant only a few seeds per pot and thin to no more than 3 or 4 plants as they germinate. Overcrowding can result in poor growth and few blooms.
5. Discuss how the floral harvest will be served, you can plan a menu while you are waiting for the flowers to grow and open.
6. If this is going to be a dinner party, plan the guest list, make and send invitations.
7. Plan the decorations for this dinner party and create these decor elements. Pictures can be cut from catalogs and magazines, recipes can be printed up, floral arrangements can be made. One group decided that since the flowers were going to be on the dinner plate, they would make the table centerpieces out of vegetables.
8. Music can be selected for the floral dining experience. The music should involve flowers, such as "Days of Wine and Roses" or "I Never Promised You a Rose Garden" or "White Sport Coat and a Pink Carnation" and your own favorites.
9. Keep a photo journal of this project, from planting to diners experiencing this meal.
10. Record comments from participants and dinner guests.

The List of Edible Flowers

PLANT	GROWING TIPS	HOW TO USE
Basil *Ocium basilicum*	Grows quickly from seed, many varieties to choose from	Garnish on salads, vegetable dishes, baked potatoes, added to soups and sandwiches
Borage *Borago officinalis*	Germinates quickly and grows rapidly	Blue flowers are great as a garnish, added to iced teas, soups, and salads
Calendula *Calendula officinalis*	Yellow or orange flowers produced weeks after sprouting	Used for color in salads, floating on soups or iced drinks. Flavor is slightly bitter
Carnation	Slower to bloom than many, but worth the wait	Red, pink, white and yellow flowers great in drinks, desserts, salads. Can be shredded

Chamomile *Chamaemelum noblis*	Easier to start from a divided clump or purchased at garden center	Used to make a tea, also a garnish on salads and drinks (Avoid if there is an allergy to ragweed)
Chives, *Allium schoenoprasum*	Easily started from seed or divisions	Use in salads, baked dishes, potatoes, soups, as both an ingredient and a garnish. Pinch off at the stem, stem is tough
Chrysanthemum	Best started from divisions or cuttings	Many colors, flavor may be strong, petals are milder than the whole flower
Clover, white *Trifolium repens*	Easily started from seeds or divisions	Scatter individual florets on desserts, ice cream, or iced teas. Can also use in baking clover bread, biscuits or cookies
Clover, red *Trifolium pratense*	Easily started from seed or divisions	Same as for white clover
Dandelion *Taxacardium officinale*	Easily started from seed or collected from a pesticide free lawn	Sweet flavor, almost like honey, great as a garnish, dandelion flower soup is delicious, use newly opened flowers for best flavor
Dianthus	Easily started from seed	Use colorful, spicy flowers on desserts, as a confetti garnish on drinks, great on ice cream
Dill, *Anethum graveolens*	Grows easily from seed, producing yellow flowers	Use in soups, salads, as a garnish on fish, mix with sour cream as a dip
English daisy, *Bellis perennis*	Easy to grow from seeds, will bloom on a sunny window in a matter of weeks	Many colors with a slightly tart taste. Great as a garnish on salads, soups, stews, potato and vegetable dishes
Fennel	Sometimes slow to start from seed, best to use small plants from garden center	A mild licorice flavor that can add so much to everything from meat to ice cream, great addition to tea or coffee
Fuschia	Best to use a started plant from your local garden center	Colorful, fleshy flowers have a sweet, lemon flavor that is great on desserts, ice cream, salads and drinks
Green beans, wax beans, snap beans	Grow with ease from seed	Use flowers as a garnish, in iced teas, in biscuits and baked goods, add to sour cream to make a great dip
Hibiscus, *Hibiscus, rosa-sinensis*	Use started plants from local garden center, or start from cuttings	Colorful flowers have a citrus flavor. Great garnish, or fill with diced fresh fruit to make an edible fruit cup

Hollyhocks *Alcea rosea*	Perennial plant easily started from seed, or grow from started plants from your favorite garden center	Makes a great tea. Gather a variety of colorful blossoms, wash and put in a sun tea jar. Steep for about four hours, add ice & enjoy
Johnny-jump-up *Viola tricolor*	Easy to grow from seed, blooms within weeks, Can also use pansies	Colorful flowers are sweet, can be candied, used as a garnish for drinks, desserts or salads
LabLab bean Hyacinth bean	This is the bean Jack traded the family cow for. It grows very fast	Use delicious flowers as a garnish, snack, main ingredient in a creamy soup, add to mashed potatoes, or drinks
Lavender	Best to use started plant from a local garden center	Use colorful florets in everything from cakes and biscuits to masked potatoes and ice cream
Marigolds, dwarf *Tagetes patula*	One of the easiest to grow from seed, blooms very early	Use colorful part of petals as a garnish or mix into salads and deviled eggs. Makes a great topping for baked potatoes, mix with sour cream as a veggie or chip dip
Mint	Most mints grow very quickly from cuttings or divisions	Use the flowers in baking, drinks, as a topping for ice cream or in icing for cakes and cookies
Nasturtiums	Grows easily and quickly from seed	Colorful and spicy flowers are great on a salad or sandwich, can also be chopped up in sour cream for a spicy dip
Peas, English	Start quickly from seed. DO NOT USE SWEET PEAS, THEY ARE POISONOUS	Flowers have a bean like flavor, make a good garnish or addition to soups
Pineapple sage, *Salvia elegans*	Grows quickly from cuttings	Bright red flowers taste like sweet pineapples. Use as a garnish on everything
Radish	Grows very quickly from seed	Small pink flowers have a spicy flavor. Use as a garnish or in breads and biscuits
Rose, miniature	Best to use started plants from local garden center	Colorful petals can have a variety of subtle flavors. Pinch off the pointed end of each petal, they can be bitter. Use in iced teas, baking, flavored butters. You can drop several petals in an ice cube tray to make colorful and flavorful cubes for drinks.
Sage *Salvia officinalis*	Best to use started plant from garden center or start form cuttings	Flowers taste like sage. Great as a garnish on salads, poultry, soups and baked potatoes

Scarlet runner bean	Grows quickly from seed	Use flavorful flowers as a garnish, add to a cream sauce, or desserts
Scented leaf geraniums	Grow quickly from cuttings	Colorful flowers can be used as a garnish for almost everything
Snapdragon *Anthirrinum majus*	Grows quickly from seed, use dwarf varieties	Use as a garnish on almost anything
Tuberous begonias	Started form tubers	Use petals as a garnish, note most begonias contain small amounts of oxalic acid and should be used in moderation
Violets, woods *Viola odorata*	can be started form seed or small plants can be collected from the wild	Flowers are slightly sweet. Can be used as a garnish, added to butter, used in baking, or candied

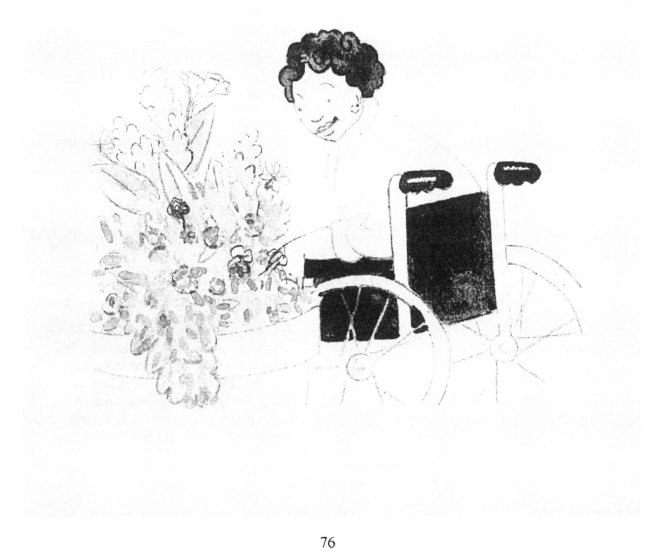

Old Shoes and Creative Energy
How About a Flower Shoe?

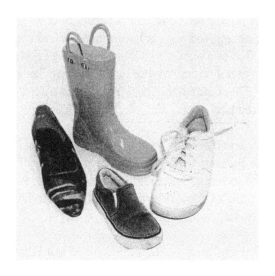 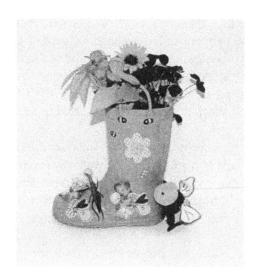

"I thought I saw a plant growin' out of a shoe," Cora said as she sat down at the dining room table. "Must be my new blood pressure medicine makin' me hallucinate."

Cora was taken by surprise by one of the first entries of the "Annual Flower Shoe" to arrive in the lobby of the assisted living center she called home. Although she claims she's not a gardener, she plans to put an old shoe or two to good use next year, "Just for the heck of it."

Horticultural therapy deals with the very essence of life and the energy of being alive. We often see programs, practitioners and facilities become so wrapped up in the book work of defining objectives and the documenting of activities and responses that the experience begins to lack the natural spontaneity that the people-plant connection should generate.

When we focus on the plants we sometimes lose sight of the real goal. It's all about the people. When we focus on the people we too frequently concentrate on the limitations, our expectations and the achievement of goals. The people-plant connection is instinctive and mentally stimulating, if we are relaxed enough to let it happen. All too often, for those of us leading our hectic lives, those of us with special needs, those of us approaching the end of life and those of us experiencing significant life changes, our existence is limited, controlled and lacking in humor and joy. There isn't time for the enchantment of discovery, the sharing of a smile or the sheer joy of creative energy unleashed. We live and work so hard that we neglect the power of whimsy.

We possess within us the tools necessary to be creative, all we need is an opportunity to use them. It is important to keep in mind that each individual comes equipped with a unique set of experiences, a viewpoint from a different perspective, a different way of functioning both physically and mentally, a different way of expressing herself or himself. We also come with our own negative baggage; inhibitions, fears, insecurities, damaged self-images and wounded self-confidence. We all need to LIGHTEN UP.

Creative energy flows best when we are smiling, comfortable with ourselves and in an environment that stimulates our senses. Isn't this what the garden gives us? We need to wear our creativity like an old shoe. In fact, that's what this is all about, old shoes.

It all began years ago when we asked a group to use "discovered containers" for their plants. Some of the participants brought coffee mugs, others used decorative tin cans, wooden boxes and a wealth of other items. One lady brought one of her husband's old work shoes. She apologized but explained that she had seen an article in a gardening magazine that showed such a shoe being used as a planter and thought it was a good idea. After some laughter and light hearted discussion about her husband's response when he found one of his shoes missing, she set about to fill it with soil and select the plants. This became the focal point of the afternoon's program. So much so that everyone wanted to do a "shoe garden."

Years later we were speaking at the American Community Gardens Association conference in Phoenix. The event was held at a school and the walkways were lined with children's shoes, painted and planted. These shoes were then sold as a fundraiser. They were decorated with faces, wiggle eyes, glitter paint and more. This was obviously creative energy unleashed and they became the topic of conversation for all those attending the conference. The greatest part of this was that everyone was smiling.

We shared this idea with people we met at other conferences and workshops. Then we received word that one horticultural therapist had taken old shoes to a new low. She held a "Flower Shoe." It became a very popular annual event and a successful fundraiser for her HT program. It worked so well for her that we stole the idea and have used it with some of our projects. This was truly an unabashed exercise in whimsy unleashed. But, the participants grew confidence, their imagination was set free and their creativity ran wild. They also had a good time doing it and laughed a lot.

Why a flower shoe?

- ❀ First, this is something we can do with our worn out or outdated footwear.
- ❀ It generates a lot of interest and conversation in senior care facilities, schools and any where else it is employed.
- ❀ It can create great publicity for your HT program.
- ❀ Holding a "flower shoe" can be a great fundraising experience
- ❀ Because it's FUN.

This is such a simple project that almost anyone can do it, even many of us with physical or mental limitations. The real beauty of this is the fact that the participants have an opportunity to be uniquely and individually creative. As one shoe artist told us, "The mind is a dangerous thing to set free."

In one facility about 15 residents participated in the creation of "shoe pots" as they were first called. These were then displayed in the lobby and the other residents were invited to vote on their favorite "shoe garden." One of the residents had a daughter who worked with the local newspaper. It was a slow news day so the color photo she took ended up on the front page. Then the TV station had to send out a crew and it was a feature on the evening news.

The next year they had over a hundred "shoe gardens" and hosted a true "Flower Shoe Show." The public was invited and paid $1.00 each for a ballot. The winning shoes were then auctioned off and the rest were sold at

$5.00 each. This project raised almost $1,000 for their HT program. The next year they had over 200 entries, many of the residents were doing two or three different shoes. They even had to raid a nearby thrift shop for their raw materials.

How creative can you be with an old shoe?

John chose a pair of old work socks as his artistic medium. After filling them with soil he painted the socks with several coats of Mod Podge so that they would hold their shape. Then ivy was planted in the top and the hole in the toe. He won the "Ugliest Non-Shoe" first prize.

Sweet, innocent Irene used an old sneaker. She told us, "It's more worn out that I am." She planted a small Weeping Fig along with Inch plant and moss in this old sneaker. She made little clay beads, painted them red and hung them in her "apple tree" to complete the "Garden of Eden in the World of Shoe." Then she went one step further and drew and cut out tiny naked Adam & Eve figures from white poster board and painted them. She pulled me aside and pointed to the first family standing under the apple tree. "Look," she said with a blush and a giggle, "They're anatomically correct too."

Six year old Dorothy was a fan of the Wizard of Oz and painted a pair of her mother's dress shoes with glitter red paint to represent Dorothy's red slippers. She planted small leaf coleus, Emerald Ripple Pepperomia and a miniature African violet along with several other plants along a yellow Lego brick road. On this yellow brick road she had placed little plastic figures of Dorothy, Toto, The Tin Man and the Cowardly Lion.

Steven spent most of his life in New York and he chose a piece of winter wear he no longer uses. This 4-buckle Arctic was filled with soil and planted with Glacier ivy, a small Snowbush Breynia, and a snowball double white petunia, to create his "Winter Wonderland." He painted the boot blue and put snowflake stickers all over it to complete the image.

Mariam chose a cowboy boot that she told us had never been comfortable enough to wear and created a beautiful cactus garden decorated with raffia and real dried chile peppers.

Bonnie planted a miniature rose in one of her husband's old dress shoes. She had painted it pale green then glued silk roses all over it. She titled her creation, "He promised me a rose garden. Now I've got one."

Anna created "A Shoe Full of Butterflies," with butterflies painted on the shoe and butterfly picks stuck in amongst the plants. Beverly painted a rabbit's head on her shoe, glued plastic ears and a plastic tail on it then planted Jelly Bean sedum and Bunny Ears kalanchoes accented with some small plastic Easter eggs.

Jack chose a sandal as his medium. He borrowed a nylon stocking from his mother and stuffed it with enough soil to fill the sandal. He then poked holes in the exposed spaces and planted weeds he found growing along the school walkway.

Others used baby shoes, spike heels, wooden shoes and the list could go on for pages. They painted them, glued various items to them and in general expressed a wealth of emotions as they converted their shoe into a garden. Some used figurines of animals, birds, insects, elves or fairies, angels and doves, even snakes and lizards. Scenes from history were created, as were historic landmarks, scenes from literature, the movies, songs, poems, seasons and holidays. During the creation of these planters there was energetic sharing of experiences, active communication and discussion. There was also a lot of giggles and outright laughter.

There were even some variations on a theme where folks have used the shoes as vases for floral arrangements, limited only to flowers they have grown. One group insisted that no silk flowers be used, while many others chose to decorate with artificial florals. The important thing is that the participants write the rules, and that they have the freedom to be creative.

What materials are needed?

✿   An over-active imagination
✿   An old shoe, boot slipper or other footwear
✿   Paint, decorations, glitter, wiggle eyes, miniature figurines and anything else that the participants can think of. Often when a need is stated, someone else in the group will have just such a treasure available, know where it can be obtained, or can have it brought in.
✿   Creativity, and the freedom to be creative
✿   Small plants to put in the shoes. Participants can be encouraged to start plants ahead of time or make a field trip to a garden center.
✿   Saucers or plastic plates to set the entries on to prevent water stains and water on the floor.
✿   Press releases and a photographer
✿   A ballot so that all the residents who didn't participate, family members and visitors can vote
✿   A place where the "Flower Shoe" can be held. It should be accessible to the public.

Flower Shoe Rules

The following is a summary of the Flower Shoe Rules that have been used by several senior care facilities and a few schools. It should be noted that these rules were established by the residents or students, not the staff or horticultural therapist. They actually formed a committee and took this very seriously. Actually, they were engaged in the entire project with an incredible sense of humor, bordering on the absurd at some times. Each facility can create their own rules, categories, and judging policies.

General rules:
✔   The shoe entries must be solely the work of the entrant, but it doesn't have to be his or her shoe.
✔   Each entry in this flower shoe must have been created with a serious sense of humor.
✔   All plants must be alive, or at the least, start out that way.
✔   All entries must be displayed in a plastic saucer or plate
✔   All entries will be displayed in the lobby, dates are given, including the date and time for the judging, sale and auction.
✔   Entries will be used for one week as centerpieces on the dining room tables.

The categories to be judged may include, but may not be limited to:
1. Best of Shoe Grand Prize
2. The most utterly, absolutely and unarguably absurd shoe, or other footwear
3. The, without a doubt, ugliest flower shoe, or other footwear, entry
4. The most original use of footwear, plants and decor
5. The most artistic expression of fashion, high or low
6. Smelliest flower shoe, or other footwear, can refer to either the shoe or the plant
7. Most colorful shoe or other footwear garden
8. The most unusual or exotic footwear
9. Special prize for the shoe that defies description or classification
10. Ugliest non-shoe, this can apply to socks, slippers or boots

Sample Flower Shoe Ballot

Please fill in the entry number that, in your opinion, is the best in each category.

____ Best of Shoe, Grand Prize winner
____ The most utterly, absolutely and unarguably absurd entry
____ The, without a doubt, ugliest entry
____ The most original use of footwear
____ The most artistic expression of fashion
____ Smelliest flower shoe
____ Most colorful entry
____ Most unusual or exotic, or downright weird entry
____ Special category for entry that defies description

Judging should be as simple as possible.
The important factor is that it be kept light and focus on fun and whimsey.

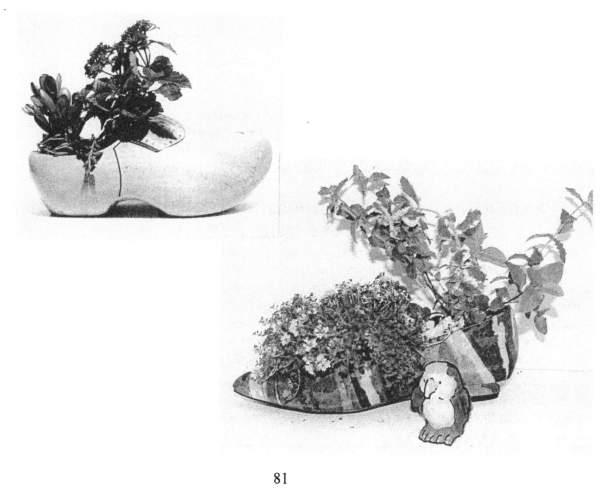

Growing a Garden of Hope

This was described as " a great project for a New Year's garden" but isn't every day a good day to plant the seeds of hope? The goal is to create a miniature garden that symbolizes the hopes each of us have for the future. This will be a very personal garden that reflects our own personal dreams, wishes and prayers. It can be as simple, or as complex, as each individual desires.

Materials needed:

1 colorful cookie tin or container of your choice
Craft paints, your choice of colors
Stickers, photos, pictures from magazines or your own art work
High quality potting soil
Colorful sand or gravel to accent the container
Seeds or cuttings of plants that symbolize hope to you
1 carefully selected stone that will symbolize our hope as a rock we can cling to when times are tough.
1 small plastic dove to symbolize peace, the universal hope of all people, everywhere. These doves can be found at any craft store.
Items selected by each gardener that symbolize their special, individual hopes and dreams.
Then select items that represent universal hopes we all share.
Hope for tomorrow, sufficient to give the gardener confidence and strength to face a new year, or another day.

Putting it all together:

1. Punch drainage holes in the cookie tin.
2. Paint in your choice of colors. You are free to use combinations of colors.
3. Apply the artwork, stamps, photos or clippings to the outside of the container.
4. Fill the newly designed planter with soil.
5. Plant the seeds or cuttings selected by each individual gardener, plants that represent HOPE to them.
6. A layer of colorful stones or sand gives a finished look to the Hope Garden
7. Carefully place the "rock of hope" and the "dove of peace"
8. The last step is to place the special hopes and dreams in your personal "garden of hope."

Some of the symbols of individual hopes and dreams
we have seen include:

- A plastic guitar was used by a woman whose granddaughter wanted to be a rock star.
- Coins were scattered on the sand by a gentleman hoping for wealth.
- A small plastic mountain from a toy set was placed in the center of the garden by a lady who hoped to one day have the strength to hike in the mountains again.
- Seashells were scattered on the sand by a young boy who hoped to someday see the ocean.
- Plastic loaves of bread were piled on one garden by someone whose hope was an end to hunger.
- One returned veteran placed broken toy guns half buried in the sand in a hope for the end of war.

> **Use your imagination and plant as many symbols as you wish. Remember, it's your garden. You can do anything you want to with it. Please share with us photos and descriptions of your gardens of hope. Perhaps your dreams can inspire others.**

The Moringa, a Tree of Hope

Moringa. *Moringa oleifera* and *M. stenopetala*, sometimes called horseradish tree or drumstick tree
Moringa family, *Moringinaceae*
Native to India, the Arabian peninsula and parts of Africa, now grown pan-tropical
All parts safe, and almost all parts are edible
Time Frame: 1 hour to initiate project, seeds sprout in about 2 weeks, tree will grow for years.
Size: Medium size project in the beginning, it will grow to become a large scale project

> This is an easy to grow plant with the potential to save thousands of lives in regions of the world racked by poverty, drought, disease and starvation. It also deserves a place in every backyard garden and should be as common as the tomato. It also deserves a place on the windowsills of everyone who hopes for a better tomorrow when there is no hunger or poverty. This is truly a tree of hope. We hope that you will grow it as a symbol of the dreams of millions of people for a better tomorrow.

Moringa as a food resource

This is a miracle tree for many areas where hunger and malnutrition are serious problems. Not only is it fast growing, drought tolerant and pest resistant, it is the ultimate in a multi-purpose plant. This is one of the keys to ending hunger, malnutrition and starvation in many parts of the world. Just in case you were curious, they call it horseradish tree because the roots actually taste like that popular European seasoning.

The leaves are delicious and nutritious, with an almost spicy taste. These leaves can be harvested daily from a few trees growing at the dooryard or along the garden path. Because this foliage is so high in protein and vitamins A & C it's literally a life saver. They are sometimes eaten raw as a salad green but most often used as a cooked green or added to soups, stews and other dishes. They can also be dried and powdered for easy storage. The powder can be added to almost any food to greatly enhance the nutritional value of a meal.

The flowers and buds are eaten raw or cooked and the bees make a delightful honey from their nectar. The flower are delicious batter fried, sauteed or used in a stirfry.

The pods, or drumsticks, are useful at several stages as they grow and mature. The immature seed pods are cooked and eaten like green beans or used in a stir fry. These diced pods can also be roasted, boiled or steamed as you would okra. The inner lining of the mature seed pod is edible and can be used much like pasta or noodles.

The seeds can be harvested when at the "green bean" stage and cooked like you would peas. They contain about 30-35% edible vegetable oil. If left to dry they can be stored for over a year and cooked as you would dried beans. This sweet tasting oil can be extracted in a simple press and used for cooking, lubrication, soaps and cosmetic creams. Because the oil burns without smoke it's also ideal for lamps. This oil doesn't turn rancid and can be used in food preservation.

The bark produces a sappy gum that is used in cooking and food preservation as well as a whole list of medicinal applications from stomach ache to the common cold. The inner lining of the bark has a spicy taste and can be diced for use in soups, stirfries, or other dishes. The bark can serve as a diuretic.

Nutritional value of Moringa oleifera

This is a plant that has been reversing many of the symptoms of malnutrition in many parts of the world. The pods are a great source of a wide range of necessary nutrients, but the fresh leaves are the most readily available to the most gardeners in first world nations, particularly those in the arid tropics. The leaves are continuously produced throughout most of the year. The dried and powdered leaves have a great advantage in that they can be easily stored for long periods of time without refrigeration, canning or freezing.

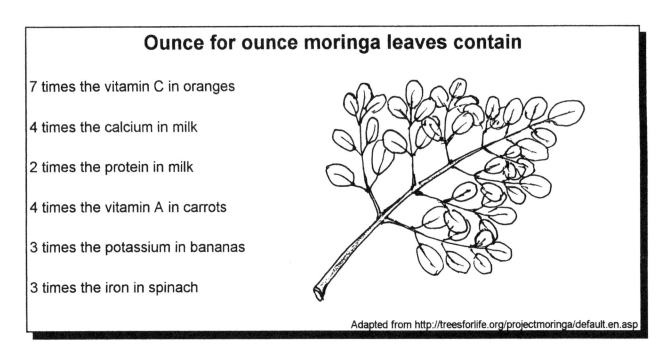

Ounce for ounce moringa leaves contain

7 times the vitamin C in oranges

4 times the calcium in milk

2 times the protein in milk

4 times the vitamin A in carrots

3 times the potassium in bananas

3 times the iron in spinach

Adapted from http://treesforlife.org/projectmoringa/default.en.asp

Other uses for this valuable plant

Clean water: The winged seeds are used to purify dirty water. Along the Nile valley it is known as *shagra al rauwaq*, or "tree for purifying." The seeds are crushed into small pieces and wrapped in a cloth and tied. This is then placed in the bucket or container of water where the seeds attract and absorb the impurities and pollutants, leaving potable water. A natural antibiotic is also released from the seed that kills most of the bacteria in the water. As our global water supply becomes more at risk this is a possible solution. Contact Hunger Grow Away at hungergrowaway@q.com or see their web site www.hungergrowaway.com for more information.

Vegetable oil: The oil has been used by artists for years. They know it as "Ben Oil." This same oil has been used in fine machinery as a lubricant, but there is also potential for its use in the production of a motor fuel that could replace petroleum derived fuels. This could make economic independence possible for many communities and impoverished nations in the arid tropics. It is also more environmentally friendly than petroleum products.

Health care: The oil has also become a popular ingredient in soaps, shampoos and skin care products. There have been numerous reports of the effectiveness of leaf powder and oil to heal rashes, lesions and minor abrasions.

Livestock: The leaves have been used very effectively as a nutritious feed for pigs, goats and other livestock.

Fencing: The trees can be used as a living fence or harvested and used as fence posts. If left to grow several years it becomes a useful lightweight lumber source.

Fuel & lumber: This is an extremely fast growing tree (outdoors it may reach 10 to 15' in the first year) that produces a lightweight wood acceptable as a fuel for stoves. The wood also has potential for carving, but isn't strong enough to be used as a building material in most situations.

Crop supports: The trees can serve as poles for beans, yams, vanilla, pepper and other vining crops, a wind break against the harsh semi-desert breezes, shade to help preserve moisture in the gardens and fields and fodder for the livestock. They can be used as living fences, privacy screens and erosion control.

Mulch: The dried pods and fallen leaves also make a valuable surface mulch on its way to becoming compost.

Crop protection: The leaves and leaf stems also provide a natural protection against the fungus that causes damping-off in seedling beds. Leaves steeped in water are reported to produce a natural fungus control that encouraged the germination and growth of seedlings.

Growing HOPE on your windowsill
Materials needed:
3 to 5 moringa seeds
A container equivalent to a six inch pot, with drainage holes
A quality potting mix with coarse sand added in a 1 part sand to 3 parts potting mix ratio
A compassionate heart

Putting it all together:
Fill the container with soil and moisten well
Plant the seeds one knuckle deep in the soil and place on a sunny windowsill
Keep moderately moist but never soggy while waiting for the seeds to sprout
While you are waiting check out the Hunger Grow Away web site, www.hungergrowaway.com
The seeds will sprout in 7 to 21 days and will grow in spurts
When they have three to five leaves they can be thinned by sharing seedlings with friends
As the tree grows you can begin harvesting a few leaves for salads, tasting and sharing.

> **It will grow quite well in a sunny winter windowsill and will grow rapidly to a height of five feet or more. During the warm months it grows well outdoors in light shade or full sun.**

Care & Feeding of a Moringa Tree
Light: Moringa likes as much light as it can get so the brightest windowsill works best. It can be a patio plant or garden plant during the summer.

Soil: While the moringa will grow in almost any well drained soil, it is at its best in a good potting mix with sand added. 1 part sand to 3 parts potting mix.

Water: This is a plant of the desert and cannot stand wet feet, but if kept evenly moist it will be very productive.

Cold: Because the moringa is a tropical plant it will freeze if kept outdoors during the winter. It will thrive and bloom indoors in a bright sunny window all winter long. It can be kept trimmed to the size with frequent pruning. The prunings can be rooted by simply sticking eight to ten inch cuttings into slightly moist soil so that at least three inches is in the soil.

Feeding: A half strength feeding with Miracle Gro once a month will make your moringa very productive.

Pests & Problems: The biggest problem is over watering. Second is over feeding which can lead to infestations of mites, aphids, scale and mealy bugs.

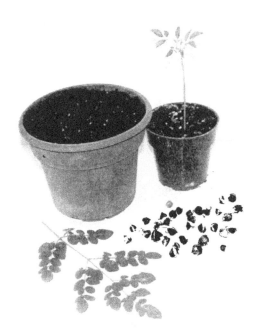

Lucky Shamrock Quiz

We are all familiar with the symbols of Saint Patrick's Day; the Leprechauns, rainbows and pots of gold, good luck charms, the wearin' of the green and, of course, the shamrock. Right now we are going to focus on the Shamrock. The following is a brief quiz. It's just for fun, and you are invited to test your friends and neighbors. Enjoy the season.

1. How many leaflets on a shamrock leaf?

2. The shamrock is really a clover.   TRUE   FALSE

3. Shamrock comes from an ancient Celtic word *seamrog.* What does the word shamrock mean in English?

4. In what song does Elvis mention the four-leaf clover?

5. What is the official national symbol of Ireland?

6. What is the difference between a four-leaf clover and a shamrock?

7. How did St. Patrick use the shamrock in his teaching?

8. In the song, "I'm Looking Over a 4-Leaf Clover" what do the four leaves represent?

9. What is the legendary connection between the shamrock and the Garden of Eden?

10. What color are true shamrock flowers?

Bonus question. What do you get if you cross a four-leaf-clover with poison ivy?

Answers on page 90

87

A Leprechaun's Garden
Four-Leaf Clovers & Shamrocks

Objective: Create a good luck planter for the day we are all Irish

White clover, *Trifolium repens*
Bean family, *Fabiaceae*
Native to Europe and British Isles, including Ireland
Rating: Easy
All parts safe
Time frame: 1 hour to initiate, 2 months from planting to showy plant
Life span: White clover is a perennial
Size: Small, 4 inch container with plant growth rarely exceeding 6 or 8 inches.

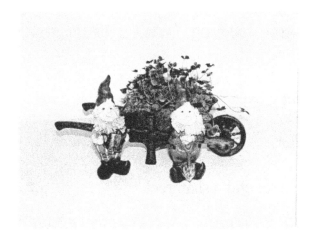 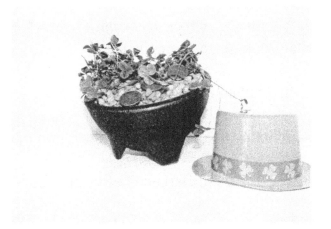

More than you ever wanted to know about shamrocks:

We find many plants marketed in March as we celebrate the day when everyone is just a little bit green. Oxalis, several varieties of clover, a clover cousin called medic and several others are all sold as shamrocks. In this project we are using what most botanical historians consider the original, one and only, genuine SHAMROCK. One of the great joys of childhood for many of us was to find a four-leaf clover. Often they were tucked within the covers of the family Bible or pressed in photo albums, or glued to picture frames to bring good fortune. Many families had specific and unique customs surrounding four-leaf clovers. It is fun to share these traditions, arts and crafts. In one of the senior care facilities where we had a horticultural therapy program the residents collected these stories and memories into a community scrapbook that received additions every year.

History: The word "Shamrock" comes from the Irish word *seamrog* which means "little clover." Among the earliest Celtic peoples the white clover was considered a source of good luck. When St Patrick came to Ireland he used the Shamrock to demonstrate the concept of the Trinity. Wonder what he did with the four-leaf clovers.

White clover is a great agricultural crop providing excellent forage for cattle, helping to prevent erosion and adding nitrogen to the soil. It is also a great colorful addition to a boring turf lawn. It will even grow in the shade. In fact it's almost as attractive in a lawn as the beautiful dandelions.

A tea made from the leaves was used medicinally by the Europeans for rheumatism and gout. This tea has also been used for fever and the common cold.

There are patented varieties of the traditional white clover that are noted for the production of many more four-leaflet leaves or colorful red bands across the center of the leaflet. The plant stays compact, rarely exceeding 4-6" in height. The flowers are white with a touch of pink, and they will flower almost all year long.

Note: if this project is started on January 17th the plants will, with the "luck of the Irish" be really impressive for Saint Patrick's Day.

Materials needed:
1 St. Patrick's Day coffee mug, or a plastic green hat party favor, or container of your choosing
A few white clover seeds, or a division from a plant growing in the yard, or one of the patented varieties
Sufficient soil to fill the official Saint Patrick's Day Planter
An Irish heritage, either real or seasonal
1 leprechaun is helpful but not essential. You can substitute a small child and make this an intergenerational program.

Putting it all together:
1. Take the Shamrock quiz on the preceding page.
2. Fill your chosen, or created, container with soil.
3. Share a good Irish story or joke.
4. Plant the seeds or divisions in the container.
5. Share some memories of four-leaf clovers.

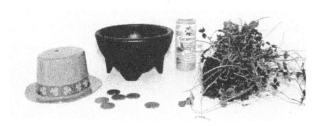

Variations on a theme:
Use as a centerpiece on the dining room tables
Make many of these shamrock planters and give them to family, friends and total strangers
Use as a fund raiser for your horticultural therapy program, family vacation or retirement fund
This is one of those projects that can move outdoors when the windowsill becomes crowded.
White clover makes a great hanging basket subject, too.

Care & Feeding of your Good Luck Plant
Light: Indoors a bright sunny windowsill is best. If they don't get enough light they will be spindly rather than compact. Without bright sun they are also reluctant to bloom.

Soil: Shamrocks will do well in almost any reasonably good potting soil. The important thing to remember is that it should be loose and well drained. Outdoors they will thrive in a wide range of soils.

Water: Shamrocks enjoy an evenly moist soil. Indoors, or grown in containers, they will suffer if the soil dries out. When planted in the ground they will take drought conditions once they are established.

Cold: This is a plant that can take freezing weather and summer heat. In areas where it gets really cold (Like Minnesota) it will go dormant for the winter.

Containers: Your "shamrock" will probably outgrow the mug or seasonal container by the end of the first year, and you will need to transplant it. It will thrive in almost any well drained container that gives it room to grow. They will do well in a hanging basket, window box or decorative planter. Outdoors they serve as a great groundcover in larger containers holding shrubs.

Feeding: A half strength solution of Miracle-Gro once month is usually sufficient.

Problems: Very few insects dine on this plant and there are no serious diseases. The biggest problem is drying out when grown in a container.

Other plants considered "Good Luck"

Many people, from many cultures around the globe have special plants they consider "good luck." In every community there are people from distant shores that would be delighted to share their stories about these plants. Some we have heard about are:

Sansevieria

Moringa

Dracena varieties

Aloe

Ask your friends and neighbors, perhaps even a stranger or two, about the plants they consider good luck. Then let us know what you have learned. Contact us at **petals_pages@msn.com** Thank you.

Answers to the Shamrock quiz:

1. Three, occasionally a leaf with four leaflets is found.
2. True, although many other plants are marketed as shamrocks, the one popular in Ireland is a clover.
3. Seamrog means "little clover"
4. "Good Luck Charm"
5. The harp, not the shamrock
6. The shamrock normally has 3 leaflets, a four-leaf clover is a rare malformation that is generally viewed as being even more lucky.
7. The three leaflets symbolized the Trinity, the Father, the Son and the Holy Ghost. When a four-leaf clover was found the fourth leaflet symbolized God's Grace.
8. Sunshine, rain, roses and the one I adore
9. The shamrock was supposedly the only item Eve carried out of the Garden of Eden.
10. White. The flowers may show a pink tint, or edges trimmed in pink. The flowers are lightly fragrant and can be dried for use in arrangements.
Bonus question. A rash of good luck (Contributed by one of our horticultural therapist friends who wishes to remain anonymous)

Lucky Bamboo

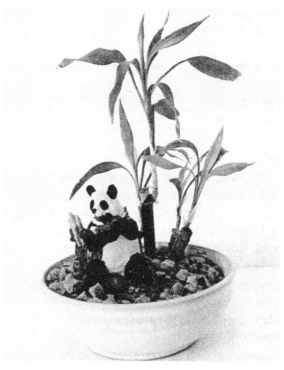

Lucky bamboo is also known as Medusa Bamboo, Chinese Good Luck Plant, Lucky Lily and Lucky Palm.
Dracaena sanderiana
Lily family: *Liliacea*
Native to Africa, not the Orient
Mature size: 2 to 4 feet, sometimes more
Safety: all parts of this plant are safe, but water must be changed frequently to prevent stagnation and the development of waterborne organisms.
Time Factor: One hour to initiate project.
Life span: It will last indefinitely if given even minimal care
Size: Small, 4 inch container; with a height of 6 to 10 inches by the end of the first year.

All you ever wanted to know about your "Lucky Bamboo"

Today we know this plant as Lucky Bamboo, although it isn't a bamboo at all (Bamboo is a grass, Dracaena is a lily). In Victorian England it was called ribbon plant or ribbon lily and was a popular parlor plant because it thrived in low light conditions. In its native Africa it is considered a roadside weed. Thailand is today the world's largest producer of this popular plant, but many of the Caribbean nurseries are now producing the plants we find in the American marketplace.

The Chinese have used this plant as a symbolic gift for the opening of a new business (it is said to bring prosperity), or the purchase of a new home (its presence in the home is said to bring positive energy). According to the principles of Fung Shui this plant brings harmony between the forces of nature. It's even claimed by those selling it that strategically placed in the home it can energize your love life. Unfortunately, we couldn't learn just where this strategic location was.

Materials needed to Grow a lucky Bamboo in water:

At least 3 cuttings of "Lucky Bamboo"

Decorative container, vase, coffee cup or dish

Colored stones or sand

Red ribbon, or other colors to demonstrate your advocacy, concerns, interests or causes. The red ribbon represents fire, passion or positive energy.

A few small chips of aquarium charcoal

Fresh water, bottled water works well

Putting it all together:

1. Begin with the container: It's your choice. A vase, bowl, coffee cup, or almost anything else that will hold water. Keep in mind that you will need a container at least 1 ½" deep.

2. Fill your container with the stones, pebbles or colored sand: your choice, match the color to your preference or decor. The stones help to balance the weight of the container with the plant and prevent spills.

3. Mix a few chips of charcoal with the stones or sand to help prevent fungus problems.

4. Place the cuttings of your "Lucky Bamboo" in a pattern you prefer. They can be bundled together, set at angles, arranged in a line, or whatever other arrangement suits you. They can be held together with a rubber band or the ribbon in the color, or colors of your choice.

5. You can use the stones to hold the plants in the position you want. After they develop roots they will usually stay in place with little difficulty.

6. Water: It is important to maintain about one inch of water in the container. It should be changed weekly to prevent stagnation. You can also add a couple small chunks of charcoal to help prevent the growth of fungi and other organisms in the water.

7. Feed once a month with a half strength solution of Miracle-Gro.

Lucky Bamboo can also be grown in soil rather than water:

1. It's best to grow them in a 4 to 6" container with drainage holes in the bottom. You can use a found container, or a hand decorated one that you have created just for your Lucky Bamboo. One of our friends used a discarded drinking mug made from a section of bamboo as the container.

2. Use a good, quality potting soil, and make certain that at least 2 inches of stem are below the soil surface.

3. They can still be bundled, tied with ribbon or arranged as you wish.

4. Keep the soil evenly moist but not soggy for best results. Frequency will depend on the temperature, humidity and size of container.

Creating a Lucky Bamboo Twist

You can create fancy shapes with your lucky bamboo. It's easy and doesn't require intricate processes or fine coordination.

Place the plant where the light is coming from only one direction. You can create a cardboard screen if necessary to control the amount of light coming from other sides of the planter

Within a week or two the plant will start to "reach" for the light.

By turning the container slightly you can cause the stem to curl or twist.

When you frequently turn the plant you can get a true spiral effect.

Notes:

We purchased a container of "Lucky Bamboo" cuttings from the clearance shelf at the local discount store for $2.00 and took it to a Green Thumb Club meeting the next week. We found that there were 23 good, healthy cuttings in this bundle, along with two that were dead. The club members became so engaged in a discussion about luck, both good and bad, that they had to wait until next week to plant their Lucky Bamboo.
One Gentleman decided to try an experiment. He added some red cake coloring to the water to see if the leaves turned red. A lady with a profound interest in the lottery glued Monopoly money and coins onto her coffee mug planter. Another selected a small blue stoneware bowl, painted white doves on it, then placed a number of the plastic mini-doves used in wedding favors on the plants themselves and made a peace tree. Use your imagination, be creative, and above all else share your stories of luck, both good and bad. Two former teachers conspired together and compiled a list of the various colors of ribbons and their meanings. This was far more extensive than we expected.

All of these plant projects provide an opportunity to share, discuss, discover, and engage in pleasant conversation. These chats among friends are a far more important form of good luck and good fortune than money. Aren't we truly lucky to have good friends, especially when some of them are green?

Goldie and the Sacred Lotus

Lotus, *Nelumbium nucifera*
Water lily family, *Nelumbonaceae*
All parts safe
Rating, Easy and fun for a wide range of ability levels
Time factor: I hour to complete the initial project, daily feeding of the fish
Life span: Lotus will live for years but will outgrow the fish bowl in a few months.
Size: Medium, the size of the container is the determining factor

The lotus, symbol of beauty

To followers of the Eastern religions, the sacred lotus is the symbol of beauty, happiness and even fertility. The Hindu faith tells us that this beautiful flower resides within each of us and represents eternity, purity and our divine connection, hence the name *sacred* lotus. Like the human spirit, the lotus is reborn each year from the mire and muck to grow and blossom. The lotus is the symbol of the human spirit rising from the muddy waters of despair to bloom in the bright light of the Creator. There are multitudes of writings on the sacred lotus, and the art produced celebrating this beautiful and dramatic flower is some of the best work ever produced by the creative spirit of humanity.

This is a dramatic water lily type plant native to Asia, from Iran to China and Japan. The leaves are large and beautiful in the simplicity of their design while the large pink flowers are held above the water surface on heavy stems that can be over three feet tall. The plant is hardy throughout USDA zone 5 and winters outdoors by going dormant. On your windowsill, it will stay green all year. The flower itself is strikingly beautiful, with simplicity of form, subtle colors and an alluring perfume. It's easy to see why this flower is a symbol of purity, beauty and divinity. It's also obvious why this has been the inspiration for some of the greatest art the world has ever known.

Both beauty and function

Not only is this entire plant a treat for the senses, virtually all parts are edible, and nutritious as well. The tubers can be harvested any time of the year and, when cooked, have a pleasant flavor and celery-like texture. These roots can be dried and ground into a starchy powder like arrowroot that has been useful in treating victims of dysentery. Slices of root can also be pickled or soaked in sweet liquids for a special dining treat. The young leaves, harvested as they are unfurling are also delicious, raw or cooked. They are sometimes used like cabbage leaves as a wrap for cooking. The stems are cooked and peeled, then diced to produce a vegetable with a flavor not unlike beets. The seeds can be popped like popcorn, or ground into a flour for baking and cooking. The seeds contain between 15 and 18% protein. The flower petals can be eaten raw or floated in drinks as a garnish. They can be dried to make a delicate tea. Dried petals can also be used to produce a ceremonial incense. The stamens alone produce a most delightful tea. Beyond the dinner table, every part of this plant has a traditional medicinal value in Ayurvedic medicine. For thousands of years Indian traditional medicine used this plant to treat various forms of cancer. Today several pharmaceutical companies are working to isolate a series of compounds that may have anti-cancer value.

You can grow one of these from seed on your windowsill for at least a year before it needs a pond to call its very own, but the fun is in starting it and watching it grow from seed. Especially when Goldie, the goldfish, is there to help.

Years ago, when one of the authors of this book was a very small child growing up on a farm in western Pennsylvania he had a most charming elderly lady as a neighbor. Everyone called her Goldie, and she was the neighborhood's universal grandmother. There were always cookies, homemade candy, fresh fruit from her backyard or flowers that she shared with a most delightful smile. One year she decided that she was going to grow water lilies in an old bathtub that sat at the corner of the garden, by the gate. We all eagerly helped her put some soil in the bottom of this tub, collect some wild aquatic plants and even a few minnows for "Goldie's Lily Pond." She ordered some seeds for the *Sacred Lotus of the Mystic Oriental Religions*" and this was our focus for the summer. The seeds arrived and she had each of us carefully nick them and plant them in the old bathtub. There were ten seeds in all. We visited daily to watch the progress. The first one sprouted in 12 days, while the last one didn't show the beginnings of life for two months. They grew quickly, the stems reaching the top of the water and unfurling. To us kids, and Goldie too, this was a thing of great beauty. On her birthday in July, we bought her three little goldfish for the lily pond. It was fun to watch both them and the seedling lotus grow together. Both occupied that old bathtub lotus pond for years. We hope that you have as much fun with this project as Goldie and all of us kids did with hers.

Materials needed:

1 or 2 small feeder goldfish
1 small aquarium, that will hold at least 2 quarts of water, can be recycled from a yard sale or thrift store
1 cup of coarse sand or aquarium sand
3 to 5 sacred lotus seeds, obtained from a lotus pod (can be purchased at any craft store dried flower dept).
1 piece of coarse sandpaper, nail file or emery board to abrade the seeds
goldfish food
a pinch of patience
a dash of childish delight
optional, other aquatic plants to provide some color while the lotus sprouts
Almost forgot, one small rubber ducky

Putting it all together:

1. Clean the aquarium and rinse thoroughly.
2. Fill with fresh, clean water.
3. Wash the sand, then pour into container and allow to settle for about thirty minutes.
4. Remove seeds from the dried lotus pod. (Many seed companies also sell the seeds). Wash seeds thoroughly.
5. Sand one side or end of each seed until the seed coat is worn through. Take care not to damage embryo inside. Many Green Thumb Club members have used a nail file or emery board.
6. Carefully place the seeds so that they are barely covered by the sand. Note: they may float at first, but will eventually sink to the bottom.
7. Add goldfish after water has been in the aquarium for at least 24 hours.
8. Take care not to overfeed the goldfish. If this is done properly you will have created a micro-environment that will use the fish to feed the young plants while the baby lotus provides oxygen for the fish. If not, you will need to refresh the water frequently.
9. You can also add the rubber ducky as the finishing touch.
10. The seeds will begin to sprout within five days, but some may take a month or more. The sprouting leaves will grow so fast as they race to the top of the water that you can almost watch them.

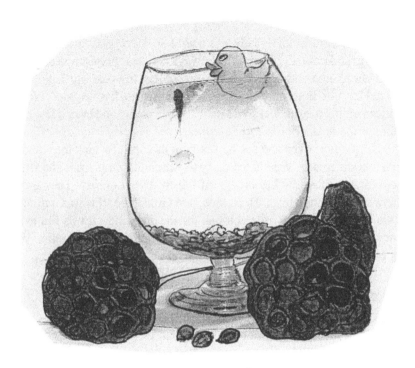

Care & Feeding of your lotus pond

Light: Indoors a bright sunny windowsill is a must if they are to do well. Outdoors they will thrive in full sun or light shade.

Soil: The goldfish will produce sufficient nutrients for the lotus for the first season.

Water: They are at their best with at least six inches of water. Keep the water fresh by adding more as needed.

Container: You will need to move the lotus plants, and the goldfish into a larger home as they grow.

Cold: These plants don't tolerate freezing weather. They are best grown as container plants that can be moved in from the cold in the winter, or given a permanent home on the windowsill. Note: There are hardy members of the lotus or waterlily family that will thrive outdoors all year, but will be dormant during the cold months.

Feeding: The goldfish will supply all the nutrients necessary.

Problems: Few insects dine on this plant. The biggest problems result from insufficient.

Maintenance: Trimming away the fading or dead leaves is a matter of good grooming. Because some varieties will get quite large this will be a short term project. Some varieties will bloom in a larger aquarium, even better in a pond or outdoor container, like a bathtub. That is, if they get enough light and you have sufficient patience.

Geranium Basket

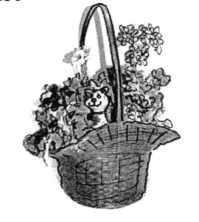

Geraniums, *Pelargonium species*
Geranium *family, Geraniaceae*
Origin, most from southern Africa
Completely safe, flowers are delicious
Rating: Very easy
Time factor: 1 hour project.
Life span: Plants will need
transplanted, but will live for several years
Size: Medium size project

A brief history of the geranium:

The geranium (*Pelargonium*) family includes some old favorites like the zonal and ivy geraniums. Some have brilliantly colored flowers in shades of red, pink and white, even burgundy. Others have variegated leaves with greens, creams, white and pink stripes or splashes. Most of these plants originally grew in South Africa, while others came from various parts of Asia. The flowers of the scented leaf types are more dainty, usually in shades of pink, white or lavender. But these geraniums aren't grown for the flowers; they are valued for the distinctive aroma and shape of their leaves.

Scented geraniums are considered herbs and have been used both medicinally and in the kitchen. There are over 200 named varieties of scented geraniums. The fragrance can range from mint to rose, citrus to spicy. Some have tiny leaves, others produce frilly, almost fern-like leaves and some have rich variegations. Some varieties grow upright and may form a small bush, others are trailing, some can be trained as a topiary and others are great in a hanging basket.

During the Victorian era the geraniums with fragrant leaves were very popular as parlor plants because the scented leaves helped to mask the scent of cigar smoke, cooking and other household odors. They were grown in decorative pots and urns, trimmed and trained into exotic shapes. The leaves were valued for potpourri, baths and pillow stuffing. Men would tuck a few leaves in their shirt pocket and ladies wrapped them in their cuffs and scarves.

In the kitchen both the flowers and the leaves can be added to cold drinks, teas and coffee. They can also be used in baking, added to salads and soups, used with chicken, fish, venison, beef, cooked vegetables, mashed potatoes, and ice cream. These geranium leaves can be used both fresh and dried.

Materials needed:

1 decorative basket left over from Easter, or found at a local thrift store
Sufficient aluminum foil or plastic film to line the inside of the basket
Sufficient good quality soil to fill the basket
3 to 5 geranium cuttings, a good mixture of zonals, ivy geraniums, scented geraniums and any fancy sorts you can find. These cuttings can be from 4 to 8 inches long
Pruning shears or scissors to prepare cuttings for planting
A sunny windowsill

Putting it all together:

1. Line the basket with foil or plastic film.
2. Fill the basket with the potting mix.
3. Prepare cuttings by using the shears to remove the bottom set of leaves so that at least 2 inches of stem is leaf free.
4. Insert these cuttings into the soil so that at least 2 inches of stem is in the soil.
5. Water lightly and avoid over watering while cuttings are rooting. Remember, geraniums are native to the semi-arid regions of South Africa and suffer from too much water.
6. As the new plants begin to produce new leaves and flower buds feed with Miracle Gro or your favorite house plant food.

Care & Feeding of your Favorite Geraniums

Light: Indoors a bright sunny windowsill is a must if they are to do well and bloom. Outdoors they will thrive in full sun or light shade.

Soil: Geraniums will do well in almost any quality potting mix. The important thing to remember is that it must be loose and well drained.

Water: They like to be kept lightly moist, never soggy. Too much water can result in fungus growth, root rot and other diseases. These were originally desert and semi-desert plants.

Cold: These plants don't tolerate freezing weather. They are best grown as container plants that can be moved in from the cold in the winter, or given a permanent home on the windowsill. Note: There are hardy members of the geranium family that will thrive outdoors all year, but will be dormant in the cold months.

Feeding: A weak solution of Miracle-Gro once a month during the active growing season is usually sufficient.

Problems: Few insects dine on this plant. Mealy bugs, white fly and mites can attack sometimes, but this is rare and they can be controlled. The biggest problems result from insufficient light or too much water.

Pruning: Frequently deadheading (removing the spent flowers), and trimming away the fading or dead leaves is a matter of good grooming. Because some types of geraniums tend to get leggy, it is a good idea to keep the stems short and trimmed to shape. The pieces that are trimmed off can be started in a pot of soil (some like to start them in a glass of water). They can also be trained into topiaries in the form of globes or other shapes. We have seen Green Thumb Club members create "Bonsai Quickies" with geraniums.

Notes from the field:

The geranium seems to be the universal conversation starter. It never fails. You can take two people who have never met, put a red geranium in front of them and within three minutes one of them will say something like, "When I lived in Michigan we usta raise 'em so big ya couldn't cover 'em with a bushel basket."

The other one would respond with something like, "My favorite has always been the ivy geraniums. My Grandma, rest her soul, grew all kinds of scented leaf ones."

And it goes on from there as two strangers become friends.

Geraniums are universally familiar and get a reactions from many who are disconnected from much of life, ranging from profound depression to demntia.

Gourd Gardens

Lagenaria siceraria and many other species
Melon family, *Cucurbitaceae*
Most likely Native to Africa
All parts are safe, some have medicinal and food value
Rating: Medium to difficult skill level
Time factor: will vary with each individual, but at least 3 days will be needed

One of the best, and most adaptable items we can use as a creative planter is the gourd, unequaled in its diversity and creative potential. You can paint, carve, use a wood burner. You can applique or glue almost anything to them. They are also fun to grow, although not indoors. They come in so many sizes, shapes and textures that you will never run out of things to do with them.

We have seen gourds made into hanging baskets, large planters, nested planters, and bird's nests. Chet, one of our Green Thumb Club members, collected clippings from the comic pages of the Sunday paper that pertained to gardening. He then glued them onto the surface of a large dipper gourd with the bottom cut out of it. Then holes were drilled around the sides and he used twine to make a quite whimsical hanging basket. The gourd was hung upside down with the neck at the bottom and geraniums in the top.

Sheila, another creative gardener, cut the front from a large gourd and painted the inside sky blue, and the outside light green with flowers from a magazine glued in place. She then cut a small hole in the back, almost to the top and inserted a seven watt bulb and holder from an old electric Christmas candle into the hole. She planted Rabbit's foot ferns and Creeping Charlie inside and placed some colorful stones she had collected from a nearby steam. She had created a living night light.

Rosa cut a series of one inch holes in the sides of a large gourd and made a 100% organic strawberry jar for her herbs.

Lenny, selected a large globe shaped gourd. He cut the top off and glued postage stamps from his collection all over the surface to make a "postage stamp garden." He planted three kinds of English ivy cuttings in it and in a few months it was overflowing with ivy vines that were accented with the colorful stamps.

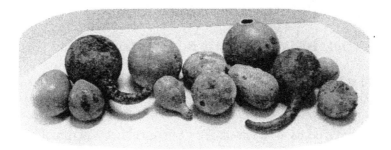

Notes from the field:

Gourds can be started indoors on a sunny windowsill and transplanted outdoors when danger of frost is past. They will grow well on a fence, trellis or even a tree. They can be made into birdhouses, bowls, dippers, etc.

You can do all sorts of creative things with a gourd, or several gourds. Set your imagination free and see what happens. Use any medium available, go through the junk drawer or the toy box. Make it uniquely yours. Gourd gardens can also make great fund raisers and gifts.

Materials needed:

1 or more gourds, dried or cured
Vinegar and kitchen pot scraper, plastic or metal
Keyhole saw, or craft saw
Medium or fine grit sandpaper
Waterproof paint or sealer
Decorative materials of your choice
Sufficient potting mix to fill your gourd or gourds
Whimsy of your choice
Plants, cuttings or seeds for your gourd planter
Healthy sense of humor

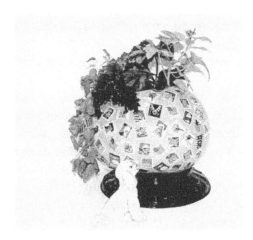

Basic tips for working with gourds:

1. Begin with a properly dried gourd that is free from decay or rotted areas. It may have some dark discoloration, peeling skin, or even patches of mold on the surface. This can easily be removed with vinegar and water. Using a small scraper such as those used for washing pots and pans works very well.

2. After the surface is thoroughly cleaned allow it to dry completely before the fun begins.

3. Decide what you want to do to, or with, this gourd. You can gather paints, materials to be glued to the surface or any other decor materials.

4. Mark out the opening, or openings, where you want to place the plant, or plants. This can be on the top, or you can turn the gourd over and use the bottom of the gourd for the top of the planter. The opening can be round, or some other truly artistic shape. Holes can also be cut in the sides.

5. Pilot holes can be drilled with an electric drill, or a knife, but BE CAREFUL. You can use a small keyhole saw to cut openings in almost any shape you wish. Care must be taken when cutting the holes so that neither you nor the gourd is damaged. Use sandpaper to smooth the rough edges.

6. You may also want to drill a hole in the bottom to facilitate drainage.

7. After you have gained access to the inside of the gourd scrape out all the seeds and as much of the dried pulp as possible. The smoother you can make the inside the better, because of what happens next.

8. After the inside is cleaned it needs to be sealed. You can use either waterproof paint or any other sealer to coat the surface. If the inside is waterproof your gourd planter will last for years, it if isn't a few months is about the life span.

9. After the inside has been coated or painted, and is thoroughly dry turn your attention to the outside surface. Give it a coat of waterproof paint before applying anything else. Let this dry for at least 24 hours.

10. Now be creative. Add paint, fabric, paper, articles from the newspaper, family photos, beads, coins or whatever strikes your fancy.

11. After the entire gourd planter is completely decorated fill with the potting mix and plant with your chosen plants.

12. You can add whimsy to the planter and plants including stones, shells, plastic insects left over from Halloween, craft butterflies or anything else you happen to find.

Global Gourd Quiz

Let's try this little test of your knowledge. These trivia questions are all great topics for conversation and further research.

1. The gourd is believed by botanical historians to have originated in
a) Africa   b) Australia   c) The Carribean islands   d) China   e) North America

2. TRUE or FALSE   The calabash pipe, made popular by Sherlock Holmes, was made from the neck of a gourd.

3. TRUE or FALSE   Gourds have been used for cradles and baby baths in Africa.

4. An African musical instrument made from a gourd and strings of small shells or beads is called
a) Rattle flute   b) sitar   c) shekerie   d) oud   e) bush harp

5. TRUE or FALSE   In China the gourd was once used as cricket cage.

6. Native Americans used gourds as
a) hats   b) rattles   c) flutes   d) a four string guitar

7. The gourd is so popular in Haiti that "gourde" is
a) the middle name of every female child   b) planted at every doorway   c) the name of the Haitian monetary unit   d) worshiped as a god

8. TRUE or FALSE   The gourd has never been used to make masks.

9. In some Asian cultures a gourd is placed by the sickbed for
a) donation from visitors to help pay the doctor   b) fresh flowers to welcome the angels   c) water for the one who is ill   d) the hastening of recovery, as an element of Feng Shui

10. TRUE or FALSE   The plastic water bottle is nothing new. Native peoples around the world have carried gourds filled with water as canteens for thousands of years.

Answers:
1. a)   2. True   3. True   4. c)   5. True   6. b)   7. c)   8. False   9. d)   10. True

Garden Trophies

Objective:

This is a project that enables you to showcase some of the plants that you have grown, shared and enjoyed. It is also an opportunity to be creative. The finished product can also make a great gift or be used as a fund raiser.

Safety: All materials selected should be safe
Rating: Moderately difficult, requires patience and coordination
Time factor: At least three one hour sessions, plus one to two weeks for the flowers and leaves to dry
Size: This will vary with the materials available. It is best to use a wood plaque that is at least 4 x 6 inches.

Materials needed:

Assorted leaves and flowers from plants you have grown
1 phone book or other large book to serve as a flower press
Photos that can be trimmed
Stickers, poems, small pictures from magazines or catalogues
Basswood round, other wood plaque, or a piece of plywood
1 sheet of fine sandpaper
Velcro tabs for hanging
White glue
Spray acrylic sealer

Optional materials can include:

Paint for background on plaque
Craft Paints for customizing
Dried flowers, seeds, pods, moss or bark
Craft butterflies, birds or other miniatures
Memories from the junk drawer

Preparing the leaves and flowers:

- Pick 1 or 2 fresh leaves, that aren't more than 3 inches long, from some of your favorite plants.
- Collect leaves from as many plants as you wish, up to 20 or 30 leaves total.
- Carefully place between the pages of the phone book, several leaves can be on each page but they should not touch.
- Wait 1 week for thin leaves to dry, 2 weeks for heavier leaves.
- Note: you can use small flowers as well, but they should be placed between pieces of tissue paper to prevent discoloration from the ink on the book pages.

Preparing the basswood round plaque:

- Sand the face of the plaque smooth with fine sandpaper.
- Wipe the plaque clean with a moist paper towel.
- If you wish to paint the face of the plaque, this it the time to do it, using craft paints.
- Place the picture hanger on the back of the plaque.

Putting it all together:

* Arrange the leaves in an artistic pattern. Experiment and select a design you like the best, after all this is your "Garden Trophy."
* Trim a photo, poem or use small stickers and pictures to finish the design. (Optional)
* Remove the leaves from the plaque and arrange on the table in the design you chose.
* Carefully brush the white glue on the plaque, covering the area where the leaves will be placed.
* Carefully place the leaves one at a time on the glued portion of the plaque. If you get glue on your fingers, wipe them clean with a moist paper towel.
* After the leaves, flowers and other items are glued in place allow the glue to dry completely
* You can now glue dried flowers, craft butterflies, or any other decor you choose on the plaque to give it some added dimension.
* Spray entire plaque with acrylic sealer. Do this outdoors to avoid exposure to fumes from the sealer.
* Enjoy your memories of gardens past; and share the stories with friends.

What Green Thumb Club members have done:

Grace arranged small dried flowers in a rainbow pattern on a plaque she had painted sky blue. The leaves were placed at the bottom to symbolize the earth, and where the rainbow touched the green leaves she had tiny butterflies.

Jerry Placed a photo of his Bichon in the center of the plaque and surrounded it with dried and pressed herbs from his herb garden.

Midgie chose to use mostly ferns and campanula flowers with some dried moss and several small angel figurines for dimension.

Barry had been a DJ for much of his life and he chose to use an old "scratched beyond redemption" LP recording as his plaque. This he spray painted gold, then glued photos of his favorite musicians. Dried leaves were painted sliver and glued in place along with flowers and items that symbolized "the music of my ill spent youth."

Sandy, chose to use her calligraphy skills, parchment paper and creative genius to write lines of poetry which she glued on the plaque. These she surrounded with fine borders of dried leaves. She produced a series of these and gave them to her each of her grandchildren.

Set your imagination free, make a statement, enjoy the process.

Growing a Christmas Tree Topiary

Objective:

To grow a Christmas tree from a creeping fig for use as a table center piece or decoration throughout the Christmas season. This is a long term project best started in June or July. This can provide stimuli for creative expression, fine muscle coordination, nurturing skills and opportunities for memory stimulation and socialization.

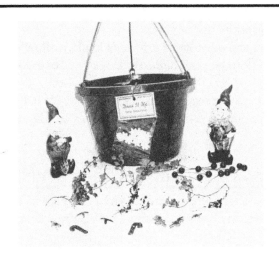

Creeping fig, *Ficus pumila*
Fig family, *Moraceae*
Safety: All materials are safe
Rating: Moderately difficult, requires patience and coordination
Time factor: 1 hour to initiate project. Five to six months to complete
Life span: With proper care this will last for years.
Size: Small to medium project. 4 to 6 inch hanging basket

Materials needed:

3 to 5 creeping fig *Ficus pumila* rooted cuttings Note: small leaf English ivy also works well.
4" or 6" plastic hanging basket with plastic hanger
Good quality potting soil
Twist ties or craft holly berries
Later in the process miniature Christmas ornaments and garlands can be created and added as ornaments.

In the beginning:

❋ The containers can be painted, decorated with stickers or decals. Creative gardeners are encouraged to set their imaginations free.

❋ Fill hanging basket with the potting mix.

❋ Strike the cuttings or plant plugs, 3 to 6 per container. Place them near the hanger wires.

❋ Water well and place in a northern or eastern windowsill. Keep moist and new leaves will begin to appear.

What you need to do to make a Christmas tree:

* Turn this planter once a week so that each side gets its sunbathing time.
* Once a month the new growth will need to be trained to the wires of the hanging basket with twist ties (or those little holly berries on a wire). Be careful not to twist so tightly that the stems are broken or damaged.
* Feed every month with Miracle Gro to encourage vigorous growth and a full Christmas tree.
* The objective is to produce a full Christmas tree shaped plant by training and trimming.
* In November you can begin making mini-ornaments, garlands and a topper for the tree.
* Now your miniature Christmas tree can be decorated and used as room decor, center pieces on the dinner table or given as gifts.

Variations on a theme

Experiment with other vining plants such as English ivy, philodendron, Swedish ivy or Creeping Charlie pilea. Use 4" or 8" hanging baskets or regular containers with a wire or dowel teepee for training.

Digging deeper

* Participating gardeners can share memories of homemade Christmas ornaments and collect ideas for next year.

* This is a great intergenerational project to share with grandchildren and grandfriends.

* Participants can do some exploring and learn more about the plants being used. This research can take place in the library or on the Internet.

* Extra Christmas trees can be created as gifts for friends, neighbors or total strangers.

* These mini-trees can be used as a fund raiser for your group, favorite charity, or community program.

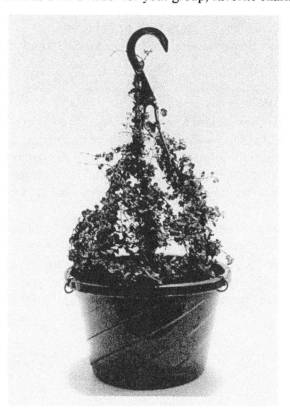

Global Herb Garden
A Windowsill Basket of Herbs

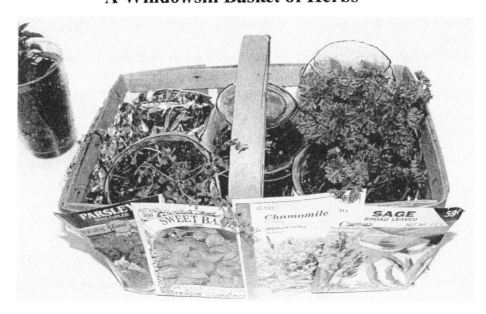

Objective:

To create a basket planter filled with herbs from all over the world. This can be both a creative activity and a learning experience. As we plant and grow these herbs we can share information about culinary, cosmetic and medicinal herbs. We can experiment with them as both seasoning and as an artistic medium, using sprigs of various herbs in everything from hair rinses to soaps and candles, potpourri and gift cards.

Safety: All the herbs listed are considered safe
Rating: Moderately easy
Time factor: at least 2 sessions to initiate, will grow for 6 to 18 months
Life span: Many of the herbs listed are annuals, others will need to be transplanted to larger containers
Size: Medium to large size project

A brief history of herbs:

Herbs were among the first plants domesticated by our ancestors. On every continent, in every culture, herbs are used to make food taste better, to preserve foods, to heal, to comfort, to make people and their homes smell better, and to simply make a difficult life more bearable and a good life even more enjoyable. Every kitchen herb has its purpose, its own history and its own mythology. We all have memories of various herbs that were a part of our meals. Each of these herbs and spices can trigger images of both foods and people from our past.

You can choose from the herbs we have listed below (or be radical and use totally different ones) for your Global Herb Garden. These are all popular herbs that are easy, safe and fun, to grow. Each produces leaves that can be eaten fresh from the plant, and each is highly nutritious, providing Vitamins A & C as well as other nutrients. This is a great sensory experience for everyone, including special needs students and elders with dementia. These Global Herb Gardens also make a great centerpiece for the dining room table.

Parsley is a native of the Mediterranean basin. Today it's the traditional garnish on the side of the dinner plate, but it has a reputation in myth and legend of increasing endurance. Greek Olympic athletes were fed bowls of parsley before there were drug tests for the games. In Medieval Europe it was said that the seeds had to descend into the earth to visit the devil seven times before they would sprout. This herb was known as the wife of garlic because it was considered a breath freshener. It's is quite easy to start from seed.

Pineapple sage is a member of the sage family that has a distinctive pineapple scent and flavor. The red flowers are delicious and both flowers and leaves are used in salads, sweet sauces, puddings, ice cream and even Jell-O as a flavoring. It is native to the Near East and was known as "sweet sage." It is also used to flavor teas, cold drinks, a wine and goat cheese. This, and most other kinds of sage, is easily started from cuttings.

Rosemary is one of the world's most popular herbs. It has been valued in the kitchen since people have been cooking. There is a story that Mary washed clothes one Monday morning and spread them on a bush to dry. When she removed the dried clothes from the bush it burst into bloom as a beautiful and aromatic rosemary bush. It was a popular strewing herb in homes, churches and hospitals in Medieval Europe. Strewing herbs were sprigs of aromatic plants scattered about the floor so that when one walked over them the scent was released and made the room smell better. This was also a traditional symbol of faithfulness and fidelity and was a part of wedding bouquets. A sprig of rosemary was also worn by the groom on the wedding day. A knight's wife would tucked sprig of this herb in her husband's coin purse when he had to go out of town on business, fight in a crusade or participate in a tournament. Rosemary starts easily from a cutting but is slow to root.

Basil is a rugged aromatic herb that has beautiful flowers and leaves. Sweet basil is a mild herb that can be eaten raw, used as a breath freshener or salad green as well as being valuable in cooking. There are basils that have deep purple leaves, basils with tiny leaves and others that have large lettuce-like leaves. There are other uses for basil beyond the kitchen. The leaves can be steeped in bath water to relieve muscle aches, heal rashes and in general soothe a tired body. It can also be scattered among clothing in closets and dresser drawers to keep moths away. Most basil varieties will start easily from seed or cuttings.

Spearmint, and other aromatic members of the mint family, has been among the most popular of herbs everywhere people and plants have grown up together. Mint has been used to soothe a troubled mind, stimulate circulation and ease an upset stomach. It was buried with the Egyptian pharaohs and strewn on the floors of European castles. It is still today one of the most popular room freshening and deodorizing herbs. The leaves can be chewed raw, used in cooking or to add flavor to chewing gum and toothpaste. Most mints (spearmint, peppermint, chocolate mint, apple mint, pineapple mint and hundreds more) are easily started form cuttings. Many of the popular spearmint varieties are native to North America.

Garlic needs no introduction. It is the single most popular and widely used herb on earth. Native to central Asia, it has conquered the world. The Romans gave it to their athletes and soldiers for greater strength and stamina. In Egypt it was used as a medium of exchange and workers were paid in garlics. During World War I garlic juice was used to disinfect wounds. The leaves can be used as a snack or in cooking. Garlic is easy to start from individual cloves separated from the bulb and planted like an onion set. Think of the garlic clove as a mouse and press the clove into the soil headfirst so that only the tail is visible.

Some more herbs from all over the world that you can grow on the windowsill

Bay leaf is a tree that will grow on your windowsill for several years
Mini Chile peppers from South and Central America
Chives from Europe
Dill from Eurasia
Fennel from Europe
Geraniums, including scented leaf varieties, from Africa
Ginger, from the tropics
Lavender from Eurasia
Lemon balm from Europe
Lemon verbena from the Carribean
Marigolds from Mexico
Marjoram from Mediterranean Basin
Mint, many varieties and scents, from all over the world
Nasturtiums, needs lots of light
Rose, miniature types will do well on a sunny windowsill
Sage, many varieties
Salad Burnett from Europe
Thyme, many varieties from Europe and Asia

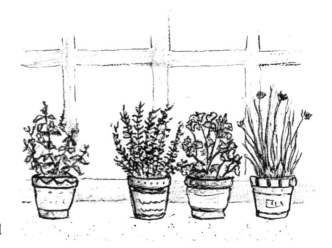

Materials needed for your global herb garden:

1 splint, or chip, basket, windowsill size
Craft paints or seed packets for the basket
Decor items of your choosing to make the basket uniquely yours
4 to 6   3 or 4" plastic pots (recycled from other projects)
4 to 6 McDonalds sundae cups
Sufficient quality potting mix to fill the plastic pots
Recycled Easter grass, any color you choose, sufficient to fill in around the pots in the basket
Membership in the National Geographic Society is helpful but not essential

Putting it all together:

1. Drill or punch a drainage hole in the bottom of each sundae cup.
2. Fill the plastic sundae cups about ½ way to the top with a good grade, moist not soggy, potting soil.
3. Take three cuttings from each herb, if using mint, basil, rosemary, sage, thyme, oregano or many other herbs that start easily this way. These cuttings should be between 3" and 4" in length.
4. Carefully remove leaves from the bottom half of the cutting.
5. Holding the cuttings for each herb in a bundle, insert into the soil until the cutting is half in the soil and half in the sunshine.
6. Water lightly and place the lid on your "mini-terrariums."
7. If starting herbs from seed, fill the sundae cup to about 1" from the top, scatter a few, (no more than a dozen), seeds on the surface and barely cover with more soil, then water lightly and place the lid on your herbal incubator. The seeds of most herbs will germinate within two weeks.
8. While waiting for roots and sprouts, paint the basket, glue herb seed packets or create an herbal collage with

white glue and clippings or pressed stems of real herbs.

9. After cuttings have new leaves the lids can be removed from the mini-terrariums. As soon as the seeds sprout, just like children, they will need lots of sunshine to grow healthy and strong.

10. Place the pots of now vigorously growing herbs in the basket and fill in around them with the Easter grass.

11. Keep in a bright, sunny window, snip & trim frequently and use to enhance your favorite meals.

12. These plants will need to be transplanted to larger containers in 2 to 4 months.

Care & Feeding of Your Global Herb Garden

Light: A bright sunny windowsill is best when growing them indoors. If they don't get enough light, growth will be weak and spindly.

Soil: Most herbs will do well in a good quality potting soil mix. The important thing to remember is that it must be loose and well drained. Most herbs don't do well in heavy or clay type soils.

Water: All of these herbs enjoy an evenly moist soil, but don't do well in a soggy (windowsill swamp) environment. The parsley and the mint will quickly wilt if the soil is too dry. This makes them a good moisture meter.

Cold: Most herbs can take anything the average windowsill can dish out in terms of cold. For some of the more tender varieties there may be some frost damage if ice forms on the inside of the glass. This potential danger applies to herb gardeners as well as the herb gardens.

Containers: You aren't limited to the basket of herbs. Your global herb garden will thrive in almost any well drained container that gives it room to grow. They will do well in a plastic bucket or decorative planter as long as there is drainage. Set your imagination free, be creative and artistic. You can paint, glue, carve, wrap, weave, use an old hat, discarded shoes, rusted skillets, or anything else that suits your fancy.

Feeding: A ½ strength solution of Miracle-Gro once a month is usually sufficient. Overfeeding can result in weak growth. Herbs are at their best when they are kept on a strict diet.

Problems: Very few insects dine on these plants, in fact many herbs are used to repel a number of species of insects. The biggest problem comes from insufficient light that causes spindly, pale, leggy growth. The family cat usually poses a bigger problem than insects.

Harvesting: If you are going to all the trouble of searching for just the right container, customizing it, planting cuttings and seeds, nursing the darn things along, feeding, watering and defending them from the family cat, you should get some benefit from this global herb garden. Don't be afraid to trim, snip and pinch sprigs of these plants to use in cooking, salads, drinks, potpourri or craft projects.

Hangin' in There

"Hanging baskets can double the garden space and put some of your choice plants at eye level."

Hanging baskets have always been popular. They make it possible to have flowers and foliage at a variety of heights, and open the door to some creative landscaping, both indoors and out. People were using hanging baskets for their flowers, herbs, vegetables and ornamentals long before the Egyptian pharaohs were building pyramids. Today we have a wide range of decorative style baskets and hanging containers to choose from. But the creative gardener can go far beyond what the garden center has to offer.

It's unfortunate that many of the garden books and professional landscapers disparage hanging plants as mundane or common place. They claim that they are labor intensive and short lived. The truth is that they provide flexibility, variety and efficiency. We can put the baskets that are in season, or at least look their best this week "on display" while others are put back for refurbishing. Having the plants suspended in mid-air also keeps them up out of the reach of most pets and small children. Hanging baskets also put the plants at an accessible level for those of us with limited mobility.

General Care & Feeding of a Hanging Basket

☞ Regardless of type, hanging baskets outdoors will require frequent watering to avoid stressing the plants.

☞ The smaller the basket, the more frequent watering it will require. A six inch diameter basket is going to dry out in the hot summer sun, long before a twelve inch basket filled with the same plant will need a drink. This is true even if the basket has one of those snap on saucers or one of those clever internal self watering devices.

☞ Successful hanging baskets begin with a high quality potting soil, not the bag of mud that you paid 99¢ for at the discount store. There are formulas specially designed for hanging baskets, but most "professional potting-mixes" will work quite well.

☞ Location, location, location, is the key to success. Sun-loving plants want you to hang their basket where the light is brightest, but many plants want some shade. That's why it is important to know your plants. Most failures with hanging planters aren't the result of watering but of insufficient light.

☞ Rotate the baskets so that each side gets an opportunity to do some sun bathing. This will help to keep the plants well rounded and healthy.

☞ Don't be shy about pruning, removing declining leaves and, in general, keeping the plants in a hanging basket well groomed.

What will grow in a windowsill hanging basket?

Almost anything that you can grow in a pot will grow in a hanging basket, but most effective are the plants that vine, drape or cascade over the edge.

❀ You can grow miniature roses in a hanging basket as long as they receive at least six hours of full sun per day.

❀ Many herbs are happy to grow in hanging baskets; parsley, chives, many of the trailing mints, oregano, thyme, creeping rosemary, and the list could go on for pages. A community of herbs in a single hanging container works very well.

❀ Many vegetables also do well in a hanging basket. Strawberries, ornamental peppers, tomatoes like the Sweet 100, even cucumbers, lettuce, and kale do well just hanging around, as long as there is lots of sunshine.

❋ Most of the common house plants such as the philodendron, ivy, and ferns will thrive in a hanging basket indoors or in a shady location outdoors in warm weather.

❋ Dinner table and ornamental sweet potatoes thrive indoors in a sunny window, or outdoors in light shade.

❋ Many cacti and succulents, including trailing jades, Christmas cactus, orchid cactus and the old favorite, string of pearls, are at their best when they can hang around.

Some more plants for your indoor hanging baskets

Asparagus fern is a rugged and vigorous sprawling plant that has small thorns.

Beans, LabLab, Scarlet Runner or any other vining type bean will do well with lots of light.

Begonias are found in many forms and colors. Some flower periodically, while others sprawl and drape over the sides of the container. The Rex begonias have dramatic leaves.

Bridal veil and cousins like inch plant are "can't fail" plants that are almost indestructible.

Ferns, Boston, as well as other types including the fuzzy little rabbit's foot, Maidenhair and Staghorns.

Christmas cactus will grow well in a hanging basket.

Coleus with its dramatic leaf colors and forms makes a great hanging basket subject.

Creeping fig, a vining member of the fig family with small leaves. Very rugged.

Donkey tail sedum and many other succulents grow very well in a hanging basket.

English Ivy boasts many leaf forms and color patterns.

Geraniums are a natural, including the ivy leaf, rose bud and some scented types that have a trailing habit.

Goldfish plant, an orange flowered cousin to the African Violet, is ideal for a hanging basket.

Grape ivy, a true member of the grape family, and **Kangaroo vine**, a cousin of the grape, enjoy just hanging around.

Orchid cactus and Night Blooming Cerus are at their best in hanging baskets.

Pepperomia is available in many varieties with unusual textures and colorations.

Philodendrons are found in many vining forms. They are almost indestructible, but should not be ingested.

Piggy-Back Plant, also known as Mother-of-Thousands or *Tolmiea,* has baby plants on the leaves.

Polka Dot Plant, *Hypoestes,* colorful leaves, vigorous grower for climbing or hanging.

Pothos, Devil's ivy, *Scindapsus,* are variegated cousins of the philodendron.

Rattail cactus is a great flowering cactus for hanging planters.

Spider plant, few plants are easier to grow in a hanging basket.

String-of-pearls, a novel member of the *Senecio* with bead shaped leaves. (Note this is toxic if ingested).

Sweet potatoes, garden variety or ornamental, are a natural for the hanging planter.

Swedish ivy does quite well just hanging around, but it is neither an ivy, nor is it from Sweden.

Velvet plant, also called Purple Passion Plant or *Gynera,* has fuzzy purple leaves.

Zebrina, Wandering Jew, many color and leaf variations can be mixed for effect.

Have the courage to experiment. Grow plants that you might not have seen in the hanging baskets at the garden center. Try mixing several plants in the same basket; caladiums and ferns or ivy make a dramatic combination. When you create a combo-basket, try to use plants that have similar needs as far as light and watering. Try creating baskets with different colors and features for different seasons and holidays.

Notes from the field:

✿   Paint, decorate, glue fabric or cover the pot with a collage of pictures.

✿   Try varying the height of the hanging baskets to give a more informal appearance.

✿   Be creative in making your own hangers. Macrame is attractive and rugged. We saw one hanging basket made from an old doggie dinner plate with dog leashes for the hangers. A small bicycle wheel was used as a tray for a large pot. This was suspended from bicycle chains.

✿   Mix and match the plants so that there is complimentary foliage color, form and texture.

✿   When securing a hanging basket make certain that all brackets or hooks are sufficiently anchored to hold the weight of a recently watered container, and withstand high winds of outdoors.

✿   Avoid using containers that are too large and difficult to handle.

✿   Use sufficiently heavy chain, macrame cord or other type hanger to support the container.

Thinking beyond the traditional plastic hanging basket

Be creative and use various found containers as hanging planters.

❦   Small galvanized buckets are popular but the most off-the-wall hanging basket we ever saw was made from a stained glass lampshade.

❦   A close second was birdsnest ferns planted in an old army helmet with a GI Joe doll peering over the rim. Whimsy counts.

❦   One of our young Green Thumb Club members used a restaurant size tomato soup can with a cherry tomato plant cascading over the rim.

❦   Mason rescued one of his wife's old purses from the floor of the closet, filled it with soil and planted petunias to cascade over the edge. Then he placed a plastic bluebird in the center and hung it outside his window. A pair of wrens soon set up housekeeping in it and raised a family there.

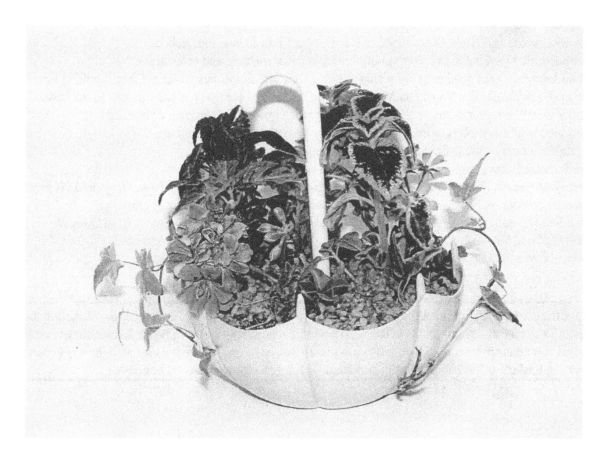

Jack & the Bean Stalk
the Lablab (or Hyacinth Bean)

Objective: To grow an "old fashioned" and relate it to a traditional story. Great for memory triggers and conversation starters.

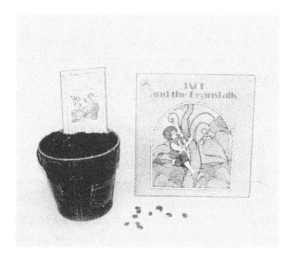

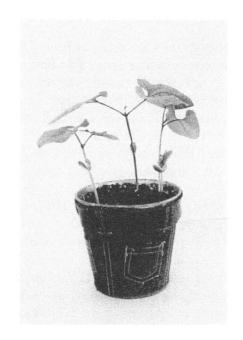

LabLab Beans, *Dolochios lablab*
Bean family, *Fabaceae*
Native to Asia and possibly East Africa
All parts safe, dried seeds should not be eaten raw
Rating: Very easy
Time frame: 1 hour to initiate the project. Two to three months for vine and flower production.
Life span: Best treated as an annual.
Size: Large scale project

Questionable moral values

Jack & the Bean Stalk is one of the most popular of our classic fairy tales. But if we look a little deeper into this story there is some serious anti-social behavior that needs to be addressed. We question whether this should be considered suitable for children, and strongly feel that this is an "Adults Only" story. Think about it. Here we have a wayward youth who is sent on a simple shopping trip by his poor destitute mother. He's lazy and trades the family cow for a handful of beans to avoid going all the way into town. This displays a blatant disregard for his family, his mother and the economic system as a whole. In a fit of anger he even discards the beans. After they grow he recklessly endangers his life, and the emotional stability of his mother, by climbing this vigorous vine. At the top of the vine he finds the estate of a famous character actor who had appeared in numerous horror movies. He then commits a number of crimes including, but not limited to, trespassing, vandalism, breaking and entering, petty larceny, grand theft, burglary and trafficking in stolen goods. As if this weren't bad enough, after he climbs down the beanstalk with all these stolen goods he commits pre-meditated murder. Is this the moral example we want to set for our children?

All about the bean:

Still this bean is fun. And, you can grow it without committing any of the above mentioned crimes. Because this vine grows with such vigor we strongly suspect that these were the beans that Jack received in his trade for the cow. You don't have to trade a cow for them though. The seeds are readily available.

This plant is also known as Hyacinth bean, Pharaoh bean, shink, bonavist & Chinese flowering bean. It is a vigorous vine reaching 12-18 feet (4-6 m) on trellis or fence and is perennial in frost free regions. It's available in both a white flowering and a purple flowering model. Both grow equally well.

If we could only grow one bean this would be it. The lavender, pink or white flowers are so spectacular that in the Orient bouquets are sold as a part of the florist's trade. Not only are these flowers beautiful, they're also delicious, tasting like sweet green beans. They make a great garnish addition to salads, soups and stews. They can be smothered with a lemon flavored cream sauce for a truly delightful side dish. You can also add a handful of these flowers to rice to enhance the flavor and give it a pink blush. The cut flowers are popular in many parts of the Orient for bouquets and as tokens of affection. The story goes that a love struck young fellow gives the girl of his dreams a bouquet of lablab flowers. If she is interested in him she invites him in to share a dinner of lablab flowers served in a cream sauce.

The young beans are a rich purple in color. They can be used raw in salads or cooked like green beans. When cooked they retain a pink color. As the seeds begin to form and the pods swell, they can be shelled like peas or limas. When cooked these beans have a good flavor. Left to dry on the vine, then shelled, the dry beans can be stored for a long time. The dried black or cream colored beans have a delightful flavor when cooked. But that's not all. A bonus for all growing this delightful vegetable is in the leaves. Young, tender leaves can be harvested and cooked as a you would spinach. With bits of bacon or ham they are delicious. They can also be cooked with slices of lemon rind for a different taste. But wait! There's still more. This remarkable plant also produces an edible tuber about the size of a turnip. Sliced in a mixed vegetable stir-fry it is delicious. Or you can boil, bake, roast or serve this tuber with a cream sauce. In mild climates this root can be stored in the ground where it was growing until you are ready to use it.

What more can we ask of a plant that grows easily from seed, thrives in a wide variety of soils and loves the summer heat and humidity. It will grow in full sun or light shade. While this bean will take a good deal of dry weather it does best with regular watering. This is an ideal summer vegetable that can begin to flower in less that 60 days. The first leaves can be harvested in 30-40 days. In frost free areas it will grow and bear for several years. Lablab beans can also be grown as a windowsill plant. They will vine and bloom with enthusiasm. This plant is too much fun to grow alone. Share it with friends, neighbors, children, grandchildren or grandfriends.

Materials needed:

1 container, approximately 1 gallon capacity (a standard 6" clay or plastic pot will also work well). Some folks find that this is a great candidate for a hanging basket.
Sufficient soil to fill the container
3 to 5 LabLab bean seeds
A copy of the traditional fairy tale, Jack & the Bean Stalk
A healthy imagination and a crafty personality because you will need to be creative
A custom made trellis or support for the vine. You can use twigs, cord, colorfully painted wood or almost anything else you find in the closet or junk drawer.

Putting it all together:

1. Fill the container with soil.
2. Raise your left hand and hold it thumb up.
3. Rotate hand so that it is now thumb down.
4. Press thumb into soil to the depth of first joint.
5 Repeat until you have made as many holes in the soil as you have seeds.
6. Place seeds 1 per thumb print, cover and water well.
7. Place on a sunny windowsill and wait, seeds usually germinate in 5 to 10 days.
8. While waiting, read the story to a friend, relative or neighborhood child, if you have parental permission.
9. As the seeds sprout make a creative trellis or support for the vines.
10. As the buds open, dine on the first flowers, fresh from the vine.

Care & Feeding of Jack's beanstalk

Light - The more light the better. A sunny window or patio is ideal.

Soil - It does best in a loose compost rich soil with a little sand added, but will accept almost any quality potting medium, as long as it's well drained.

Water - The soil should be kept lightly moist but too much water will do it in. Lablab beans are moderately drought tolerant.

Feeding - half strength Miracle-Gro about once every month or two is a good diet. Over feeding can produce weak growth and less bloom.

Training - This is a natural climber and will twine its way around a windowsill, or over a trellis.

Containers - A one or two gallon container is ideal. We have also seen them grown well in a galvanized bucket turned into a hanging planter.

Pests - Fortunately there are few pests that bother these beans. The biggest problem indoors is insufficient light. Over watering and poor drainage can also be a problem.

Part of the joy of growing uncommon plants is in the sharing. You can share the delicate flavor of these blossoms with friends, family and guests. The leaves can be cooked like spinach and the young beans are great used as you would green beans. The dried beans are flavorful. Mature Lablab beans should not be eaten raw because uncooked they are difficult to digest.

A Christmas Tree for All Seasons
Norfolk Island Pine

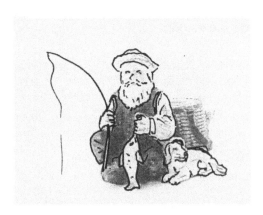

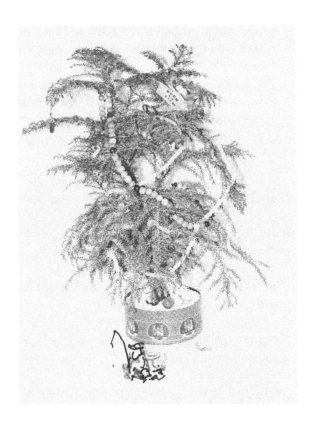

Norfolk Island Pine, *Auracaria heterophylla (A. Excelsa)*
Araucariaceae family, closely related to the pines
Native to the South Pacific
All parts safe
Rating: Very easy
Time frame: 1 hour to initiate the project
Life span: These "trees" will continue to grow for years
Size: Medium size project

A tree with a story:

The Norfolk Island Pine is a majestic native from a tiny island, appropriately named Norfolk Island, located off the east coast of Australia. In fact, it is a territory of Australia. One of the major exports is seeds from the tree that has made this island famous. It was settled by Pitcairn Islanders, descendants of the Bounty mutineers. You do recall the classic movie version of Mutiny on the Bounty, don't you? In that movie from 1935 Fletcher Christian, was played by Clark Gable and Capt Bligh was played by Charles Lauton. They just don't make 'em like that anymore. The tree will grow from 150 to 200 feet tall and the trunk can exceed 10 feet in diameter. Relax, it won't get that large on your windowsill. Other members of this family can be found in South America, Australia, New Zealand and the South Pacific. The seeds are eaten raw, roasted and used in cooking. The tall straight tree trunks were use as masts for sailing ships in earlier times.

They are often sold as "living Christmas trees" and are decorated with lights and ornaments. They were once marketed as *house pines or parlor pines*. This is appropriate since this is the only pine that will grow well indoors. It was the darling of Victorian parlors because it was easy and accepted cool temperatures in the winter.

Materials needed to start this project:

1 small Norfolk Island Pine, best from a 4" pot
3 to 5 cuttings of English ivy (any variety, variegated, needlepoint, traditional, etc.) These should be between
      4 and 6 inches in length

116

Scissors or small pruning shears
A Christmas tin or pot decorated for Christmas
Sufficient quality potting soil to fill the container
Recordings of your favorite Christmas music
A DVD of Mutiny of the Bounty, to watch while the trees grow

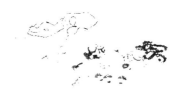

Getting started:

1. Select an appropriately festive container, a Christmas cookie or candy tin works well if you punch a couple holes in the bottom.
2. You can use a standard 6" clay or plastic pot and decorate it with whatever comes to mind; paint, glitter, beads, sequins, ribbon, silk flowers, even credit card bills from Christmas gifts you purchased last year.
3. Play some of your favorite Christmas music while decorating the container. You can sing along if you wish. Don't worry if you are doing this long before the Christmas season, Christmas music is fun any time of the year.
4. Fill the container with soil and place your tree in the center, planting at the same depth it was in the nursery container.
5. Snip the leaves from the bottom 1 to 2 inches of each ivy cutting
6. Strike cuttings of English ivy around the edge of the pot.

As the tree grows:

1. Add hand made decorations.
2. As the tree grows through the years you will need to give it a larger container, and add more ornaments.
3. Add ribbon or yarn garland. Be creative with this as well.
4. A short string of miniature Christmas lights can be added to for a holiday touch. Don't keep lit for prolonged periods of time, it can burn the foliage and is also a fire hazard. Never leave unattended when the lights are on.
5. These "Year 'round Christmas trees" can be used when young as a table decoration.

Care & Feeding of your Norfolk Island Pine

Light - The Norfolk Island Pine is quite comfortable on the average windowsill. It can be outdoors during the warm months. There it enjoys light or filtered shade when young.

Soil - It does best in a loose compost rich soil with a little sand added, but will accept almost any quality potting mix, as long as it's well drained.

Water - The soil should be kept lightly moist, but too much water will do it in. Avoid soggy soil. If the foliage turns yellow and the new growth looks sickly it is probably getting too much water.

Feeding - Miracle-Gro half strength about once every month or two is a good diet. Over feeding can produce weak growth that is open to fungus and insect attack.

Pruning - This is a moderately slow growing evergreen that requires little pruning. When it's pot bound it grows even slower. Indoors it rarely exceeds five or six feet in height. If the central leader is trimmed, it will almost always produce a twin trunk immediately below the cut. It can even be trained to make an effective bonsai specimen.

Containers - As mentioned above, you can use almost anything as a pot for your Norfolk Island Pine, as long as there is good drainage. Clay, plastic, metal, wood, ceramic, decorative or found. One of our friends is growing hers in a small wheelbarrow, conveniently placed in front of the bay window in the living room. It is has lights, crafty ornaments and the most recent photos of her grandchildren on it. Now she has started hanging hand-painted blown eggs on it. "Not just for Easter," she told us.

Pests - Fortunately, the Norfolk Island Pine has few insect pests. Sometimes you will find mealybugs or scale but early intervention with a Q-Tip dipped in alcohol can solve this problem. Drying out can cause wilting and tip die back. There are few diseases that will affect this rugged plant when its growing on your windowsill or patio and most of these are a result of improper watering.

Propagation - Unfortunately, Norfolk Island Pines can't be started from cuttings. They are started from the seeds, which have a relatively short shelf life. Seeds remain viable for only a couple months.

Indoors or Out - This is an ideal plant for indoor cultivation. You can move it outdoors for the frost free months and it will thrive in the fresh air. If it has been grown in a low light situation it should be kept in light shade outdoors. If you live in a mild or subtropical climate it can even go outdoors for good. It's even salt tolerant and can be grown along coastal areas.

Digging Deeper:

Joni dried some leaves and painted them with gold and silver paint. These served as the ornaments.

Gracie used beads from Mardi Gras past and star stickers to decorate her tree.

Lenny, being addicted to fishing, carefully selected some choice lures as ornaments and placed the tin can pot in an old fishing hat.

As a Green Thumb Club project the families of the participating gardeners provided handcrafted ornaments that had special meaning. Another club member made ornaments from school pictures of the grandchildren.

In a classroom project the students made origami ornaments for their trees.

One windowsill gardener made a money tree by gluing fine ribbon hangers to assorted coins.

Many change the decorations with the season, from small silk flowers and Easter eggs to mini flags and even Halloween pumpkin ornaments.

Pauline used the opportunity to teach a group of visiting children how to make ornaments out of straw and ribbon.

A Pot of Gold on Your Windowsill

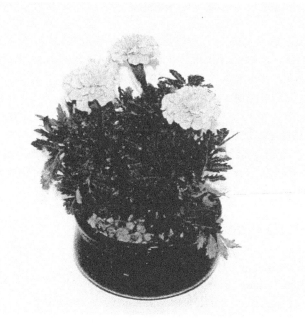

Marigold, *Tagetes patula*
Daisy family, *Asteraceae*
Native to Mexico
All parts safe
Rating: Easy
Time frame: Six to eight weeks for the first blossoms
Life span: Marigolds are annuals
Size: Small scale project

History of the marigold

Marigolds are easy to grow on a bright windowsill, even though we usually grow them outdoors in a sunny location. While they are often called French, African and Irish lace marigolds they are all American, originating on the deserts of Mexico and the American Southwest. It became very popular in Europe after the Spanish priest, Fray Marcos, introduced it in the 1540's. The original was a rugged plant producing a multitude of small yellow flowers. Today we have an amazing variety of colors, forms, sizes and shapes to choose from. In the sixties the Burpee Seed Company staged a great contest encouraging gardeners to produce a white marigold. This made everyone a plant hybridizer and did much to make this plant so popular that Senator Everett Dirkson promoted the marigold as the national flower.

There are some marigolds that are lemon-scented, some have no scent at all. There are perennial shrubs in the family like the Copper Canyon Marigold, and an anise flavored perennial marigold, *Tagetes lucida*, called Mexican or Spanish tarragon.

Herbal uses of the Marigold

Marigolds were used medically by the Native Americans. Teas were brewed from the leaves and flowers to reduce fever, soothe an upset stomach or ease a sore throat. A hair rinse made from the leaves was said to discourage head lice. The leaves were dried and crushed to repel insects where food was stored. They also used the leaves and flowers as a seasoning in their soups, stews, meat dishes and breads.

In Europe and in the missions of the Spanish conquest marigolds were used as a strewing herb. Clothing and bedding were rinsed in marigold scented water. Candles and incense contained dried marigold flowers and leaves. One article states that marigold flowers and leaves were fed to farm animals to keep them healthy, and the flowers were fed to chickens to produce eggs with a deeper yellow yolk and more flavor.

Marigolds have traditionally been valued by organic gardeners because the scent discourages insects in the garden. The roots release a chemical that discourages or kills nematodes in the soil. Outdoors marigolds can be planted with cucumbers or squash to keep the squash beetles away. Marigolds planted among the beans keep the bean beetles away, and marigolds planted among the potatoes control both nematodes and potato bugs.

Materials needed:

Your choice of marigold seeds, dwarf varieties are the best for this project
A black caldron left over from Halloween, or brass spittoon, to serve as the pot for this floral gold
Sufficient potting soil or soilless mix to fill the container

Putting it all together:

1. The container will need some drainage holes drilled in the bottom, three 1/8" holes work well.
2. Fill the pot with your potting mix.
3. Sow between 10 and 15 seeds and cover lightly.
4. Place on your sunniest windowsill and keep evenly moist.
5. Seeds should begin to sprout in about seven to ten days. Thin to between three and five plants as they grow. Note: thinned plants can be potted up in Styrofoam cups and shared with friends.
6. Rotate your "Pot of Gold" once a week so that it will grow evenly.

Care and Feeding of Marigolds

Light: Indoors marigolds need to be on your brightest, sunniest windowsill. If they don't get enough light the plants will be spindly and refuse to bloom. If they have a place in the sun they will be in constant bloom. Outdoors they will thrive in full sun or light shade.

Soil: Marigolds do well in a loose compost rich soil, but will grow in almost any soil with a little encouragement. Indoors use a quality potting mix for best results.

Watering: Marigolds don't like wet feet, but you do need to keep them evenly moist. This encourages a healthy root system and they will reward you with many blooms. If they dry out they will wilt, and sometimes the buds will fail to open.

Containers: These delightful plants will grow in almost anything. Be creative and use them in found containers, old shoes or creatively personalized pots.

Feeding: Marigolds, as is the case with many flowering plants, are heavy eaters and respond well to a regular, monthly feeding of Miracle-Gro Bloom Booster, or a slow-release plant food like Osmocote.

Companions for marigolds: Marigolds willingly share their space with such delights as dandelions, coleus, Bells of Ireland, lettuce and carrots. You can experiment and discover other botanical friendships.

Problems: There are few problems, other than mites and these usually infest plants that are under stress from lack of water, insufficient light, or over feeding. In fact, marigolds are used as insect repellents in the garden.

Most marigolds are annuals: To keep them blooming longer you will need to deadhead the spent flowers. As they complete their life cycle the plants will decline and die. This is their nature, not the result of anything you have done. Save the seeds and start the process again.

Marigolds, Great for Crafty People and Creative Chefs

Marigold flowers can be picked when at their best and dried for bouquets or a potpourri.

The flowers, fresh or dried, can be steeped in hot water to make an aromatic tea or a room freshener.

The petals can be separated and dried, then used in paper making.

Fresh marigold petals can be added to a salad or used as a topping for ice cream, cereal or biscuits.

Parrots and parakeets enjoy the flowers as a snack.

The dried flowers can also be added to a soup for a different and lively flavor.

The colorful flat part of the petal has a pleasant flavor, but the pointed tip, the part that is inside the green part of the flower can be quite bitter. It's best to use only the flat part of each petal.

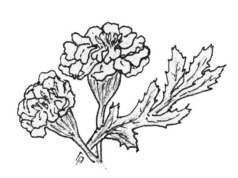

Friendship Gardens,
A Good Old Days Tradition

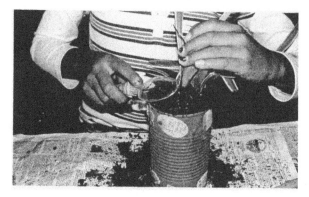
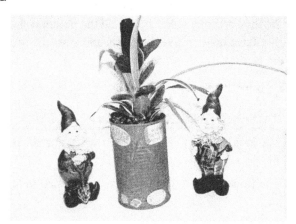

Safety factor depends on the plants selected.
Rating: Very easy
Time frame: 1 hour to initiate, 1 to 2 months for completion, value goes on for generations
Size: Small scale project

In the good old days:

It was once the custom, back in the Good Old Days, to share snips and sprigs of plants with family, friends, guests and casual visitors. It was usually something that grew easily from a cutting. This was a token of friendship and a way of sharing. It was also a way, in days that were perhaps a little less commercial, to obtain something new and different. Sometimes it was something commonplace, sometimes it was a rare, almost one of a kind plant that had been in the family for generations. Often the official names of these plants were lost through the years that it had been a botanical family pet. They were often given names that seemed appropriate to the owners. The once very popular blue flowering Iris *Neomerica gracilis* from South America was known as the Walking Iris, Apostle's Iris, Apostle's sword, Kitchen Iris, Weeping Iris and Smiling Grass. A member of a Green Thumb Club that met at Leu Gardens in Orlando, Florida proudly provided each of the other members a starting from a plant that had been her great-grandmother's.

Sometimes these friendship plants were only cuttings shared, other times Mama or Grandma had little plants started in old tin cans. Sometimes this was a project for the kids on a rainy day. The idea was to share a living plant as a symbol of friendship. It's possible to populate your entire windowsill with such shared plants, tokens of friendship, a living scrapbook of acquaintances or a botanical journey down memory lane. The following is a "just for fun" project for home or classroom designed to promote friendship and re-discover a great tradition from the past.

Materials needed to start a Friendship Garden:

An assortment of tin cans or other found containers. This is recycling at its best.
Paint or decorative materials
Blank gift cards on which you can record care instructions
Sufficient soil or potting mix to fill these cans
Cuttings from three of your favorite easy-to-start plants
A tray or saucer to preserve the windowsill from water damage
Ribbons to make bows for the tin cans when they are being shared

Putting together a Friendship Garden:

- ❤ Wash cans, remove the labels and punch 2 or 3 holes in the bottom for drainage.
- ❤ Paint or decorate the cans.
- ❤ Fill each can with potting mix.
- ❤ Take cuttings or offsets and strike them in the soil, mixing the textures colors and growth habit.
- ❤ Place on saucers or tray and keep watered.
- ❤ While waiting for the plants to grow and the guests to arrive, write simple care instructions, a creative poem, or a picture on the card, then sign it so they will know next year where it came from.
- ❤ When a friend, guest or even the Avon Lady comes calling, give them a plant, but first tie a bow around the can to give it a festive flair.

Some plants that make easy Friendship Plants

African Violet
Aluminum Plant
Angel Wing Begonia
Basil, many varieties start from cuttings
Begonias, many colors, shaped and leaf forms
Boston Fern, started from divisions
Bridal Veil
Christmas Cactus
Coleus
English ivy
Geraniums, a multitude of varieties
Hens & Chicks
Hoya, Wax Plant
Inch plant
Jade Plant
Kalanchoes, flowering types
Maternity plant, Mother of Many
Peace lily
Pepperomia
Philodendron, many types
Purple passion plant
Rabbit's Foot Fern
Sansevieria, Snake Plant
Swedish ivy
Spider plant
Wandering Jew
Zig-Zag cactus, also called Ric-Rac cactus

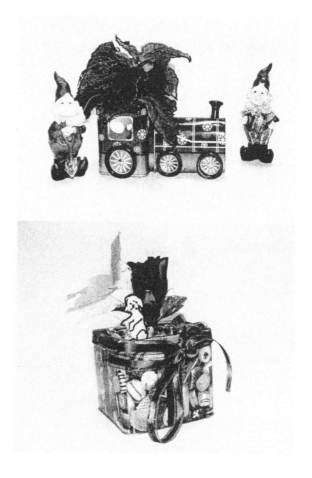

Note: these are all tender plants that do well indoors on the windowsill.

The Great Green Thumb Club Sing-Along Quiz

Music and flowers just seem to go together. From the Yellow Rose of Texas to My Wild Irish Rose or perhaps you have been Lookin' Over a Four-Leaf Clover or pondered along with Peter, Paul & Mary about Where Have All The Flowers Gone? Can you put the plants and flowers back in these lines from songs popular in the 20th century? Note: you can get extra points if you can recall the artist who sang the song, and even more points if you are willing to sing a few lines.

1. *Days of Wine and* _____, was written by Henry Mancini.

2. If mares eat _____ then little Lambs must eat _____ is from a popular children's song.

3. _____ *Fields Forever*, was a complex song that became the name of a memorial garden near Central park in NYC dedicated to the song's composer.

4. *Tie A Yellow Ribbon 'round the Ole* _____ _____ has several myths about its origins.

5. *Don't Sit Under the* _____ _____ *with Anyone Else But Me.*

6. I'm a Lonely Little _____ in an _____ Patch.

7. *I Never Promised You a* _____ _____.

8. *Green Grow the* _____ was a popular folk song in the 19th century.

9. *Yes, We Have No* _____.

10. _____ *Weep for Me.*

11. *A White Sports Coat and a Pink* _____.

12. The _____ *Blossom Special* holds a special place in American music.

13. *In them Ole* _____ *Fields Back Home.* Do you know what state these fields located in?

14. John Denver sang about one America's favorites in the song *Homegrown* _____.

15. Stevie Wonder did a unique album titled *The Secret Life of* _____.

16. *Waltz of the Flowers* and *Waltz of the Sugar Plum Fairies* are both from the _____ Ballet by Tchaikovsky.

17. Waylon Jennings sang about growing up poor on the farm in the song, *Where the* _____ *Don't Grow*.

18. Then, of course there was *Second Hand* _____, a song as ageless as its artist, Neil Diamond.

19. The _____ *Cantata* was a classical wake up call composed by Bach.

20. _____, _____, _____, *and Thyme* were apparently popular at Scarborough Fair.

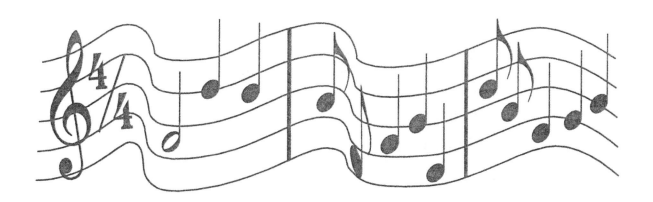

Answers: No fair peeking
1. Roses, 2. Oats, ivy, 3. Strawberry, 4. Oak Tree, 5. Apple Tree, 6. Petunia, Onion, 7. Rose Garden, 8. Lilacs, 9. Bananas, 10. Willow, 11. Carnation, 12. Orange, 13. Cotton Fields, 14. Tomatoes, 15. Plants, 16. Nutcracker, 17. Corn, 18. Rose, 19. Coffee, 20. Parsley, Sage, Rosemary

OOPS! There Goes Another Rubber Tree Plant

Objective: Pure whimsy in the form of an old familiar plant and a popular song

Rubber tree, *Ficus elastica*, *'decora or robusta'*
Mulberry & fig family, *Moraceae*
Native to India
All parts safe
Rating: Very Easy
Time frame: 1 hour to initiate, with little effort
Life span: Yyour rubber tree will grow and thrive for years
Size: Medium scale project

High Hopes

The song was titled 'High Hopes,' and it was originally written for a short run Broadway musical. We know this because during a horticultural therapy session at a nursing home in Florida we were doing a project using liners of these rubber trees. We mentioned the song and asked if anyone could remember the lyrics. A gentleman in the group stood and began to sing. His voice was strong and he delivered all the words perfectly, and he was every bit as entertaining as Frank Sinatra. When we complimented him he explained that he had been the assistant stage director during the play's "very short run." It was a joy to encounter him in the group and he spent most of the hour answering questions about the play, his job, Broadway plays in general and the history of this piece of music. When we give others the opportunity to speak, we can all learn a lot. This is why we stress in our classes that one of the most important things we do as horticultural therapists is listen. It was a popular song performed by many artists but it was Frank Sinatra that made the ant and the rubber tree immortal. Just in case you don't remember the lyrics, the complete music and words are available all over the internet. The best part of this upbeat tune, the verse about the rubber tree plant is included here to get you started.

High Hopes written by Cahn/Van Heusen

Next time you're found with your chin on the ground
There's a lot to be learned so look around.

Just what makes that little ol' ant
Think it can move that rubber tree plant.
Anyone knows an ant, can't
Move a rubber tree plant.

But he's got high hopes . . . he's got high hopes,
He's got high apple pie in the sky hopes.
So any time you're getting low
'Stead of letting go,
Just remember that ant.

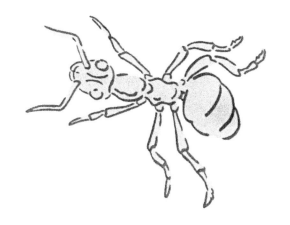

Oops there goes another rubber tree
Oops there goes another rubber tree
Oops there goes another rubber tree plant

The Rubber Tree Plant throughout history:

In generations past it was a rare home indeed that didn't have a rubber tree. We have all sung the song about the ant with high hopes moving that rubber tree plant. This native of India and the Pacific islands became popular in Europe in the 1700's and became an American tradition in the early 1800's. This and other members of the fig family are gaining new importance today as botanical air conditioners because they can filter so many impurities out of the indoor atmosphere.

This is a large family including many popular house plants and food resources like the edible figs, mulberries and breadfruit. There are even some black sheep in the "fig" family, like the "strangler fig" from South America. Figs are found throughout the tropics and most of the temperate regions of the world. While this isn't the primary source of rubber, the milky sap was once used to produce a waterproofing material for umbrellas, raincoats and even canvas overshoes that came to be known as "rubbers." A form of paper, *amata*, is made from the bark of one member of this fig family in Mexico. Well over a thousand years ago the Mayans dyed very thin sheets of this paper bright colors, glued them together to make a large paper bag with the opening at the bottom, tied a lamp filled with oil to it and lit this "lamp." As the oil burned and heated the air in the bag this colorful balloon rose into the air. They created the first hot air balloon, and this was centuries before the French thought it was their idea.

In south Florida, southern California and other frost free areas this will grow to be a tree, but for most of the country it's a container plant. It grows moderately fast but can be a great windowsill plant for a several years. This is one of the most adaptable and foolproof plants we can grow, and all the time it's sitting there it is cleaning the air we breathe. There are many varieties, named because of their leaf color. Some have solid green leaves, but burgundy, red, golden and variegated forms are also available. As they grow they will get aerial roots like their famous cousin, the banyan.

They can be grown in containers to whatever height you choose. They also make an interesting semi-bonsai and work well as a windowsill plant in a whimsey container with pot decor of your choice.

Materials needed:
1 small rubber tree plant. Most garden centers will have pots with between 3 and 6 plants in them at a reasonable price.
1 four inch, or larger, standard flower pot or found container with drainage holes
1 pkg of novelty plastic ants to glue on the planter, or one large ant. These are found everywhere during the Halloween season.
Sufficient potting mix to fill the container

Putting it all together:
- Wash and dry the container.
- Fill with soil.
- Plant the rubber tree in the center of the container.
- Glue ants onto this container.
- Water well and place in a sunny window.

Care & Feeding of Your Rubber Tree Plant

Light: Indoors a bright sunny windowsill works, but they can take subdued light and simply grow a little slower. Outdoors in warm climates they will thrive in full sun to medium shade.

Soil: Almost all members of the fig family will do well in any good potting mix. The important thing to remember is that it must be loose and well drained.

Water: In containers they should be kept evenly moist. Outdoors they are moderately drought tolerant and can survive with limited watering if necessary.

Cold: They will take a mild frost with some leaf damage, but temperatures dipping into the 20's will freeze them to the ground. They are best grown as a container plant in frost prone areas.

Containers: Any container will work for your rubber tree plant. It is best to use a container with good drainage holes. If you use a large container the rubber tree will grow into it. A smaller container will keep the plant compact.

Feeding: A weak solution of Miracle-Gro once a month during the growing season (spring, summer & fall) is sufficient. Feeding with a slow release fertilizer, such as Osmocote, twice a year also works well.

Problems: Very few insects dine on this plant, other than scale, easily controlled with a Que-Tip dipped in alcohol. There are no serious diseases to worry about.

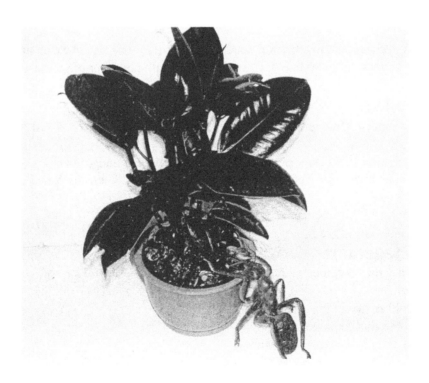

Quiz for the Peanut Gallery

> When I was young, I said to God, "God, tell me the mystery of the universe."
> But God answered, "That knowledge is for me alone."
> So I said, "God, tell me the mystery of the peanut.
> Then God said, "Well, George, that's more nearly your size."
> George Washington Carver, scientist, artist and great human being

1. One of the classic children's shows from the golden age of TV was the Howdy Doody Show. It began in the late '40's and continued into the '60's. It recorded a number of firsts in children's broadcasting. The live studio audience was called the _____ _____.

2. Peanuts are most closely related to: a) cashews, b) chocolate, c) peas, d) pistachios

3. Which American president was a peanut farmer?
a) Abraham Lincoln, b) Jimmy Carter, c) Lyndon Johnson, d) Andrew Johnson

4. The United States produces how much of the world's peanut crop?
a) 60%, b) 35%, c) 18%, d) 6%

5. Peanuts originated in: a) South America, b) Spain, c) India, d) China

6. TRUE or FALSE. Peanut butter was invented by an American doctor to provide nourishment to frail elderly patients.

7. TRUE or FALSE. Peanuts are sometimes called 'Goobers' from the Congolese name for the nut, *nguba.*

8. TRUE or FALSE. In a recent survey it was found that men prefer smooth peanut butter while women would rather dine on crunchy.

9. George Washington Carver developed over 300 uses for the peanut. Which of the following uses did he not develop?
a) Peanut butter, b) Printer's ink, c) Toothpaste, d) Glue, e) shoe polish

10. TRUE or FALSE. The Mr. Peanut symbol of Planters Peanuts was first drawn by a 13 year old boy as an entry in a logo contest.

Answers to the Quiz for the Peanut Gallery

1. Peanut Gallery
2. c) Peas. Peanuts are in the bean (Legume) family and are also first cousin to green beans, limas & lentils.
3. b) Jimmy Carter is the peanut president, although some give Thomas Jefferson credit for being one of the first to grow the peanut in the colonies at his plantation in Virginia.
4. d) The United States produces about 6% of the world's peanuts. India and China are the top producers.
5. a) South America is where the peanuts we know and love today originated. The Incas and their neighbors were growing them for thousands of years before the Spanish discovered them.
6. TRUE, peanut butter was developed in the 1800's as a nutritious food source that could be consumed without teeth and easily digested.
7. TRUE, The name popular in the anti-bellum south, goobers was a corruption of the central African name for a similar legume, *nguba*, that grows there (known today as Groundnuts or Bambara groundnuts).
8. TRUE, men prefer their peanut butter smooth and women like theirs crunchy. Wonder why.
9. Peanut butter was not one of the George Washington Carver's creations. It had been in use before he began his research.
10. TRUE. In 1916 Antonio Gentile entered his 'Peanut Man" drawing in a contest sponsored by the Planters Peanut Company. His design won and he was awarded $5.00.

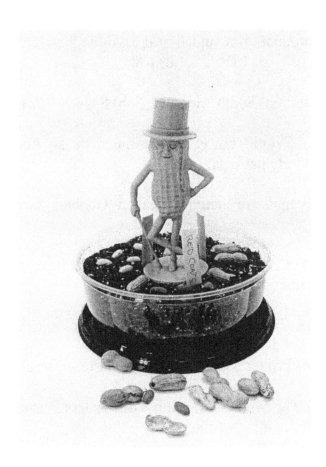

Planting a Pint Size Peanut Patch

Peanut, *Arachis hypogaea*
Bean family, *Fabaceae*
Native to South America
All parts safe
Rating: Very Easy
Time frame: planting to harvest about 12 to 15 weeks
Life span: Peanuts are annuals
Size: medium

"I'm Bill McGee from Tennessee," was how he identified himself to the group during introductions at the beginning of the new horticultural therapy program at the long term care center. He went on to explain that he had been a farmer, preacher man and a banjo player, until the eyes failed him and his legs gave out.

Another Black gentleman in the group, about the same age told us he was Justice Carter, "I'm from just north of Dothan, GA and been a peanut farmer most of my life, that is 'til ole Father Time caught up with me."

At that point Bill McGee turned in his wheelchair, "Where at near Dothan? I was born and raised there myself. Did my share of peanut farming too."

As this conversation progressed these two gentlemen discovered they had lived about two miles from each other, went to school together. They even courted the same girl for awhile. Bill had changed his name when he went on the stage, and later stepped behind the pulpit. They had been in the same senior care facility for almost two years and didn't recognize each other until that afternoon in the horticultural therapy session. From that day on they became the best of friends. By the way, neither of them got the girl.

The common thread through all this was the peanut farming, and peanuts are an interesting project for your windowsill, too. Peanuts are fascinating because they grow from yellow flowers that, once pollinated, bury themselves in the soil to produce the seeds we refer to as peanuts, which are really beans.

Planting a pint size peanut patch
This is a scientific experiment, and just plain fun. This is also a great intergenerational project. This exercise in peanut cultivation began after a discussion between Billie McGee and Justice Carter. They were discussing various ways of growing peanuts and the rest of the group wanted to see who was right. Now you too can join in this experiment. Great for the classroom as well.

Materials needed:
Raw peanuts in the shell, enough to share
Clean plastic clear container, like a deli or cake container from your local supermarket
Sufficient good quality potting soil to fill the container
A package of peanuts or crackers and peanut butter, for nourishment during this project
3 labels to mark the scientific part of this experiment. These can be made out of any material at hand, be creative.

Putting it all together:

1. Punch, or drill, 1 to 3 drainage holes in what was the top of the container. The former bottom can now serve as a saucer.
2. Fill the container with soil.
3. Carefully remove the peanuts from 3 or 4 shells, do not remove the red seed coat from half of the peanuts, remove from the other half so that these seeds are naked. Save 2 others still in the shell.
4. Create 'uniquely yours' labels for

> Naked seeds
> Red Coats
> Peanuts unshelled

5. Divide the soil surface into 3 roughly equal parts. You can use the empty peanut shells as dividers.
6. Using the index finger on the left hand, make a hole in the soil, about 1 joint deep, for each seed.
7. Plant naked seeds in one third, plant those with seed coat in another and plant the 2 in-the-shell peanuts in the other third and use the labels to mark each section.
8. Place in a sunny windowsill and keep watered
9. Design a journal page to track the progress of this the three planting methods in your Pint Size Peanut Patch. Record the germination times, size after first month, first flowering, etc.
10. As the peanuts grow, thin, leaving the most vigorous seedlings until you have one plant in each section.

Variations on a theme

Keep a photo log of the progress of your peanuts, from planting, through bloom to harvest
Be creative and write a poem, short story, song or do art work on the subject of peanuts
Explore various peanut recipes, such as chicken satay or peanut cookies, or peanut pudding. George Washington Carver's collection of 105 recipes can be found at

> aggie-horticulture.tamu.edu/plantanswers/recipes/peanutrecipes.html

Care & Feeding of your Pint Size Peanut Patch

Water: Peanuts should be kept evenly moist but not soggy.
Light: The more sunlight the better. Peanuts will grow well in a south or west facing window or a patio.
Soil: A good quality potting soil with just a little sand added works very well. The important thing to remember is that it must be loose and well drained.
Cold: Peanuts are annual and usually complete their life cycle in about 3 to 4 months.
Feeding: A weak solution of Miracle-Gro once a month during growing season is sufficient.
Problems: Very few insects dine on this plant, other than an occasional white fly or a few mealy bugs. There are no serious diseases when you are growing on this scale.

Just for the fun of it

In one classroom peanut project the teacher had each of his students create "Peanut People." They each selected several peanuts in the shell. Then with paper, cloth and colored markers designed hats, dresses, cowboy outfits, Darth Vader costumes and so much more. Faces were painted on with fine tip markers and they even used twigs and moss to create a landscape for the tabletop community of Peanutville.

Salad Days Garden

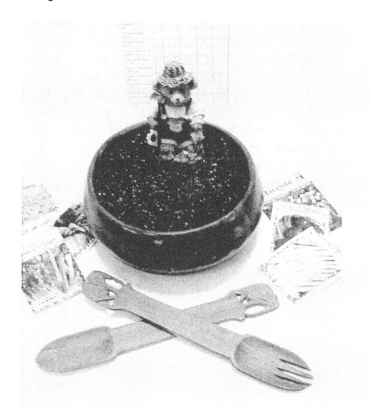

Many species of plants from many families
Native to various regions of our planet
All listed plants are considered safe
Rating: Very Easy, some dexterity required
Time frame: planting to first harvest is about 3 to 5 weeks
Life span: This is a short term project. One season at most.
Size: Medium scale project

History: We think of a salad as a lot of lettuce and a few other vegetables tossed in for color. But a salad has a world of potential. In a six inch flower pot you can grow a whole garden, and nibble on some plants that you may never meet in the average dinner salad. Many of the plants you will be growing in this salad garden are common, but you may not have eaten the leaves before. Some of these plants may be totally new to you. But, for most of these salad greens, you can start harvesting the tender leaves in 3 to 4 weeks after planting the seeds, and the harvest can continue for months.

Materials needed:
1   6" or 8" container and saucer, be creative
Soil sufficient to fill this container
Seeds for at least 5 different salad vegetables from the list on the next page
½ cup colored craft sand
Hand made labels for the varieties of seeds you have chosen
Saucer for the Salad Days Garden to protect windowsill surface
A copy of the Salad Days Garden Log on the next page
Your favorite salad dressing

Putting it all together:

✿   Select salad vegetables to be grown from the list and make labels for each one.

✿   Fill the container with good quality potting soil.

✿   With your thumb make three slight depressions on the soil surface for each variety of salad green you have chosen. Or, you can mark out rows with a pencil.

✿   Carefully place two or three seeds in each depression.

✿   Place label and make entry on the Salad Days Garden Log.

✿   Lightly cover with colored sand, or soil, and water well by placing the container in a saucer of water so that the water is absorbed from the bottom. It may be necessary to add more water to the saucer until the colored sand is moist.

✿   Place in a sunny window and keep watered. Seeds should begin to sprout in about 5 to 10 days.

✿   You can begin to harvest by thinning out the extra plants when they have leaves about 2 or 3 inches in length. Continue thinning until one plant of each variety is left in the pot.

✿   These plants will continue to produce leaves for snacks and salads for months if you do your part.

Care & Feeding of a Salad Garden on a Windowsill

Light: The brightest windowsill available, or a screenroom or patio. These salad greens will also grow under a Grow light.

Soil: This will do well in any quality potting soil mix.

Water: Keep evenly moist. Watch for wilting to indicate a need for watering.

Feeding: A weak solution of Miracle-Gro once a month is usually sufficient.

Containers: There is usually no need to transplant these salad greens into larger containers, but you can create other salad gardens in found and customized containers as you wish.

Problems: There are few problems with salad greens. The biggest problem is overcrowding because you didn't harvest often enough.

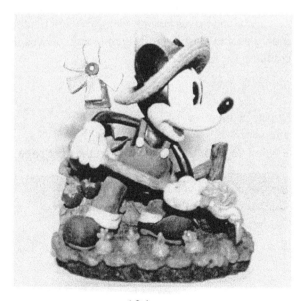

What I planted in My Salad Days Garden

Name _____

Vegetable	Date planted	date sprouted	Date of first harvest	Rate the Flavor
Lettuce, common leaf lettuce				
Spinach, European type				
Chrysanthemum, leaves				
Malabar Spinach, leaves				
Cress, watercress or upland cress				
Kale, for the tender leaves				
Beets, for the leaves and roots				
Rainbow Chard, for the leaves				
Snap peas, leaves & pods				
Sorrel, leaves				
Marigolds, leaves & flowers				
Nasturtiums, leaves & flowers				

Amaranth, leaves				
Lambsquarters, leaves				
Purslane, leaves & stems				
Arugala, leaves				
Mache (corn salad)				
Radishes				

Comments, thoughts, ideas and observations:

_____

_____

_____

my salad garden photo

The Pumpkin Parade

A short story to share, and perhaps set the mood for the fall harvest season. Hope you enjoy it.

Parker and Betty were driving their grandchildren, little Julia and her brothers, Alex and Ethan to school. It was less than a week before Halloween.

"My, how time changes the neighborhood." Betty commented. "No farms left now, just rows of neat houses and condos."

Parker was wistful, almost pensive as his eyes scanned the neighborhood. "Medical complexes and shopping centers now occupy the space where we played baseball in the summer sun. Paved streets have replaced all the dirt roads, and the new high school sits where the old Fedak farm once served as a magnet for all the children in what we called Punkin Hollow back then."

This was a season with a multitude of memories for Betty and her husband. After all, they had first met at a harvest festival held at the Pumpkin Center Grange Hall on the Sunday afternoon just before Halloween. The most beautiful girl in the world had just moved into the old Fedak farmhouse. Parker could still see her in that dark blue dress and that flowered straw hat. But most of all he could remember that delightful smile and the sparkle in her sixteen year old eyes. Good Lord, that was fifty-one years ago today. He took his hand from the steering wheel and patted her knee. She looked at him, and that smile was still there. He took his eyes from the road for just a moment to confirm a suspicion. Yep! Years couldn't dim it, nor could the bifocals hide the charm that still lived in her eyes.

She was also remembering that same day. She could still recall the embarrassment of first seeing this incredibly handsome lad, and there she was wearing old blue jeans and an apron. She could see as clearly as if it were only yesterday the unkempt hair and the red bandana that flowed from his hip pocket. She sorted through the fondest of recollections to paint this mental picture of Parker as a seventeen year old farm boy climbing down from the old John Deere tractor. She could remember the conversation that flowed as they shared a bottle of Cherry Fizz and the shade cast by the massive oak. She could see them leaning against the wagon load of pumpkins he had brought to give away to the neighborhood children.

He became somewhat embarrassed as the next mental image came into focus. Still, it's difficult to pick the memories that flash across the movie screen of the mind. And this was another memory of that afternoon. He could almost smell the fragrance of fall leaves and ripe fruit. Yes. There he was, stealing a pumpkin from Old Bert Ware's pickup. Then, behind the elderberry bushes, with Betty watching, he carved a toothy, smiling face into it with his well used pocket knife. He used that same knife to cut a bouquet of goldenrod and wild asters that he put in the top of newly created Jack-O-Lantern. With a shy giggle he handed the first floral arrangement he had ever created to her. He desperately wanted to press his lips against that charming smile, but lacked the courage.

On the way to the new education complex they passed huge piles of pumpkins. The garden centers, supermarkets, and church parking lots were all filled with pumpkins. There were big pumpkins, little pumpkins, all kinds of pumpkins. There were far too many of these orange symbols of the season. It seemed such a waste. It was so sad. They all knew that many of these wouldn't be chosen to become Jack-O-Lanterns.

137

No one would ever paint scary faces on them, or happy faces either. Not a single one of these was likely to ever become a vase for a wildflower bouquet.

Little Julia was sad. So sad that she had a tear in her eye. She was sad for all these unwanted pumpkins. Then, Julia spotted an old lady across the street. She was pushing a shopping cart full of soda cans. She saw this old lady pull a discarded sandwich from the trash and began to eat it. Now there was a tear in Julia's other eye. It was a tear for the hungry old lady.

She asked, "Why are there hungry, homeless people?"

Alex thought for a moment then spoke up, "Because they are so poor that can't buy food to eat?"

Ethan added, "I don't want anyone to be so hungry they have to eat garbage."

"Yeah," Alex said, "There's got to be a way to help them."

As Parker eavesdropped on the conversation in the back seat an idea began to form in his mind.

Obviously Betty was thinking the same thoughts. Not uncommon for these two perennial love birds. "What do they do with all the left over pumpkins?" she asked.

Parker thought for a moment, not sure what happened to them. Finally he answered, "I think they are thrown in the big dumpsters and hauled to the landfill."

"Can we eat pumpkins?" Julia asked again.

Alex laughed, "Of course we eat pumpkins. Where do you think pumpkin pies come from?"

Ethan added, "Don't you remember the pumpkin bread Mommy made last year?"

Betty was thinking now about the pumpkin seeds she used to eat when she was a child. "I'm certain there are many ways to cook and eat pumpkins."

Julia's mind was racing ahead, "You can take these pumpkins and make pumpkin pies for all the homeless people."

Betty was imagining the house full of pumpkin pies. Pies on the table. Pies on the chairs. Pies on the sofa. Pies on the bed. Even pies on the TV. These mental images were interrupted by the line of cars waiting to deposit children and grandchildren at the Greene Valley Elementary School.

Betty patted Parker's arm as they slowly maneuvered their way out of the school parking lot and back onto the street. "Do you think we need to do some research?" she queried.

Parker pulled into the lot at the community library. They went inside to find out more about pumpkins as food. They told the librarian what they were contemplating. She said, "I have an old recipe my grandmother gave me years ago for pumpkin soup."

The lady standing behind them waiting to check out a couple books chimed in, "My mother makes pumpkin pancakes. They're delicious."

"We used to roast pumpkins on the grill with onions and peppers," Alonzo, a library volunteer added as he too joined in the conversation. He paused, then added, "I bet you can get a lot of recipes down at the retirement home. There's folks there from all over the world."

Soon Betty and Parker had copies of a dozen or more recipes and were on their way to the Apple Lane Senior Center. They spent the rest of the day there, visiting with residents, talking with staff and filling a notebook with recipes, stories, ideas and suggestions.

Meanwhile Juila, Ethan and Alex were sharing the idea with their classmates and teachers. It seemed that everyone in school knew of a special fact, history, trivia or a story about this special fruit. But no one knew much about putting pumpkins on the dinner table, except for pumpkin pie. Soon it was agreed that each student would ask their parents, grandparents and neighbors for pumpkin recipes and pumpkin information. This was becoming a fun project.

Alex was thinking about all of those pumpkins and wondered how they could possibly haul all of them to wherever it was they were going to take them. One of his friends offered a solution. "My dad has a pickup truck. Maybe we can haul the pumpkins to the food pantry in it."

"But what about the Soup Kitchen on 4th Street?" one of Ethan's friends asked.

"There's the homeless shelter down by the train station," Margo entered the conversation. "They could use a lot of pumpkins."

Soon Alex was writing a list of all the places that could use pumpkins. And that's the way the entire day at school went for the three grandchildren. Their friends and teachers were all excited about the prospect of putting all these pumpkins to good use.

Parker and Betty reviewed all their notes while they sat in the pickup line waiting for the kids to be set free. When they burst through the doors and climbed into the back seat they were all taking at once.

Julia was so happy about saving all the pumpkins and feeding the hungry that she invented a little song about them.
> Pretty orange pumpkins piled to the sky,
> Hungry people, I don't know why.
> I want to make them all a pumpkin pie,
> Don't know how, but I think I'll try.

Alex was so excited about hauling the pumpkins that he sat down and drew a picture of a pickup truck filled with bright orange pumpkins. He showed the picture to his grandfather and told him that all the other kids in his class were drawing pictures too. "We have stacks of pictures showing pumpkin pies with Jack-O-Lantern faces, pumpkins on vines, pumpkins on plates, all kinds of pumpkins in all kinds of ways. "Oh Yeah! There's a lot of pictures of Jack-O-Lanterns too. Our teacher was really happy to see everyone working together."

Betty was looking at the picture her grandson had drawn. "I have an idea," she said, "We can use the pictures like this one to illustrate a Pumpkin Book."

Ethan asked, "Where do pumpkins come from?" Then before his grandparents had a chance to answer he fired more questions at them. "Who grew the first pumpkins? Who made the first Jack-O-Lantern? Are pumpkins nutritious? What's the biggest pumpkin ever grown? What's the difference between a pumpkin and a squash? Are all kinds of pumpkins good to eat?"

Then, just as Betty was starting to answer the first question Julia added one more. "What are pepitas? One of the kids in my room said she liked to eat pepitas."

Alex suggested that they could make up a pumpkin quiz to put in the recipe book. Each of the students would make up three questions for the quiz.

Ethan laughed and said, "I have another idea. Why don't we make this a test for the teacher to answer? She's always giving us tests, now its our turn. She can take the test, then we can pick one question each to put in the Pumpkin Book."

Parker thought about this for a moment, then responded, "I don't think the teacher will think this is much fun."

By the next morning everyone in the neighborhood had heard about the pumpkin project. Parents from every classroom offered the use of their pickup trucks. Owners and managers of stores, garden centers and organizations who thought they would have pumpkins left over were calling the school. The residents of the Apple Lane Senior Center invited the students to a Pumpkin Party where they could share their recipes and tell the children stories and memories about pumpkins.

By the end of the week Betty, Parker and several residents from the Senior Center had helped the students put together the Pumpkin Book. One of the residents had been a layout artist for a magazine, another had been a farmer who raised tons of pumpkins, and still another was a nutritionist who shared information about how good pumpkins were to eat. Everyone had recipes and stories to share. What a delight it was to have these elders and the school children working together on this book.

The local newspaper printed a thousand copies of the Pumpkin Book to be given to everyone who got pumpkins from the food pantry. The newspaper also printed a special Pumpkin Edition with photos and stories about the kids and the seniors writing the Pumpkin Book. There was a special article about Parker, Betty, Alex, Ethan and Julia and how the idea came to be and how it grew.

Early Saturday morning, the day after Halloween, the Pumpkin Parade began. There were pickup trucks all lined up at the school. All the students, their parents and neighbors were there too, some with wagons, others with wheelbarrows or lawn carts.

The parade started down the street, being led by the high school band. Julia was next. She had been declared the Pumpkin Princess, and she was dressed in a bright orange pumpkin costume. The wagons and trucks stopped at each place that had been selling pumpkins. The kids, parents and neighbors all worked to load the pumpkins into the trucks, wagons & carts. Soon they had a dozen trucks loaded and all the wagons and even shopping carts from the supermarket.

They had picked up every left over pumpkin in town.

This was more pumpkins that anyone could imagine. It was a mountain of pumpkins. A total of 12,000 pounds of pumpkins had been collected. The Apple Lane Senior Center residents and the elementary school students and their senior friends had put together a 64 page Pumpkin Book with recipes, poems, pictures, memories, stories and pumpkin facts. But it was really a community project. Everyone, of every age, from many traditions took part.

This project gave each individual, every family, classrooms, businesses, places of worship and the entire community the opportunity to make Halloween a time of caring, sharing and gaining in understanding. It is also an opportunity to discuss hunger, its causes and its effects. They all came to understand how everyone in the community is affected when someone is poor, hungry or homeless. This was also an opportunity to discover what everyone can do to help end hunger all over the world, and homelessness in every community.

Notes from the field:
More information on pumpkins, including some recipes can be found at the following web sites.
http://www.pumpkin-patch.com/recipes.html The Pumpkin Patch provides a great wealth of information on pumpkins
http://pumpkinnook.com/cookbook.htm The Pumpkin Nook is also a great source of information
http://www.urbanext.uiuc.edu/pumpkins/recipes.html University of Illinois Extension Service. You can also consult your own state extension service for local information.
There is the potential for many intergenerational projects that can enrich the community and provide an opportunity for everyone to be a part of the solution.

One senior center made their own Jack-O-Lanterns from small pumpkins and filled them with a harvest of dried flowers, fall leaves and a few silk flowers. These were used as centerpieces in the dining room. Another intergenerational group took the "Pumpkin Bouquets" to the local hospital. A group of residents from an assisted living center took their pumpkins and some of their favorite stories to a children's hospital and spent a delightful afternoon with interesting and amusing Halloween stories from all over the world.

Draw on the collective memories and powerful imaginations of the elders and children you know. If you are so inclined, please share what happens with us at petals_pages@man.com

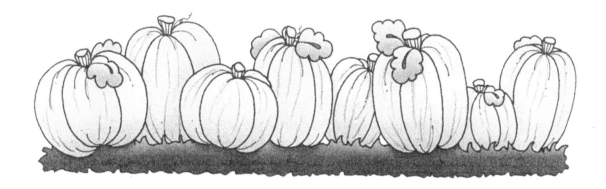

Spiders & Snakes

This is a can't fail fun project for Halloween that involves two of the easiest plants to grow. No green thumb required here. You will combine two very common plants with common names that go well with the season when we love to scare ourselves, and others.

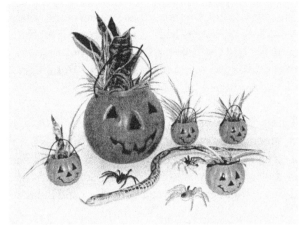

Snake Plant, aka Mother-in-Law's Tongue, bowstring hemp, Rope Grass and Good Luck Plant, to list a few
Sansevieria trifasiata
Yucca family, *Agavaceae*
Native to much of southern Africa, now naturalized throughout the tropics and subtropics
Considered safe although some sources regard the leaves as mildly toxic if ingested
Rating: Very, very Easy
Time frame: 1 hour. Life span: Almost forever
Size: Small to medium scale project

This rugged, adaptable plant was used for thousands of years by the people of Africa, from Zaire to South Africa as a source of bow strings, cord, fishline and the heavy thread for nets to catch fish and birds. There are over seventy species and the International Sansevieria Society now lists over 130 named varieties. Some are short, birdsnest types, some have cylindrical leaves, and the common Snake Plant has leaves that may exceed two feet. They bloom but the flower spike is not strikingly impressive.

They can be started from the offsets that are produced with reckless abandon, or by sections of leaf about three or four inches long. Note, plants growing from the leaf cuttings rarely have the variegation that the original leaf had.

Spider Plant, aka Ribbon Plant, Airplane Plant, Spider Ivy & St Bernard's Lily
Clorophytum comosum
Lily Family, *Liliaceae*
All parts safe
Rating: Very, very easy
Life span: generations

This is another of those South African plants that have claimed the world's windowsills. They are found in a variety of sizes, some solid green, others variegated. All produce a fleshy root that helps it survive drought on the windowsill. They will flower and even produce seeds but are usually propagated from the plantlets that form at the ends of the flower stalks.

This is one of the most efficient "air conditioner" plants, effectively removing formaldehyde, benzene and carbon monoxide, to name a few chemicals it absorbs.

Materials needed:
offsets or plantlets of your snake and spider plants
a plastic pumpkin bucket, or other hollow pumpkin shaped container about the size of a six or eight inch pot
Sufficient potting soil to fill the container
Aquarium gravel in the most ghastly color available.
Plastic spiders and snakes (they will stay put much better than the real thing).
Any other seasonal decor you have available
A good spooky story, preferably about snakes and spiders, but any Halloween theme will work

Putting it all together:
+ Fill the pumpkin, or container of your choice to the rim with the potting soil.
+ Place the Snake Plant toward the back of the planter because it will grow the tallest.
+ Place the Spider near the center or closer to the front of your planter.
+ cover the soil surface with the aquarium gravel.
+ Place the decor items where you wish. It is, after all, your Halloween garden.
+ Share a good story about spiders or snakes.

Care and feeding of Spiders & Snakes:
Light: Both of these plants are adaptable and will take low light to sunny window.

Soil: Almost any soil will work with spiders and snakes, but a good indoor potting soil or soilless mix will serve you well.

Watering: Neither of these plants likes soggy soil. We suggest that you test the soil moisture with your finger before watering.

Feeding: A light feeding with Miracle Gro once every two or three months is usually sufficient.

Problems: Almost no insect problems. They may suffer if the soil is kept too moist.

Maintenance: Spiders and Snakes are low maintenance. Check about twice a week to determine watering needs. Trim off all yellowing or dead leaves.

Notes from the field:
One Green Thumb Club member used the theme of a haunted house in an old galvanized bucket. He used some second hand spider web material from a party goods store and a couple ghost candles along with spiders, snakes and even a bat or two.

Use your imagination and have the courage to be original.

Sand Art Planter

This is a fun project for a gift, or as an element of windowsill decor for yourself. It's a two part project that can be as easy or complicated as you wish. It was suggested by one of our horticultural therapy clients at Leu Botanical Gardens in Orlando, FL when the group was faced with the challenge to "create a unique and original container using your crafty nature and artistic talents." Mercedes was in her late seventies when she suffered the stroke that she thought was the end of a meaningful life. Two years later she was raising vegetables for a neighborhood soup kitchen and volunteering at a nearby head start program as a cookie baker extraordinaire. She was doing this all from a wheelchair. Recently she tackled sand art as her newest craft adventure. This is her project. Thank you Mercedes.

Rating: Difficult, Much fine work and dexterity required
Time frame: Initial project will take 1 to 3 hours. The project will remain viable for a year or more
Size: Small to medium scale project

Materials needed:
1 clear glass, or plastic, container, such as a rose bowl, goldfish bowl, brandy snifter or other unique item that has at least a four inch opening.
1 small plastic drinking glass, 4 to 6 ounce size (McDonald's sundae cup works quite well)
2 or more colors of craft sand
1 chopstick
1 long handled iced tea spoon
Sufficient quality potting soil to fill the drinking glass, with about a teaspoon of aquarium charcoal added.
3 cuttings from one or more of the plants below, or your favorite, or what ever happens to be available
1 small bottle of diluted waterproof white glue
at least 2 colors of craft sand
1 handful of colored aquarium gravel
optional, sea shells, polished stones or other decor items to place against the glass as you fill with sand
An incredible amount of patience

Putting it all together:
1. Fill the drinking glass with soil mix and press firmly so that soil is about ½ inch below the rim.
2. Place the soil filled cup inside the clear container. There needs to be sufficient space between the two to pour the sand and work with it.
3. If the outside container is significantly deeper than the soil container you may have to place some gravel or sand in the bottom to elevate it to the rim.
4. Carefully add layers of sand, teaspoon at a time, either in layers or to create ripple effects.
5. Use the chopstick to shape and contour the layers of different colored sand to create your desired effects.
6. If you wish you can carefully place the shells or other decor as you fill the container with sand.
7. Once the sand is in place pour the dilute waterproof white glue carefully on the sand surface until it is completely covered. This holds the sand in place and prevents water from getting into and discoloring it.
8. After the sand pattern has been completed, you are ready to prepare the cuttings and strike them. Use the chopstick to make three holes in the soil and place the cuttings you have selected.

144

9. You can place colored aquarium gravel on the soil surface to add a finishing touch. This also prevents soil from washing into the sand.

10. You will need to water very carefully, because there is no drainage. Avoid over watering.

Some have placed whimsy figurines on the top of this planter. Don't hesitate to be creative, whimsical & original.

Suggested plants for your sand art planter

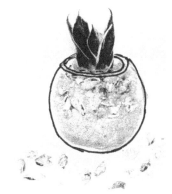

English ivy	Pepperomia
Swedish ivy	Philodendron
Jade plant	Bridal veil
Hens & chicks	Rabbits foot fern
Creeping fig	Sansevieria, birdsnest type
Inch plant	Spider plant
Cryptanthus, earth star	Zebrina
Lucky Bamboo	**many others will also do**
Peace lily	**well**

Care and feeding of a Sand Art Planter

Light: Exposure will depend on the plants you are growing, most of those from the above list will take a wide range of light conditions.

Soil: Because there is no drainage in this planting space it is important to use a good quality potting mix. We recommend that you add a teaspoon of aquarium charcoal to the soil to help prevent souring or the growth of soil fungus.

Watering: Water sparingly to avoid the problems that can arise from soggy soil. We suggest that you test the soil moisture with your finger before watering.

Feeding: A light feeding with Miracle Gro once a month is usually sufficient for the plants you will be growing. Over feeding can cause problems such as spindly growth and lead to insect and disease problems.

Problems: If the plants dry out they will wilt and you know it's time to water them. Unfortunately, if the plants are getting too much water and the roots rot they will also wilt. This is why we recommend that you test the soil with your finger, or a moisture meter, before watering.

Maintenance: This is a low maintenance project once completed. Check about twice a week to determine watering needs. Trim off all yellowing or dead leaves and watch for such critters as mites, scale and mealy bugs.

In the Cancer Center

Because soil borne organisms can pose a threat to cancer patients, some think that horticultural therapy is out of the question, but the benefits of engaging in some gardening activities can be great. Using sterile colored sands rather than soil or soilless mixes can reduce the risk considerably. The Jack's Classic formulas, Peters mixes or Miracle-Gro can also be helpful. The use of terrariums can also minimize risks. In one horticultural therapist's program he had his clients make pickle jar terrariums with sand art for soil and a wealth of creative decor items to make each one unique. The resulting terrariums were almost as beautiful as the cancer patient's smiles.

Sweet Potato Science Experiment

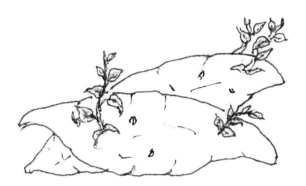

Sweet potato, *Ipomoea batatas*
Morning glory family, *Convolvulaceae*
Native to South America
All parts safe
Rating: Very Easy
Time frame: from starting to first roots is about 2 weeks
Size: Small to medium scale project

Objective:

Engage in a scientific experiment to resolve the question "Does a cutting root faster in a blue bottle or a clear bottle?"

A few years ago we were doing a program at a senior center and one of the participants wanted to start her cuttings in a blue bottle. When asked why, she told us, "Because, everyone knows cuttin's will take root quicker in a blue glass than clear one."

Disturbed by that fact that everyone knew this except us, we decided to do an experiment and had half of the group use clear plastic water bottles while the other half used fancy blue plastic water bottles. She seemed to be right, but the results were close. We have since repeated this scientific experiment hundreds of times. The results do seem to indicate that a blue, green or brown bottle does tend to root cuttings faster than a clear one.

Materials needed:

❦ Sweet potato cuttings, of vines, not the tuber. Several varieties of ornamental sweet potatoes will work. You can also use a garden variety sweet potato.
❦ Two plastic (or glass) bottles, one clear and one blue
❦ Water & a sunny windowsill

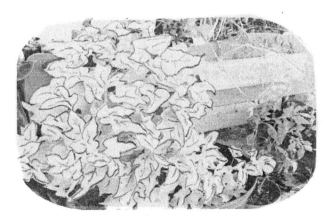

Putting it together:
1. Remove the label from the bottle. This is a good exercise in problem solving and coordination.
2. With markers create a new lable. Write the date, and, if this is a group project, you can also write your name on the label too.
3. Fill bottles with water.
4. Take cuttings, two or three per bottle. They can range from 6" to 15" in length.
5. Examine cutting for signs of insect or disease.
6. Remove the bottom leaf or two so that the cutting will fit easily into the bottle.
7. Place the cuttings in bottles so that at least two or three inches of stem are in water.
8. Watch closely to see which cuttings develop roots first, those in the blue bottle or the clear one.
9. This information can be recorded and notes compared.
10. Water should be changed once a week to prevent spoiling.

Note: As they outgrow the bottle, they can be weaned into a planter or hanging basket, see below.

Variations on a theme:
- Try using various nutrients in the water.
- Try cuttings from other kinds of plants.
- Place rooted cuttings in a larger container of water and use as a major windowsill plant.
- Examine the developing roots with a magnifying glass.
- Taste the new leaves as they begin to unfold. Sweet potato leaves are nutritious and delicious.
- Try other ways of growing a sweet potato vine, such as starting with a small tuber in a jar of water, just like Grandma used to do.
- See how long your vine will actually grow. This can become a contest.
- Can you get your sweet potato vine to bloom on the windowsill? They produce beautiful morning glory blossoms.

Notes on the sweet potato

This vigorous vine produces one of the most nutritious tuberous vegetables we can eat. The sweet potato is rich in Vitamin A and a number of other vitamins and minerals. It can help prevent childhood blindness which is rampant in many parts of the world. The leaves, ounce for ounce, contain about two times the Vitamin A that the tuber does. In many parts of the world varieties of sweet potatoes are grown for their leaves. In the Orient water spinach is an aquatic sweet potato vine that doesn't even produce tubers, but provides great quantities of nutritious leaves.

The sweet potato is in the morning glory family (*Convolvulaceae*) and has been a part of the tropical American Native diet for thousands of years. This is one of the first American foods Columbus dined on when he landed in the Caribbean. It is now grown and enjoyed all over the world because it is easy to grow. The tubers can be baked, boiled, fried, mashed, fermented into *awamori, shochu, masato* or *chicha*. The sweet potato can be made into pies, puddings, cookies, jam, candy, breads and ice cream. The stems are made into *kimchee* in Korea and in Japan the leaves and stems are used in some soy sauces. In the Isle of Majorca it's the sweet potatoes that make "black pig" such a delicious meal.

There are hundreds of different kinds of sweet potatoes. Many of them are grown as ornamentals. These will also produce edible tubers and leaves. Ornamental sweet potatoes make a great ground cover, hanging basket plant or windowsill specimen.

Going from the bottle to pot

After this project has rewarded you with a jungle of vines and a bottle full of roots, its time to transplant it into a large pot or hanging basket. The following are some suggestions for keeping your sweet potato happy.

Light: They will enjoy vining around almost any window and they do need lots of sunlight.

Soil: Sweet potatoes thrive in almost any soil, including sandy soil, but the better the soil, the better the plants.

Water: They like to be kept evenly moist and growth will suffer in a prolonged dry spell.

Containers: Sweet potatoes can be started in a container of water and will grow well that way for months, but usually won't produce tubers. They thrive in a hanging basket and will grow with enthusiasm if kept watered. They can be planted in the soil of large container where they will drape over the edges. In the landscape they will become a natural, living, growing groundcover. You can be creative and use a choice found container, galvanized bucket, coal scuttle, peck basket lined with plastic, or almost anything else.

Problems: Few insects bother the sweet potato other than mealy bugs and white fly. They are resistant to most fungus problems.

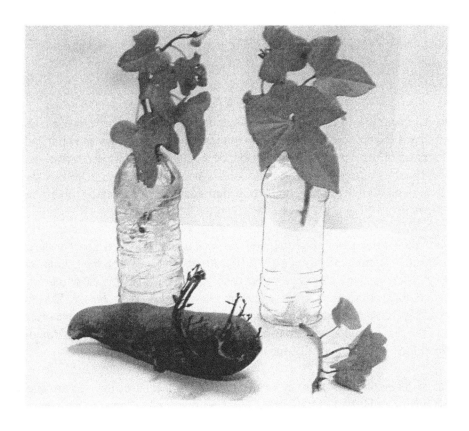

Terrariums,
or What Can You Do with an Old Pickle Jar?

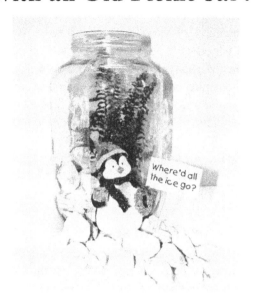

As safe as you choose to make it
Rating: Moderate to difficult, requires
coordination and dexterity
Time frame: 1 to 3 hours to initiate project
Life span is approximately 1 year
Size; Medium to large scale

A terrarium is a sealed container for a single plant or a collection of plants. Terrariums can be made of everything from plastic bags to second hand aquariums, soda bottles to pickle jars. They can be complex artistic creations, low maintenance gardens or a showcase for rare plants. They can be as simple, or as involved as you desire.

Terrarium decor:

Terrariums can require great precision. When you plant a garden in a bottle, it's sort of like creating a ship in a bottle. Miniature landscapes can be created using hand crafted items, thrift store finds or your own special whimsy. We have seen terrariums that recreated scenes from great works of literature, movies or personal experiences. One lady was so enthralled with her Hawaiian vacation that she created her own paradise island out of a pickle jar and Hawaiian plants. Joseph Wood Krutch, a naturalist and author of many books including *The Desert Year*, kept a terrarium made from an old aquarium that refused to hold water. He placed it on his desk, then filled it with various plants native to his Arizona home and added a spadefoot toad. An elderly lady who had spent most of her life in the diplomatic corps in Japan created a "bonsai in a bottle" collection by planting seedlings in assorted bottles, trimming and maintaining them with pieces of wire, knitting needles and long forceps. Carl is from Roswell, New Mexico. He planted a jar placed on its side, with sand and desert plants. Then he crafted a flying saucer from aluminum foil, then added the saucer and a few small alien figures to complete his Roswell in a bottle.

Set your imagination free, be creative and use your sense of humor. We have seen everything from driftwood and dried seedpods to crystals and geodes, action figures from fast food kid's meals to rusted tin cans used to create a setting for specific plants or to convey a message. One classroom painted background scenes on their terrariums while others glued beads, sequins, ribbon, pressed leaves and flowers on the outside of a varied assortment of plastic jars and containers.

What to grow in a terrarium:

A terrarium can be specially designed for desert plants, or it can be a micro-rainforest. It can be grown under lights, on the windowsill, or even used as a night light. Keep in mind that whatever you plant in a terrarium will not live in this confined space forever. Plants will outgrow the limited space, complete their life cycle, drop leaves, get spindly, grow too well, or too poorly. It will be necessary to recondition, refurbish, or rehabilitate a terrarium periodically. Plants can be changed out seasonally, or when you discover a new specimen that needs a home. We had one friend who had been diagnosed with lung cancer. He filled his pickle jar terrarium with dandelions planted in a rainbow of colored sand. They thrived and bloomed for him on his windowsill. He claimed that it was the cheerful, defiant flowers of this common weed that gave him hope and sustained him on his journey toward a successful recovery from his surgery.

Some people include animals or insects such as ladybugs or a praying mantis, frogs, toads, lizards, snakes, turtles, even tarantulas, with the plants in their terrariums. While this adds interest, it also complicates things for the gardener.

Materials needed to start a terrarium:

A clear container, with an opening or lid large enough to let you do the creative work necessary
A good growing medium; colored sand, aquarium gravels, soilless mix or quality potting soil
Crushed charcoal to keep soil from becoming sour
Decor items that match the theme of your terrarium. Don't hesitate to use whimsy
Plants, cuttings or seeds that match the scale of the terrarium you are creating

Your terrarium tool kit can include:

Knitting needles
Crochet hooks
Long tweezers or forceps
Small scissors
Long handled spoon, such as an iced tea spoon
An oven baster, to use for selective watering and feeding
A long handled artist's paint brush, to keep leaves and decor clean

Putting it all together:

- Plan before you begin, select a theme and develop some ideas.
- Find the container that will fit the space you have available and matches your talent for detail work.
- Clean the container thoroughly, do any painting, gluing or external decoration before you plant.
- Collect the decor elements, make certain that they are clean and free of insect eggs, molds or salt accumulations.
- Mix the fine gravel and crushed charcoal and place a layer about ½" deep in the bottom of your container.
- Add the soil or growing medium to a depth appropriate for the space available and the type and size of the plants you are using. Usually a minimum of 2" of growing medium is needed.
- Determine the front and back of the terrarium and place medium accordingly. You can contour the growing medium, make miniature hills and valleys.
- Place the largest plants and the background plants first. Note: you can trim the root mass if these plants are coming out of grower pots.

- Place smaller plants and cuttings. Use the forceps and long handled spoon to place and arrange.
- If you are using ground covers like mosses, creeping Charlie, needlepoint ivy or creeping fig, place them next.
- Now place the rocks, driftwood and other decor elements
- Use the long handled artist's brush to clean soil and assorted debris from the leaves and non-plant materials.
- Water using an oven baster so that the water goes where you want and doesn't wash out the plants.
- Put the lid on it and place your now completed terrarium when you can best show it off and it can get appropriate light.

Terrariums and the health factor

Terrariums can be of benefit to a gardener with immune deficiency, someone who is on chemo-therapy or has severe reactions to soil borne organisms. Because this garden is self contained and can be sealed for extended periods of time you don't have to be in frequent contact with the soil and the micro-biota that inhabit a conventional windowsill ecosystem. Because the terrarium, growing medium and plants can all be virtually sterile the safety factor is greatly enhanced.

Care and Feeding of your terrarium

Light: It is usually best if the terrarium isn't in the brightest window because this can cook the plants. Usually a northern or eastern exposure works best. One terrarium artist we know placed his creation, a series of pint and quart milk bottles, under his fluorescent desk lamp and grew quite successfully a wide variety of woodland plants native to his Canadian birthplace.

Soil: Use a quality soilless mix for best results. If there is a problem with allergies or risk of infection from soil borne organisms you can use play sand, or colored craft sands, rather than the packaged soils.

Watering: Once sealed they need little attention and watering is usually a monthly affair. If moisture condenses on the sides of your terrarium open the top and let the contents dry out for a day or two, reseal and watch for more condensation.

Feeding: Feeding is also done sparingly. A ½ strength Miracle Gro solution every couple months is usually adequate. Many experts suggest that no feeding be done, but this depends on the soil mix you are using and the plants you are growing.

Problems: Terrariums are incredibly low maintenance. Because this is a sealed growing environment there is little risk of insect infestation. Check your plants thoroughly before planting to avoid introducing a problem.

Going one step further

One teacher working with a class of troubled and at risk youth encouraged her students to create small terrariums using mini African violets, ferns and variegated creeping fig, all planted in a quart jar placed on its side. They added miniature wild animals found at a dollar store and gave them to patients at a local hospital, calling them "a jungle in a bottle." This little gift of whimsy was so appreciated by the patients and so empowering to the students who received positive feedback that it became an ongoing project for her classes.

The opportunities abound to make the simple, but incredibly powerful human connections. Sometimes, all we have to do is give the "problem" children an opportunity to be responsible, and hear a kind word rather than always having their shortcomings pointed out to them, and they will do the right thing.

We all have the power to enrich and empower lives. It is such a simple thing to catch these opportunities in a bottle and share the delight.

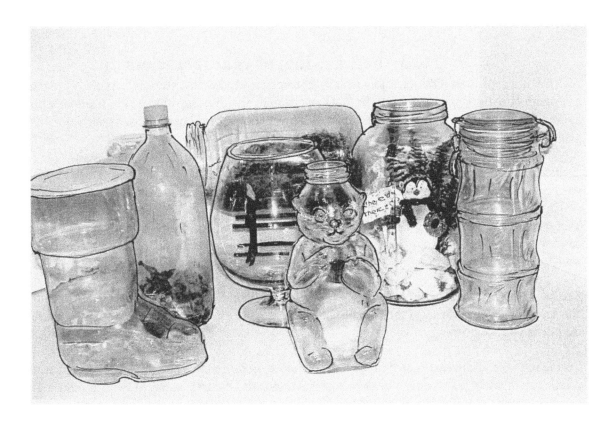

Tree in a Teacup
(Bonsai Easy)

"A bonsai, like a person, is never finished. It is always a work in progress."

"In bonsai, like life, we are both the artist and the art."

All parts safe, care should be taken with tools. Certain plants can pose a problem, choose carefully
Rating: Moderate to difficult
Time Frame: 1 to 3 hours to initiate, most bonsai will continue to grow for years
Size: Small scale

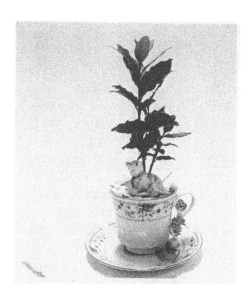

About bonsai

The practice of creating the impression of aged trees and ancient forests in small containers began in China as an art form and focus for religious meditation about 2000 years ago. It came to Japan about 1000 years ago and was a novelty in Europe in the 1800's. Bonsai became popular in the US after WWII.   The term *bonsai* means tray-planted.

For the Japanese a bonsai is a lesson in patience, with the plants being handed down from generation to generation. Originally, these were naturally dwarfed trees taken from nature. Now these landscapes in miniature are created like a work of art. The art of growing a dwarfed tree by carefully pruning the roots and the branches has taken on a distinctly American style with the focus on ease, speed and low maintenance. There are many common trees, shrubs and plants that can be trained into a bonsai form. These include azaleas, sago palms, bamboo, fruit trees, many herbs, house plants, junipers, pines, elms, oaks, English ivy and lantana.

The Japanese, and the English, have very strict rules on the creation, form and presentation of these living sculptures, with a well defined catalog of shapes and forms. We were told by a bonsai master, "Relax. If you like the way it looks, it's a good bonsai. If you don't, like a bad haircut, it will grow."

153

Materials needed:

1 small tree seedling, rooted cutting or prepared specimen, your choice of species
1 tea cup or coffee mug
Sufficient high quality potting soil to fill the container
1 tsp of aquarium charcoal
Live moss is optional, but can be effective
Stones, figurines, or other decor of your choosing to make this bonsai truly yours
Diluted waterproof white craft glue

Bonsai tools you may need:

Fine small scissors or pruning shears
A teaspoon to use as a trowel in planting and maintenance
A table fork with the tines bent to make a mini-rake
Wire to use in shaping trunk and branches

Putting it all together:

1. Clean and dry the tea cup or coffee mug of your choice.
2. Mix the charcoal and the soil, then fill the container.
3. Trim, prune, and remove damaged leaves from the seedling, rooted cutting or plant you have chosen for this project.
4. For many of the plants listed below you may want to trim the roots back slightly. This is usually optional but may help to create balance between top growth and the root system.
5. Carefully place the young plant in the container, smooth the soil around it and firm into place.
6. Water carefully. Because there is no drainage, it's important to avoid over watering.
7. If you have decided to use decorative sand or gravel, this is the time to spread it over the surface.
8. Pour diluted white glue over this gravel to keep it in place.
9. Place larger stones and/or other decor items where you want them.
10. If you chose to use soil and moss rather than sand and gravel, you don't need to use the glue.

Some plants that make great Teacup Trees

Herbs & house plants	Hardy plants for the patio	Pits and peeling bonsai
Scented geraniums	Juniper, creeping or procumbens	Lime or tangerine seedlings
Ficus benjamina	Boxwood	Chili peppers
English ivy	Myrtle, dwarf or variegated	Pear and apple seedlings
Schefflera	Dwarf holly	Grapes
Rosemary	Chinese elm	Pomegranate
Lantana	Japanese Maple	Lychee
Fukien tea	Ginkgo biloba	Coffee
Lavender	Camellia	Cherry, ornamental or fruiting
Jade plant	Surinam cherry	Sage, common garden
Calamondin orange	Australian brush cherry	Flowering quince
Dwarf schefflera	Wisteria	
Gardenia radicans	Witch Hazel	
Bay Laurel	Azaleas	

Use your imagination and experiment. Even if it fails, at least you learned something and had fun in the process.

Bonsai terms that make you sound like an expert

MAME - a miniature, or seedling, rarely more than 2 or 3 inches
SHOHIN - a small bonsai ranging from 2 to 6 inches and beginning to take form, may be 10 years old or more.
CHU - an average size bonsai, ranging from 6 to 12 inches
DAI - may exceed two feet in height or breadth. May be less than four years old or over 200.
CHOKKAN - is a formal upright form, or a single 'tree'
MOYOGI - implies an informal growth pattern
SHAKAN - means slanting form
KENGAI - cascading
NEGARI - exposed roots
SAI-KEI - a planting recreating a landscape Also known as a PEN-JING
YAMADORI - collected material, now frequently included the personalized decor items
TOKONOMA - traditional Japanese display area

Care and feeding of a tree in a teacup

Light: All plants need light and your tree in a teacup will thrive on a bright windowsill, but outdoors they are best on a screen room or in light shade. Morning sun is best. Most bonsai will also thrive under florescent lights. Because there is limited space for soil and roots, full sun can dry them out very quickly.

Soil: use a good grade potting soil. A cheap soil can be disastrous.

Watering: This is the most important factor because you have a small confined space. Check frequently for dryness and water lightly. Indoors this means it may need water two or three times a week. Outdoors daily watering may be needed. Be careful not to over water. This can create serious problems.

Feeding: A bonsai isn't just a plant on a starvation diet. A regular feeding with Miracle-Gro or any other liquid plant food, about once a month is a good idea. A timed-release fertilizer like Osmocote twice a year is another option.

Repotting: With a bonsai, it isn't always a process of transplanting the plant into a larger pot. Sometimes we can even work the plant down into a smaller and smaller size container.

Top pruning: is a two fold process. You prune to encourage the desired shape, as well as control the size of the plant. The top should be pruned several times a year to achieve this.

Root pruning: The roots of your tree in a teacup will need to be trimmed every year or two. This will involve cleaning away much of the soil, removing 25 to 30% of the roots, and repotting.

Shaping the branches: This is where the art comes into bonsai. Work with the plant to determine the form and shape, the size and image. Like a sculpture of marble the goal is to bring out the potential of the raw

155

material more than display the skill of the artist. A bonsai is a partnership with nature. The branches can be shaped with wire, weighted with stones, bent with rubber bands or tied into place with fishline.

Decor and the personal touch: Much of what we do with bonsai in America is a personal statement. We use statuary, stones, moss, miniature living plants and other items to create our own personal work of art. Think of the teacup or bonsai tray as a frame and all that goes into it as your artistic creation.

Displaying your bonsai: The Japanese frequently use a *takonoma*, or formal display area. This is often at the entryway of the home, or an outdoor tearoom. They may be on shelves, benches or pedestals. The area may have works of art, family memorabilia, a seat for meditation and space for quiet conversation. In the United States and Europe we frequently use the bonsai as a focal point surrounded by other decor plants. Remember: It is your plant; it is your work of art. You are the boss.

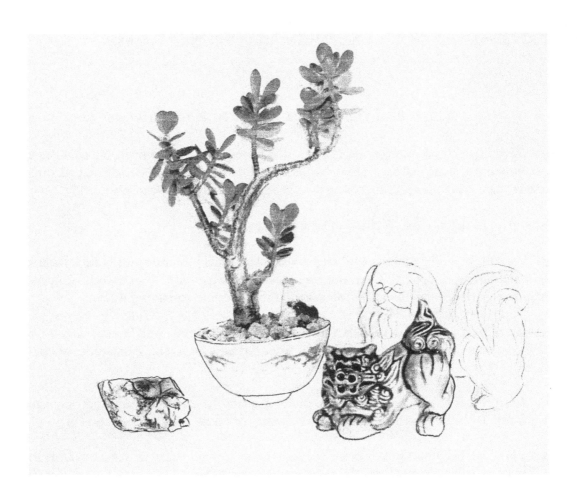

Twigs, Sticks and Stuff

All plants listed are safe
Rating: Very easy, great classroom project
Time Frame: 1 to 2 hours to initiate project, 2 to 4 weeks for bloom
Size: Medium scale project great for the classroom

During those dark days of late winter we can make spring happen by harvesting a few dormant twigs from the snow covered trees and shrubs in your landscape (see list below), then growing a spring garden bouquet to grace the windowsill or table. The bonus is a possibility that many of these dormant twigs will not only give you green leaves and colorful flowers, but take root and become new plants as well.

Materials needed:

Overcoat, gloves, warm socks and insulated boots
Pruning shears, and snow shovel
Flowering trees and shrubs as a source for cuttings
Vase suitable for a bunch of dead looking sticks

Putting it all together:

1. Dress warm and step outside with your pruning shears.
2. Gather between 5 and 20 twigs, sticks and branches. They can be from a variety of different trees and shrubs or a single specimen. Cuttings should be between 15 and 30 inches in length.
3. Bring these sticks inside, take off your boots, gloves and parka. Enjoy a cup of hot chocolate and relax.
4. While you are getting warmed up from your arctic trek fill the vase with water.
5. Make a fresh cut on the base of each twig, then put them in the vase, arranging them artistically, at least as artistically as you can when dealing with leafless sticks.
6. Place on a sunny windowsill, finish the cup of hot chocolate and enjoy a good book.
7. Check for buds breaking dormancy and change the water once a week.
8. Share the first flowers of spring with friends and family.
9. Don't discard these sticks after the flowers fade and fall. The green leaves are also a sign of spring. There is another possible bonus. These sticks may be forming roots.
10. By the time healthy roots are present it may be warm enough to plant these new trees and shrubs outdoors. You can also pot them up and give them to friends.

Time frame for your first flowers of spring:

❋ In about a week, if you have kept the vase full of water, you should see the buds swelling, perhaps even a little green will be showing.
❋ By the third week flower buds for many of these trees and shrubs listed below will be visible, perhaps even the first pussy willows and forsythias will be opening.
❋ By the fourth week you should have lots of bloom, quite a few leaves and perhaps the first hint of roots forming.
❋ Within six weeks you should have roots on many of these branches, at this point we declare them real rooted cuttings ready to pot up into real soil.
❋ They will still need to stay indoors until the snow melts and freezing weather is only a memory.

Some trees and shrubs that can be encouraged to bloom when bribed with a warm bath and a vacation on a sunny windowsill.

Apricot
Cherry, fruiting or ornamental
Corkscrew willow
Crab apple
Hydrangea
Peaches
Plums
Pussy willow
Red twig dogwood (Osier dogwood)
Viburnums
Witch hazel
Red maple
Forsythia
Flowering quince

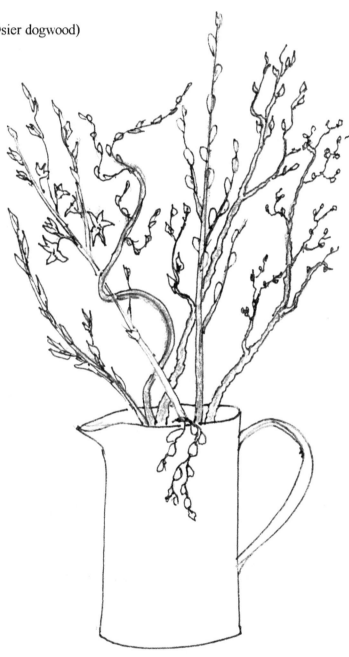

How the Pussy Willow Got Its Kittens

Katcha wasn't much of a cat, as cats go. No long silken coat of a Persian, no aristocratic swagger of a Siamese, not even a particularly beautiful color. In fact she was, plain and simple, nothing more than a barn cat. Gray and dusty tiger stripes covered her sides while a splash of tan covered part of her face like paint splatters. Even her left front paw looked as if she had stepped in a can of dull tan paint. She was preparing the nest in the corner of the barn where the grain bin stood. There was lots of hay and chaff in the narrow space between this old wooden bin and the stone wall. This would be her second litter of kittens, and she would do better this time. She was a much wiser cat now.

Stavo was a gruff old Polish farmer. To the rest of the world he showed a total dislike for the cats that occupied his barn. He would joke that he only tolerated them because they kept the mice honest. But when he was in the barn alone he would talk to them, even pet them and when he sat to do the milking Katcha was frequently the recipient of a stream of fresh, warm milk. Katrinka, Stavo's wife, was also a bit rough-edged in her speech and often scattered the cats with the harshest of language and much waving of the handmade broom that seemed to always be at her side. Yet, when no one was around, not even family, she would mix bits of bread crust with some sausages and left over gravy and leave it for the 'wee beasts' as she usually called them.

It was Katrinka that first noticed Katcha's round tummy. It was shortly after one of the last snows of March. She had been sweeping a path to the wood pile. Katcha was sitting patiently, as cats will do, waiting for a mouse to become careless enough to venture out into the snow to sun itself.

"Oh, Katcha, not more kittens." she grumbled and made the tisk task sound that was her way of showing disapproval. After she carried the armload of wood into the kitchen she returned with a pan of warm gravy, with an extra sausage broken into it. While the cat enjoyed the warm meal, much better than a mouse would have been, and a lot easier to catch, Katrinka felt her belly and scratched her behind the ears.

"Six little ones." She stroked the cat's arched back and shook her head. "Stavo don't like cats, you know. He'll drown every one of these if he finds them." She patted the cat's head as it licked the last of the gravy from the pan. "He complains that we got too many cats now, and still he sees mice."

Katrinka whispered to the soon-to-be mother cat that this would be their secret, "I promise Katcha. I won't tell Stavo, but it's up to you to keep them well hidden."

It was almost dark as Stavo entered the barn and hung the ancient kerosene lantern from the post. He put some oats in a bucket for the cow, and, while she ate, forked hay into the manger and straw into the stall. He saw the cat sitting by the corner of the old cow's stall, patiently waiting, licking her face and paws.

"You're getting fat. I must be giving you too much milk." he joked, then the truth dawned on him. "Oh, no! Not more kittens." He patted her on the head with his rough and calloused hand, then rubbed her chin with his index finger. "Don't let Katrinka see you like this. She thinks there's too many mouths to feed as is. She'd make me drown your kittens."

As he did the milking, Katcha got a couple extra squirts of milk and an extra pat on the head. He watched her as she strolled over to the grain box and back to where her nest was. Stavo took off his old woolen sweater and spread it out in the space she had chosen for her kittens. She curled up on the ancient and moth eaten sweater and dreamed cat dreams, smiling in her mind about Stavo and Katrinka, about how they were such nice people, even when they couldn't let anyone else know that they talked to cats.

It was bitter cold that night, the night the kittens were born. The wind was vicious and sharp, carrying the snow from one place to the next, breaking the beautiful crystals so that each flake was ground into fine pieces that were driven through every crack between the wood of the windows, under the eaves of the old barn so that even the old cow was covered with a dust of snow and the horses stomped their feet and shook their manes trying to keep warm.

Katcha was warm in the old sweater that Stavo had given her. As she washed each of the bundles of life she promised God she would not let anything happen to these precious gifts. They were a variety of colors. The first born looked much like her, and the second was almost all white, with some tan markings on the ears and face. One was gray striped, while another was yellow like the morning sun and yet another was a calico blend of colors. The last one, the runt, was small and a silver gray color that almost glowed in the early morning light. "They are like the sunshine of a fine spring day," she thought to herself as they began to nurse and she dozed off to dream whatever it is that cats dream.

The morning dawned cold but bright and sunny, the wind was still strong, as is to be expected in March. "Has to be a strong March wind to blow winter up into the mountains so we can plant our wheat, cabbages and turnips." Stavo always told Katrinka. It was the way of the Polish country folk to be optimistic in their view of nature and the cycle of the seasons, and the cycle of life. Stavo stood in the powdery snow and let the rising sun warm his body. When he looked out across the rolling hills and the stone wall he could see, in his mind, the wheat sprouting and the cabbages ready to cut for the kraut. He could see the mustard in bloom down by the stream, and taste the turnips, plump and hot on his plate. Life was good for a farmer in this far away valley in the foothills of the mountains.

He knew the snow would be gone by noon. He also knew that it was time to scrape and sharpen the plow, check the seeds and test the soil to see if it was ready to till and plant. The lengthening days gave him the strength to work the fields again, to plant, to move the sheep to the far pasture and prepare for the lambing that was the annual proof that spring had arrived.

In the barn he fed the cow and patted her forehead, "Soon, I think, you can go with me to the field and get the first spring grass."

He pulled the three legged milking stool over and sat the wooden bucket in place. Then he saw Katcha, lean where she had been so plump the day before. He walked over to the grain bin and peered down along the side of the wall. "Ahh, how nice." he said as he patted her on the head. "Quite a family you got here." He paused and studied the dust floating in the sunlight coming through the window. "I think we best not tell Katrinka about this family of yours. She thinks we feed too many mouths already. Yaah, this will be our secret." He patted her head and rubbed her chin. When they returned to the old cow and the milking, she got a couple extra squirts of warm milk.

Katcha was so happy she purred.

After Katrinka and Stavo had a hearty breakfast of Polish sausages, bread and carrots, he did take the cow out to the pasture by the stream and drove the sheep into the spring pasture up the hill. While he was doing this

Katrinka fed the chickens and geese. She stood in the sunshine and watched the snow melting into the soil of her garden. She closed her eyes and saw the turnips and rutabagas, the carrots and the Russian kale, the mint and the dill, all the herbs and even the roses on the bush that now stood still leafless by the kitchen door.

It was Katcha rubbing against her legs that brought her from this journey of the mind back to reality. The moment she saw the cat she knew the kittens had been born. As is the case with all country folk, the birth of any animal is viewed as a miracle and a cause for rejoicing. Katrinka had brought with her a plate of sausage and gravy and followed the mother cat into the barn. Katcha led her right to the grain bin and the nest that contained her six kittens.

"Ahh, Stavo is going to be so angry." she said when she saw the tiny kittens curled up on her husband's old sweater. "This is his favorite. I knitted it for him so many years ago I forget how many. It must have fallen from this grain bin and now it keeps your babies warm." She patted the cat on the head and scratched its ears. "This must be our secret. If Stavo saw this he would drown the kittens and chase you from the barn." She smiled and bent closer to see the kittens better.

And so it went, Stavo and Katrinka keeping the secret of the kittens from each other. Katcha would sit warming herself in the sun and purr as she thought about how strange these people were.

It was April and the wheat was being planted, the lambs were being born and the robins were building nests in the apple trees that would soon be in bloom. The kittens eyes were open and they were becoming more active now, venturing out from behind the grain bin, strolling boldly from one end of the barn to the other. They spent time playing and tumbling, chasing beetles across the floor and trying to catch the flies that somehow always eluded their tiny paws. April is a month of rain showers and sunshine. One afternoon Katcha decided it was time to take her kittens on a journey out by the stone wall and teach them how to catch mice.

All of the kittens tumbled and wrestled with each other, chased leaves blowing in the breeze and tried to catch the robins as they searched for worms in the grass by the wall. The mouse that did venture from the stones was far quicker than Katcha and watched silently from the cracks in the wall as the kittens played with the joy of being alive.

They were so curious about everything, from the nodding spring flowers to the beetles scurrying through the leaves and up the stones. Birds and butterflies were a great puzzlement to them. The little silver colored one was small in size but always the first to claim the top of the field stone wall when they played 'lion of the mountain.' She was the one that ventured into the dangerous unknown corners of the field, tried to climb the apple trees, even explore the hen house to see what was in their water pan. That resulted in an almost disastrous attack by the rooster. The kitten was only saved by Katcha who growled and fluffed up her tail so that she looked as big as the dog that lived down the lane, the one that frequently chased chickens and sometimes caught them.

One warm afternoon they all followed Stavo as he walked down the path through the apple trees, past the stone wall and into the pasture. They watched as he swung the axe to cut the brush and bushes that were growing along the edge of the stream, now swollen and running fast with the melted snow from the mountain. Katcha explained that he cut out the useless bushes so that the cows and sheep could get to the water when they were thirsty. He had chopped out almost all of the bushes with their dull bark and unimpressive stature when the head came loose from the axe handle. While he walked back to the barn to fix it the kittens stayed to play in the sunshine. They had never been this far from home before. Katcha curled up and took a nap while they tumbled, chased each other and did all those things that kittens do.

While she slept in the warm noonday sun the kittens became curious about the churning and gurgling sound of the water rushing down the stream. They cautiously tiptoed closer to the edge, first one, then another until soon all six of the kittens were standing on the very edge of the stream bank peering into the water. It all started with the little, silver-gray runt trying to catch a twig that was being carried along in the swiftly moving water. She reached just a little too far and tumbled into the stream. As the others attempted to rescue her they also fell into the water. Their yowls and screams awoke Katcha.

When she saw her kittens being carried away by the angry water she panicked and began calling for help. First she ran up to Fox who was sunning himself by the stone wall.

"Please! Please! Help! Save my Kittens!" she screamed at him.

He stood to see better what the fuss was about, then nodded his head. "I'm sorry. I would like to help, but they are too far out from the edge, I would get my feet all wet, and that water is sooooo cooold."

Next she ran to the flock of robins by the apple trees. "Please! Please! Help! Save my Kittens!" she screamed.

The robins remembered other cats and how they had often considered robins as little more than lunch. In unison they chirped, "We're so sorry, but it wouldn't be appropriate for robins to rescue cats." With that they flew of to the top of the nearest apple tree to watch the kittens, all secretly hoping that someone would save them.

The old mother hen was walking through the pasture and Katcha ran up to her. "Please! Please! Help! Save my Kittens!" she pleaded.

Mother hen, all in a tizzy raced to the stream bank, then came to a halt. "I, I, a... I can't swim." she said as she turned and scurried back from the water. "I'd like to help, but. . ."

Next Katcha begged the big old oak tree that grew by the bank, "Please! Please! Help! Save my Kittens!"

"I would really like to help, but if I leaned over any further I'm afraid I would fall into the water myself and be washed away." With that he pulled his branches back even farther from the water and ignored the cat's cries.

The sheep said that they would get their wool all wet, the rabbit was afraid that she would drown, the wild lilies growing along the bank said they weren't strong enough.

It was a voice Katcha hadn't heard before, a sad voice that almost apologized for speaking up. "I think I might be able to help. Here, over here." It was the last remaining bush. The one willow left along the stream's edge. Its branches were so sad as it anticipated its fate, so obvious in the pile of fallen branches that had been its neighbors.

"Please, climb up on my longest branch, the one that leans out over the water."

162

Katcha did as this shrub said. Her weight bent the branch just enough to touch the water, and this was at the moment the kittens were being carried by in the swift current.

The first born, the one that looked much like Katcha, was the first to grab the tip of the branch. The kitten that was almost all white, with some tan markings on the ears and face, was saved by grabbing the tail of the first, finally grasping the branch with its tiny, but extremely sharp claws. The gray striped and the yellow ones were next, both being scooped from the water by Katcha. The calico grabbed the branch, but slipped. Frantically it splashed and floundered. It disappeared beneath the water. The small silver gray runt was its only hope. Katcha was holding her paw out to the littlest kitten, but she ignored it and dived under the water to find her sister. Finally she felt the fur of the calico and pushed it to the surface just in time for Katcha to scoop it to safety. It seemed that the runt would be lost. The water was too cold and she was too small. The shrub made one last effort to bend another branch into the water. Just in time the tip of this branch was within reach of the little kitten. She grabbed it and was pulled to safety. The little silver gray kitten, shivering and cold, patted the shrub and thanked it for saving her life, and the lives of her brothers and sisters. Katcha hugged the bush and thanked it too.

Stavo returned from the barn just in time to see this last rescue. He was also in time to see what happened next, as Katcha tried to lick all of the kittens dry in the warm afternoon sun.

It was a soft and gentle voice that seemed to come from the clouds, or perhaps it was the sun itself. Stavo claimed later that it came from the water, or the earth. Regardless it was, all agreed, the voice of God.

"Because you were so compassionate and put the universal love of life into action I have a gift for you. So that everyone will know that love is what life is all about, you shall bear the greatest symbol of spring, the season of new life."

With that a cloud fell over the little shrub. When it lifted, every branch and each twig was covered with miniature silver colored kittens. This neglected and ignored willow became the universal sign of the hope and joy of spring. To this day we call these first spring flowers catkins.

And, that's how the pussy willow got its kittens.

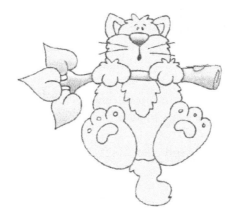

163

Pussy Willow Bouquet

Pussy Willow, *Salix discolor*
Willow family, *Salicaceae*
Native to North America, Europe & Asia
Safety: All parts safe, some edible
Rating: Easy to start, moderately easy to grow
Time frame: Less that 1 hour for first stage, rooting will occur within two weeks. When planted outdoors the pussy willow will grow for years
Size: Small to medium size windowsill project

About the Pussy Willow:

This is one of those great, familiar friends of childhood, a popular landscape shrub and a universal symbol of spring. There are many members of the willow (*Salix*) family that produce the fuzzy catkin-type flowers. One from Japan (*Salix yezoalpina*) grows only 6 to 12 inches tall while the Giant Pussy Willow will exceed 30 feet in height. One variety has flattened fan shaped stems, others have pink, black, silver or white catkins. Male and female flowers are produced on separate plants and the pollen is carried from flower to flower by both bees and butterflies.

In medieval Europe the branches of pussy willow were carried in a parade through the village and each neighbor was tapped on the shoulder to assure good health and happiness. In some parts of eastern Europe there was a symbolic flogging with the branches on Palm Sunday to symbolize how Christ softens the blows of life. It was also the custom in parts of Asia to present each newborn infant with a pussy willow tree started from one that belonged to a family member. One of the first catkins from that shrub was preserved in a "keepsake box."

The Native Americans used the bark and catkins to make a tea for fever and pain relief. Willow bark is a traditional source of Salicin (Aspirin). The tender leaves have also been cooked and eaten as we would spinach. In Asia several types produce a succulent flower bud that is also cooked and used as a vegetable. The branches are popular throughout the world for basket making.

Care & feeding of your Pussy Willow

Starting cuttings: Few plants are easier to start than pussy willow. A cutting of almost any length will root in water or moist soil, usually in a matter of days. Once there are roots, leaves will begin to form and the plant will grow rapidly. Begin with two or three cuttings about 6 to 10 inches long or longer. Plant so that at least 3 inches of the cutting are in the soil and at least 2 or 3 buds are exposed.

Light: Outdoors they will thrive in full sun to medium shade. Indoors they need a bright sunny windowsill. Note that they can only survive indoors for a few months.

Soil: Pussy willows will also grow in sandy soil outdoors if some compost is added. The better the soil the better the bloom. They don't like clay soils.

Water: In containers, or in the ground, they like to be kept evenly moist. These are not drought tolerant shrubs.

Containers: Pussy willows will grow in almost any well drained container that gives it root room. They can even be grown as a Bonsai, or a large container plant if kept pruned.

Feeding: A weak solution of Miracle-Gro once a month during the active growing season is usually sufficient.

Problems: Summer stress is the most serious problem. Pussy willows aren't drought tolerant and will suffer if they dry out. There are few problems other than mites that attack willows temporarily growing indoors.

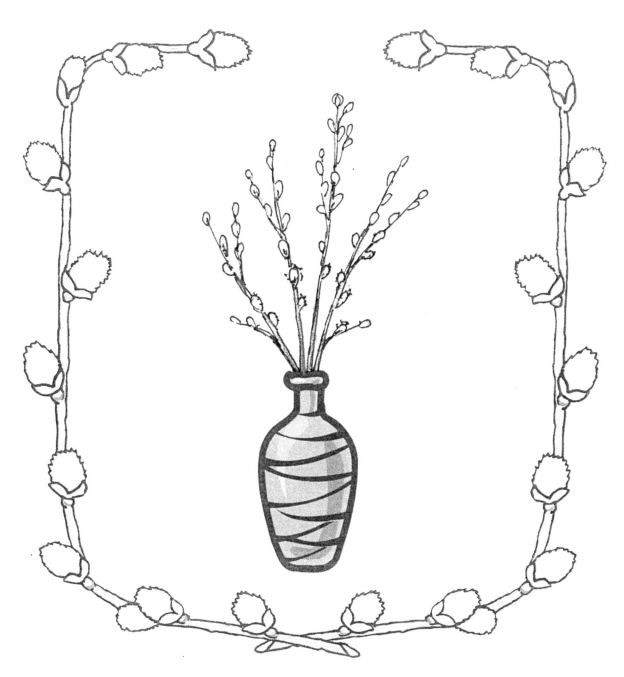

St. Valentine's Day Quiz

Can you complete these famous couples?

1. Romeo and _____

2. Mickey and _____

3. Scarlet O'Hara and _____ _____

4. Popeye and _____ _____

5. Marc Anthony and _____

6. Napoleon and _____

7. Robin Hood and _____ _____

8. Petunia and _____ ___

9. Tarzan and _____

10. King Louis XV and _____ _____

11. TRUE or FALSE   This 'lovers' holiday is based on a Christian martyr from 3rd century Rome.

12. Emperor Claudius II had an indirect influence on this holiday because be:
    a) issued a decree that all residents of Rome should be married.
    b) established specific rules for courtship that involved wine and roses
    c) outlawed marriage because "married men make poor soldiers."

13. The rose is the universal floral symbol of Valentine's Day. But in France there is another flower that is commonly given on this day in honor of a jailer's daughter who was healed of her blindness. This flower is: a) the iris,   b) the aster,   c) the dandelion,   d) the carnation

14. TRUE or FALSE   Valentine cards didn't become popular until the price of postage was reduced to a penny in the 1800's.

15. Who was the first American manufacturer of Valentine cards?
    a) Miss Esther Howland, a student at Holyoke College
    b) Reginald Hallmark, a New York book seller
    c) President Franklin Pierce

Answers on page 168

A Living Valentine

Objective:

To train a vining plant onto a heart shaped wire frame. This can become a gift item for friends, relatives, and total strangers who might become friends.

English Ivy

Hedera helix
Aralia family, *Araliaceae*
Native to Europe & British Isles
All parts safe
Rating: Moderately Easy, strength and dexterity are needed to shape the framework
Time frame: planting to finished tree, 4 to 6 mo.
Size: Small to medium scale

or

Creeping fig

Ficus pumila
Mulberry family, *Moraceae*
Native to East Asia
All parts safe
Rating: Moderately Easy, strength and dexterity are needed to shape the framework
Time frame: planting to finished tree, 4 to 6 mo.
Size: Small to medium scale

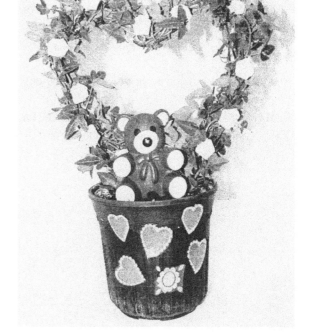

Materials needed:

A 6" clay pot (new or well cleaned), or a found container.
Craft paints in assorted colors
A lightweight wire clothes hanger, or medium weight floral wire
Sufficient good quality soil to fill the pot
Two or four vining plants, or cuttings, either of the above work well
Several twist ties from bread wrappers

Putting it all together:

♥ We start with the pot and the paints. Begin by washing the pot to remove dust. Then you can paint any design or pattern on the pot you so desire. It can pertain to Valentine's Day or a birthday, or any other momentous event, holiday, or occasion. Note: if you would rather glue photos, pictures, used postage stamps, napkins, wallpaper or gift wrap onto the pot, that's ok too. After all, this is your project.

♥ Open the wire coat hanger and bend into the shape of a heart. Set aside until the plants are comfortably planted in the pot. (You can also use floral wire).

167

- ♥ Fill the pot with soil.
- ♥ Using the index finger of your left hand, make two holes on opposite sides of the pot.
- ♥ Put cuttings or small plants in the holes and firm into place.
- ♥ Place the wire heart in the pot to provide a topiary frame for the plants to climb.
- ♥ Use the twist ties to attach the vines to the heart shaped wire. This will need to be repeated every week or two until the entire wire is covered with vines.

Care & feeding of your Living Valentine

Light: For the two plants listed above, almost any exposure will work well. They will tolerate moderately low light so a northern or eastern windowsill is acceptable.

Soil: Any quality potting mix will work well for this project.

Watering: Both of these plants like to be kept evenly moist.

Feeding: Because you want this to grow quickly, a feeding with Miracle Gro every other week is ideal.

Problems: Damaging the vines by twisting the twist ties too tightly is the biggest problem we have encountered. The second greatest problem is letting the soil dry out. Both the ivy and the ficus need to be kept evenly moist.

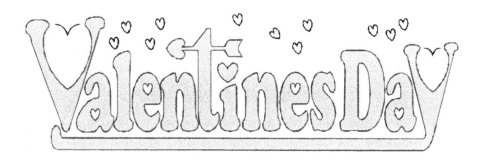

Answers to the Valentine's Day Quiz
1. Juliet
2. Minnie
3. Rett Butler
4. Olive Oil
5. Cleopatra
6. Josephine
7. Maid Marian
8. Porky Pig
9. Jane
10. Marie Antoinette
11. True
12. C
13. D
14. True
15. A

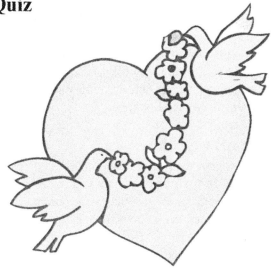

Tillandsia In a Sea Shell

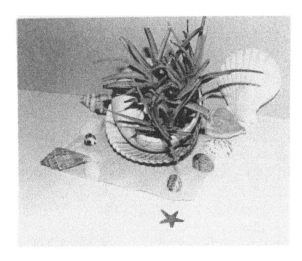

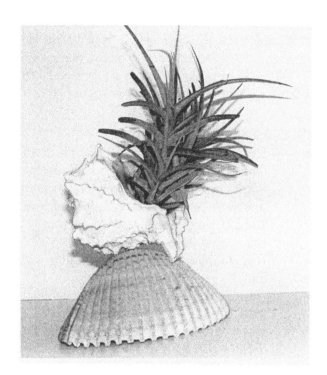

Air plant, *Tillandsia var.*
Pineapple Family, *Bromeliaceae*
Native to South America
All parts safe
Rating: Very easy
Time frame: 1 hour to initiate project
Life span: If misted frequently tillandsias will last for years and bloom, otherwise this is a short term project
Size: Small scale project

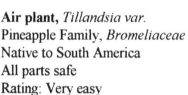

What's a tillandsia?

This is a cousin of the pineapple and Spanish moss. Bromeliads are classified as either terrestrial or epiphytic. Terrestrial species live, like any other self respecting plant, with roots in the ground and leaves in the sunshine. Epiphytic bromeliads live up in trees, on rocks, or on the ground, but they derive their moisture and nutrients from the atmosphere and rain water. Most tillandsias are tree huggers, footloose and fancy free.

These tillandsias are called air plants , or airplane plants because they don't need to be potted and can get along quite well without soil. Some varieties are among the smallest of the bromeliads, rarely growing over a few inches in diameter. Others will reach several feet in diameter. These plants multiply by producing offsets called "pups" around the base of the plant. Left on their own they will form a clump. They are slow growing and extremely rugged, but they are living plants that need light, air circulation and water. They will bloom, often with bright pink or blue or yellow flowers emerging from a flattened bract. The flowers can sometimes last for months.

This is the Timex watch of the plant world, "It takes a lickin' and keeps on tickin." Tillandsias are safe, non-toxic plants everyone can enjoy

Materials needed:

1 Tillandsia, or other small bromeliad

Several sea shells, conchs, oysters, cockleshells, use your imagination.

Waterproof craft glue (you can use Liquid Nails too)

Small colorful shells, or other decorative items

An old Beach Boys album, just to set the mood for playing with seashells

A touch of whimsy, a miniature monkey, a plastic lizard or perhaps a pair of wiggle eyes

Putting it all together:

* Listen to the Beach Boys, if you are doing this project alone, you can even sing along as you sort through your collection of sea shells and pick out just the right ones for this project.
* Wash the seashells in soap and water and rinse well. This will remove any salt residue that may be present. The salt can harm the tillandsia plants.
* Use a conch type shell as the planter and glue it onto a cockleshell or oyster shell that can serve as a base. Allow to dry.
* Rinse the tillandsia in room temperature water to remove any debris, potential insect problems or other dirt.
* Next place a dab or two of glue inside the conch and position the tillandsia the way you want it to grow.
* If you wish to glue small shells, or any other decor items on the shells this is the time to be creative. This is also the time to place your whimsy where it will have the greatest impact. Use your imagination.
* Relax and listen to the Beach Boys again.

Care & feeding of your tillandsia

Light: Tillandsias will do best on a northern or eastern windowsill indoors. Avoid full sun. Just like us, they will sunburn. They will take a shady location quite well.

Soil: These plants don't need soil. Instead they thrive glued to sea shells, driftwood, refrigerator magnets or any other object that you might find. In the wild many varieties will grow on electrical wires, the siding of a house or anything else that stands still long enough.

Water: While these plants can go for months without a drink, they are at their best with a misting every few days or a dunking once a week. They do not like standing water and will rot out if kept too wet. They should dry within four hours to prevent decay.

Feeding: These plants aren't heavy eaters and can do quite well with the nutrients that are floating through the air and contained in the water that you are misting with periodically.

Temperature: Tillandsias are cold sensitive and most will suffer in a frost or freeze. They are at their best when the temperature is between 50 and 90 degrees.

Pests: Almost nothing eats it, fungus doesn't grow on it, but in its natural habitat it can be home to birds, insects, reptiles, mice and other plants.

Tiptoeing Through the Tulips, Spring on the Windowsill

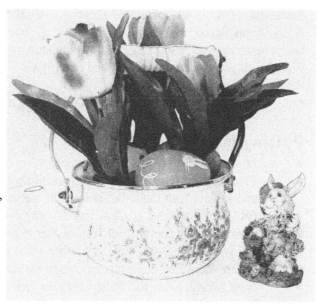

Tulips, *Tulipa* varieties
Lily family, *Liliaceae*
Safety factor: Tulip leaves and bulbs are toxic and care should be taken that they not be ingested
Rating: Moderately easy
Time frame: 2 or 3 1 hour sessions to initiate project, 3 to 4 months from start to bloom
Size: Small to medium scale project

Objective:

To grow colorful spring tulips on a windowsill
This is a project that takes about six weeks after the bulbs have chilled. Started in Early January the bulbs should flower around Valentine's Day.

Tulips throughout history:

While several varieties of tulips have grown wild in Central Asia and the Holy Land for thousands of years it was the Turks who first domesticated them. In fact the name tulip is from the Turkish word *tulpend* which means "turban." This move from mountain sides to garden beds took place about 1000 AD. It made its way to the University of Leiden Botanic gardens sometime in the 15th century. By the 17th century tulips had become highly prized elements of the European landscape and they were also a major item of commerce. Soon it was a craze that rivaled Hula Hoops, Beanie Babies, and Harry Potter. At its peak, tulip bulbs were selling for thousands of dollars each.   There was intense market speculation and the era of "Tulipmania" was underway. As is usually the case, soon everyone was growing tulip bulbs and they were no longer a rare commodity to be traded. This soon led to the "Tulip Crash." Investors lost their fortunes, homes and families. They may have also developed a certain hostility toward tulips in the process.

Today there are thousands of named and often patented varieties of tulips to choose from in a rainbow of bright colors. It is interesting to note that some of the frilly and multi-color varieties that often sold for such high prices were in fact the result of a virus infection. Today the multi-colors and parrot tulips are genetically stable hybrids, not diseased stock.

Materials needed:

3 to 5 Tulips, or more, in your favorite color and form
A paper bag
1 refrigerator vegetable drawer
1 four or six inch clay pot or bulb pan, or a found container of equal size with drainage holes
Sufficient soil to fill the container. This can be quality potting mix, topsoil or a mixture of sand and compost
A label to mark date and variety
Decor items such as beads, sequins, paints, pictures from a bulb catalog or magazine & an active imagination
Waterproof glue for beads, stones, and other trims
Waterproof sealer to cover decor
A cool place to keep the pot filled with bulbs while they grow, away from grazing cats.

Putting it al together:

- First select the bulbs you want to grow.
- Place them in a paper bag, like a lunch bag, then put them in the vegetable crisper in you refrigerator and forget about them for six to eight weeks. Be careful not to store them near apples or any other fruit. Fruit releases ethylene gas that can damage the bloom.
- Customize the container of your choice to make it truly yours.
- Fill your uniquely designed container about half full of soil mix. Then select 3 to 5 tulip bulbs.
- Determine which is the top and which is the base end of the bulb. The base end goes down.
- Next we will place the bulbs about an inch apart and fill with the soil until only the tip showing.
- Place in a sunny window and rotate pot every few days to keep the plants growing straight and tall.
- There is no need to add plant food during the growing process.
- Water when the soil begins to dry but don't keep the soil soggy.
- Your tulip garden will bloom 4 to 6 weeks after first leaves begin to show. This will depend on temperature, sunlight and tulip variety.
- After your tulips have flowered they can be planted outdoors in a shady location. Feed with a good bulb food and they may bloom again next year.

Digging deeper

☺ Gardeners can share memories of other bulb plants like tulips, daffodils, crocus, narcissus.

☺ This can be a great intergenerational project.

☺ The curious can explore the Dutch bulbs in mail order catalogs, magazines, the library or on the Internet.

☺ Plant pots of tulips as gifts. You can be creative and design special pots for special friends.

☺ Potting up bulbs at bi-weekly intervals you can have tulips in bloom for an extended period of time.

☺ One Green Thumb Club member used a large Christmas cookie tin and planted two bulbs every week for a month. She was quite proud of the fact that her garden was in bloom for a month and a half.

☺ Another club member planted three different types of tulip bulbs in the same container and also had an extended blooming season.

172

Hyacinth in a Teacup

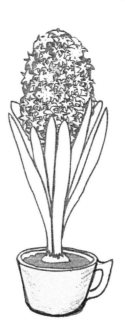

Hyacinth, *Hyacinthus orientalis*
Lily family, *Liliaceae*
Native to the Mediterranean, Holy Land and Eurasia
Note: the bulbs of hyacinths, daffodils and tulips are toxic
 and care should be taken that they not be ingested
Rating: Moderately easy
Time Frame: 6 to 12 weeks

Hyacinths in History and Legend

This is a member of the lily family native to the Mediterranean and the Holy Land. Botanical historians tell us this may have been the "lilies of the field" referred to in the Bible. The name, hyacinth, comes from Greek Mythology. At an earlier Olympic Games a Spartan athlete was struck and killed by a discus poorly thrown by Apollo. It was at the spot where he fell, the Association of Ancient Greek Bulb Producers claimed, that the first hyacinth grew. They were named for a famous Polish saint, St. Hyacinth, who saved a statue of the Virgin Mary from a fire in the 1300's. The statue was singed, but saved. It became a famous icon and thousands made a pilgrimage to see this "Virgin of the Fire." Because of the delightful fragrance and bright colors of these flowers they were placed around the statue. Hyacinths, and other fragrant flowers and herbs, were popular in the musty and dank old European castles, churches, monasteries and homes. They were forced into bloom throughout the winter months to give hope and good cheer to the people in an age before electricity, central heat and running water, TV, video games or MP3 Players.

They bloom in colors including white, yellow, pink, blue, lavender and red. The super fragrant flower spike will range from 8" to 12" tall and last for about 10 to 15 days. Many of the hyacinth bulbs found in your local garden center have been "pre-chilled" and will bloom in about 6 weeks from planting. If the bulbs you grow haven't been chilled, see the chilling method used for the tulips on the preceding page.

Hyacinths are grown commercially almost exclusively in Holland. They can be grown from seed (it takes 5 to 8 years to produce a blooming size bulb from seedlings), or bulblets that form on the sides of the "mother" bulb. Growers will cut the base of the bulb with a knife before planting to generate the production of more bulblets. From a bulblet to blooming size is about 3 years.

Materials needed:
1 teacup or ivy bowl for each hyacinth bulb
Colorful aquarium gravel or marbles
Hyacinth bulbs, your choice of color, pre chilled if available

173

Procedure when using pre-chilled bulbs:

→   Fill the teacup or ivy bowl about 2/3 full with fine stones or gravel or marbles.

→   Place the pre-chilled bulb firmly in the gravel.

→   Fill in around the bulb with more gravel, until it is almost to the rim.

→   Fill with water almost to the top of the gravel.

→   Place the now planted hyacinth bulb in a sunny window.

→   Turn the ivy bowl every few days to keep the plant growing straight and tall.

→   You will need to add water frequently, but don't add so much that the bulb is sitting in the water. Just the roots should be wet.

→   The cooler the temperature the longer the flowers will last.

→   There should be no need to add plant food.

→   After the flowers are done, the bulb can be planted outdoor in a shady location.

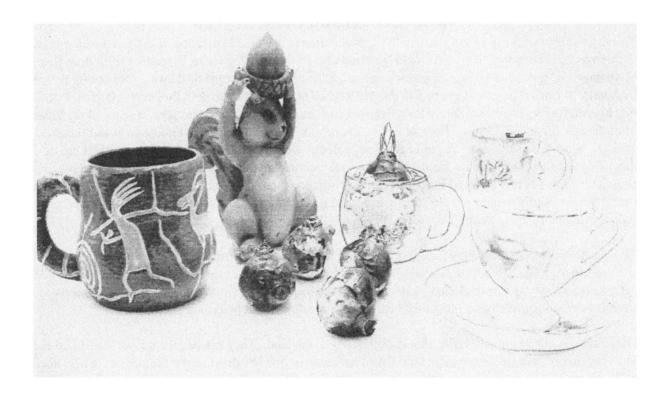

174

Everything's Coming Up Roses
A quiz about songs with roses in the title

There's a multitude of songs written about roses. Some are a tribute to a true love named Rose, while others use the rose as a metaphor. Some simply have roses in their titles. The following are only a few of the many "rose" songs that have been popular through the ages. If we include different languages and cultures the list of rosy songs is well over four thousand long. Let's see how well you do with this little quiz. Note: you get extra points if you can sing a few bars of the song. This is a great group quiz, cooperation counts, and everyone wins.

1. Nat King Cole sang of the _____ *Rose* as a musical metaphor.

2. Country music legend _____ _____ waxed poetic with *Roses are Red, Violets Are Blue*.

3. The Irish have been particularly enthusiastic about roses with even more classics including the beautiful ballad, *The Banks of the Roses*. They also gave us *To a ____ Rose* and *My ____ Irish Rose*.

4. These Irish romantics also gave us *My Lovely Rose of Clare* and *Sweet Rosie O' _____*.

5. Barbara Streisand sang about a lady from Second Avenue called _____ _____ _____.

6. _____ _____ made an impassioned declaration of love with *Rose, Rose, I Love You*.

7. The teeny-boppers danced to *Roses & Lollipops* while Bobby Darren sang about _____ *Yellow Roses*.

8. Then we can fast forward to the hard rock of Guns & Roses and their album, _____ *Roses*.

9. Roger Whittaker made the Christmas song _____ *Like a Rose* a seasonal tradition. We also have the classic hymn, *Lo 'ere a Rose Is Blooming*.

10. Neil Diamond gave us _____ *Rosie*.

11. Nelson Eddie sang his heart out to *Rose* _____.

12. And, of course, there were roses at Ricky Nelson's _____ *Party*.

Answers:
1. Ramblin' Rose, 2. Jim Reeves, 3. Wild . . . Wild, 4. O'Grady, 5. Second Hand Rose, 6. Franky Lane,
7. Sixteen, 8. Stolen, 9. Mighty, 10. Cracklin', 11. Marie, 12. Garden

Were You Ever Promised a Rose Garden?

Rose, *Rosa, varieties*
Rose family, *Rosaceae*
Origin in dispute
Completely safe, except for thorns
Rating: Moderately easy
Time frame: Approximately 4 to 6 weeks for cuttings to root, 3 to 4 months for the first bloom

A brief history of the miniature rose

The rose family is a large and varied one that includes strawberries, apples, pears, tea roses and briars. Almost all wild roses came from the northern hemisphere. The oldest evidence of roses is found in the fossil shales of Montana and this dates back millions of years. The earliest record of miniature roses is from the Island of Mauritius in the Indian Ocean. They were found there and taken back to England in 1810 where they were grown as a popular novelty. In 1917 A Swiss army officer, Dr. Roulet, contacted a friend, Henri Correvon, about a dwarf rose that was said to have been growing in a pot for over 150 years in a village at the foot of the Jura Mountains. This rose became known as "The Jura Lass" and its decedents are still sold today. Now there are hundreds of miniature roses in a wide variety of colors, shapes and growth habits. Some produce flower buds little larger than a grain of rice, others produce flowers with soft velvet petals. Some minis are climbers, others will stay compact for years. Many miniature roses are very fragrant, although some of the popular market varieties have no scents at all. Still, most of the ones marketed in your local garden center bloom with enthusiasm and tend to be more rugged than many hybrid teas. Most miniature roses will grow and bloom well on a sunny windowsill or in a patio garden.

Starting miniature roses from cuttings is easy and there are many ways you can encourage the cutting to become a blooming mini rose bush on your windowsill. Note: many varieties of miniature roses are patented and these should not be propagated without paying the royalty, especially if you are going to sell them.

Materials needed:

A clear plastic sundae cup from MacDonalds
A small amount of moist, good quality potting soil, some prefer moist sand
3 to 5 cuttings from your favorite mini rose bushes, about 3 to 5 inches in length
Rooting compound such as Rootone

Putting it all together:

1. Empty the sundae container and wash well.
2. Put about 2 inches of moist potting soil in the plastic sundae cup.
3. Prepare the cuttings by trimming off the leaves on the bottom 1 to 1 ½ inch of stem.
4. Make a fresh clean cut with pruning shears or a scissors and dip end of the cutting in the rooting compound.
5. Place the cutting in the soil to a depth of at least 1 inch, while singing a few bars from your favorite song with 'rose" in the title. Then put the cap on your micro-terrarium.
6. Place the mini-greenhouse where it will get filtered light and wait until you see new leaves forming. Singing a rosy tune to these cuttings daily is rumored to encourage them to root sooner.
7. After the cuttings have become baby rose bushes you will need to transplant them from the nursery into a home of their own.

Notes from the field:

While you are waiting for roots and leaves you can be preparing "uniquely yours" containers for the time when they are ready for you to let them out of the bag. This can be a clay flower pot painted or decorated with your own personal creative touches. You can use a brass or tin container, an old shoe or almost any other found container that you can punch drainage holes into. One of our Green Thumb Club members used a large tin can that had at one time held some Red Rose Tea Bags. Feel free to use your imagination.

Care & Feeding of your Miniature Rose

Water: In containers, planters or in the ground, they like to be kept evenly moist but not soggy.

Light: Indoors a bright sunny windowsill is a must if they are to do well and bloom. Outdoors they will thrive in full sun or light shade.

Soil: Mini roses will do well in almost any quality potting soil. The important thing to remember is that it must be loose and well drained.

Cold: This is a plant that doesn't mind freezing weather, and will even bloom with a light frost, but will go dormant if it is outside during seriously cold weather.

Containers: Your mini roses will thrive in almost any well drained container, or hanging basket, that gives them room to grow. They will do well in combination with low growing herbs or creeping ground covers.

Feeding: A weak solution of Miracle-Gro once a month during the active growing season is usually sufficient.

Problems: A few insects, like aphids and thrips dine on this plant. Spider mites can be a big problem if the plants are stressed. There are some diseases such as Black spot and powdery mildew that can cause leaves to drop, but mini roses are considered by many experts to be far more rugged than the bigger hybrid teas. Powdery mildew can often be controlled by misting with a mixture of cider vinegar and water. We use a 1 part vinegar to 9 or 10 parts water. Removing any leaves that begin to yellow or drop is one of the best ways to prevent the spread of insects and disease.

Pruning: Your mini rose will bloom throughout most of the year, but it can be pruned back each February and again in late summer to make it fuller and more compact. Constantly deadhead, (removing the spent flowers) to keep it in bloom.

Conversations:

Everyone has a favorite rose. The story of this favorite rose can be fascinating. When we started a little roundtable discussion at an adult day care center some years ago we were surprised with some of the comments. One gentleman, with a smile on his face and a sparkle in his eyes told us his favorite rose was the one he gave his future wife on their first dinner date. Tristan spoke up with a memory of the rose she was given as she held her first daughter for the first time. Stella told us she still had the dried bouquet she was given when she won a skating competition. Gil leaned forward and shared a story of the development of a new rose variety he had been responsible for when working with a major rose grower. What's your favorite rose?

Green Air Conditioners

Objective: To create a unique container and plant it with house plants that filter the air we breathe.

Assorted plants from many different families
Safety: Note that the plants from the list on page 179 with an (☹) are considered toxic if ingested
Rating: Very easy
Time frame: 1 hour to initiate project, the plants will last for years with minimal care
Size: This is a medium to large scale project.
Note: This project was first done in a classroom with special needs children. They then did a presentation at a parent-teacher meeting.

Oxygen:

When you take a deep breath you inhale oxygen, then you exhale carbon dioxide. When a plant "breathes" it takes in carbon dioxide and releases oxygen. When we spend time in the company of our favorite plants we enrich their atmosphere and they return the favor by elevating the oxygen level of the air we are breathing. It's a great system, and this may be one of the reasons why people who work, play and, yes, even talk with their plants seem to be more alert, experience less depression and tend to live longer.

Air filters:

Plants make great air conditioners. They filter a lot of the junk from the air we breath including tars and nicotine from tobacco smoke, formaldehyde from carpeting, wall coverings and other building materials, and carbon dioxide. At the same time they are busy putting oxygen into the air we are using. NASA has done extensive research on the value of plants as an environmental control and oxygen supplement for space travel. This has some potential for the space we live in, as well as a space station. A simple philodendron is so efficient at removing the poisons contained in cigarette smoke that in about three months a philodendron leaf may actually contain more nicotine than a tobacco leaf.

Plants have a number of advantages as air conditioners:

★	They are 100% organic
★	They are silent
★	They don't require expensive service calls
★	They are very energy efficient
★	There are no dangerous moving parts
★	They are more attractive than the average air conditioner or air purifier
★	They are considerably less expensive to install.

While all plants trade oxygen for carbon dioxide and trap dust particles and other junk on their leaf surfaces, some plants actually absorb and chemically break down certain pollutants. For some plants the process is a little different. They absorb the pollutants and store them in the tissues of the leaf. When the level of toxins becomes too high the plant discards that leaf and installs a new filter in the form of new leaves. All you have to do is discard the old ones that have yellowed or fallen.

The following are some of the indoor plants that make efficient air cleaners

Areca palm	Philodendron (☺)
Boston fern	Pothos (☺)
Cast iron plant (☺)	Pygmy date palm
Coffee	Rabbit's foot fern
Coleus	Rubber tree
Dracaena	Schefflera
English ivy	Spider Plant
Geraniums	Swedish Ivy
Grape ivy	Sweet potato vines
Peace lily (☺)	Weeping fig

This is by no means a complete list: Sansevieria, aloe, even African violets and begonias are great air filters. Most plants will trap dust particles and all plants enrich your oxygen supply. Enjoy your green friends. These are all easy to grow and have common needs. This means that you can create a community of plants that will work together to clean the air you breath. The possibilities are almost endless, but we are suggesting a custom made window air conditioner. You can substitute a hanging basket if you wish. A large container on a plant stand or pedestal also works quite well.

Materials needed:

3 to 5 organic air conditioners selected from the list above, or others you prefer

1 container, such as a window box, large square cookie tin or other found container

Sufficient quality potting mix to fill your container

A vigorous imagination that can devise whimsy items as trim for the air conditioner. You don't get to decorate those expensive mechanical air conditioners, do you?

Putting it all together:

1. Clean the container and make certain there are drainage holes.
2. Decorate the container to make it uniquely yours. Go ahead, make a statement. Landis, a very creative member of one of our Green Thumb Clubs glued color pictures from air conditioner advertisements on the sides of his wooden box planter. Others have attached silk flowers, pieces of air filter, Baggies filled with dust and an amazing array of other items to their chosen planter. This is between you and your imagination.
3. Fill the container with the potting soil.
4. Using the index finger of your left hand make a hole for each of the cuttings, plugs or plantlets.
5. Arrange the plants, with lower growing ones toward the edges and the tallest growing ones in the center
6. Firm into place and water well.

Care & Feeding of your Green AC

Light: Note that all of the plants on the list above are happy in relatively low light and don't have to be on that sunny windowsill. They can even be set back from the window if necessary. Flowering plants such as African violets and begonias will need more light.

Soil: Any quality potting mix will work well for these plants. Not only are they effective air filters, they are rugged, tough survivors.

Watering: Most of these plants like to be kept lightly moist. If the soil is soggy it encourages the growth of soil fungus organisms and this can cause allergenic reactions. This defeats the entire purpose of creating a green air conditioner.

Feeding: All of these plants are at their best on a limited diet. We recommend a ½ strength Miracle Gro solution once a month, or Osmocote twice a year.

Problems: Because these are among the most rugged plants for the average home there are few problems. Over watering can create the most serious difficulties, but under watering comes in a close second.

Maintenance: We recommend that you wipe the dust from the leaves once a month using a damp paper towel. Do not use Mayonnaise, vegetable oil or any of the commercial leaf shines. They aren't necessary and can seriously limit the plant's ability to filter the air you are breathing.

Digging deeper:

Using plants as air conditioners is nothing new. Herbs were used before written history to brighten the home, make it smell better and in general make life more pleasant and healthier. The Victorian era used house plants extensively to make the home more tolerable.

There were studies done by NASA about the potential for using live plants as air conditioners during long trips into space, or on space colonies. Much of this research was put into a readable book by one of the people most involved in the project. This book can be found in many libraries, as are several other works by Dr. Wolverton. *How to Grow Fresh Air: 50 House Plants that Purify Your Home or Office* by B. C. Wolverton.

Tin Can Garden

Assorted garden vegetables
Various plant families
Native to the planet Earth
Safety factor: All of the vegetables mentioned below are safe unless otherwise noted
Note: Tomato leaves are toxic if eaten
Rating: Easy
Time Frame: 1 hour to set up, 6 to 12 weeks for first harvest
Great classroom or intergenerational project

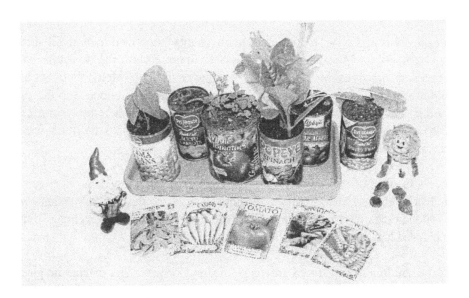

Lunch Is on the Windowsill

Melody was a young lady who walked with difficulty and supported herself with leg braces and a most beautiful smile. Glenda was Melody's next door neighbor, across the hall in the apartment building where they lived.   Glenda's life changed forever when her car was struck by a drunk driver while she was on her way home from the supermarket one evening. These two formed a rather informal support group and spent a lot of time together that winter.

Glenda was entertaining her young friend one afternoon when they decided to have some lunch and Glenda took a can of beets and another of spinach from the cupboard. Melody was fascinated with the labels on the cans and began asking questions. Neither had ever grown vegetables before, but they both became quite curious about where their food came from. They sat down at Glenda's computer and began the quest to learn all they could about each of the vegetables in Glenda's kitchen pantry.

It was while they were searching for information on spinach that Melody got the idea that started a project that took the rest of the winter and into spring. "Can we grow some of these on the windowsill?" she asked with that smile broader than ever.

"We can try," Glenda responded. "Let's see what happens."

Melody picked up the Popeye's Spinach can and studied it, turning the can from side to side. "We can use this can for the pot, can't we?"

It was agreed that they would try to grow the vegetables in the can that had contained them. Glenda and Melody went back to the computer and went to the web site of a mail order seed company. The rest of the afternoon was spent preparing an order for seeds that matched the cans of vegetables. They ordered tomatoes, green beans, yellow wax beans, beets, carrots, peas, turnips, and, of course, spinach. They even ordered cabbage seeds to plant in the sauerkraut can. When they came to the can of sweet potatoes they couldn't find any seeds listed. Then Melody found an ornamental one with purple leaves, advertised as a started plant. They ordered one of them too.

While they waited for the seeds and sweet potato plant to arrive they continued to learn all about the vegetables they would be growing. Melody drew pictures of each one for a scrap book Glenda found in the closet. The anticipation was almost as much fun as the planting would be. Melody's father had already gotten them a bag of potting soil and a big tray to put the cans on. This tray, along with the empty cans sat on the windowsill waiting for the seeds to arrive. Finally the big day came when they found a package in the mailbox. The seeds were here, and they were both so excited. They planted the seeds, watered them well and waited, and waited, and waited.

Finally, in about a week, the first of the pea and bean seeds sprouted. In a few days every can had little seedlings growing in it. Glenda and Melody turned the pots each day so that the baby plants would grow straight and strong. Glenda took photos of each one of them every week. And everything from seed packets to photos to pressed leaves ended up in the scrap book.

Soon Melody had all the children at her school growing Tin Can Gardens. Her teacher taught them all about nutrition and why it was good to eat vegetables. They had a farmer visit the classroom and talk about how vegetables are grown, then they collected recipes from their grandparents and neighbors. Soon every windowsill in the school had a Tin Can Garden and many of the apartments had vegetables growing in their window boxes. All because of a little girl with braces on her legs and an old lady in a wheelchair.

You can create your own Tin Can Garden. Enjoy the experience of growing your own vegetables. Oh, by the way, eat your vegetables. They're good for you, and they are even better when you share them with a friend.

The following are great vegetables for your Tin Can Garden:

Beets	Spinach
Cabbage	Sweet potatoes
Carrots	Tomatoes
Chiles	Turnip greens
Garbanzo beans	
Green beans	
Mustard	
Onions	
Peas	
Peppers	

Where the Wild Things Grow

Lambsquarters, (wild spinach)
Chenopodium album (and other varieties)
Amaranth, *Amaranthus*
Purslane, *Portulaca oleracea*
Native to the planet Earth
All parts safe
Rating: Very easy
Time frame: from seed to sprout 6 to 21 days,
dining begins in about 3 weeks
Life span: these are all annual plants
Size: Small to medium scale

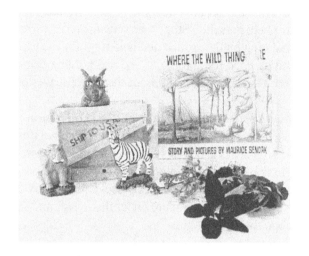

Where the Wild Things Grow

Within us all is an instinctive fear of the unfamiliar, the wild things that surround our existence. But we also possess an incurable curiosity, the drive to learn and understand. These two forces, fear and the yearning to know, are always dueling within us. Unfortunately we all too often give in to the fear rather than seeking to learn. Sometimes this fear is based on logic, but usually it is based on our own ignorance, our lack of understanding, and our feeling that we aren't in control. Still, some of our most wonderful discoveries occur when we let go, when we permit ourselves to go "in search of the answers to questions unknown" as John Denver sang in *Calypso*, his musical tribute to Jacques Cousteau.

We all too often accept without questioning, without opening our minds to the wisdom of others, other generations, other cultures, our planetary neighbors and the folks next door. We are particularly fearful about the wild things around us. We willingly accept all sorts of chemicals, additives, preservatives and artificial flavorings in the food we eat. We limit our diet to a handful of plants that are easy to grow, harvest and market while ignoring many of the plants that are most nutritious. The typical American diet is based on less than a hundred species of plants, yet the world contains over 25,000 edible species. When we were doing the research for our first exploration into hunger and food issues we grew and tasted over two hundred uncommon vegetables. Much of what we learned about these food resources came from the global community that could remember what their grandparents grew, or gathered. This is a knowledge that is fading, but it is wisdom that is well worth rediscovering and sharing with each other. It is not only a valuable part of human history, it is also a key to understanding who we are today, and how we can survive tomorrow.

"Weeds," she said as she began to pull the offending little plants from the raised bed that contained her student's lettuce, carrots and a few struggling beans. "I hate these things. They're the monsters that ate our garden." Ms. Claire is a special-ed teacher and this was the classroom garden that the children were supposed to be tending, but she found it was easier to weed and water herself, so that in reality it was her garden. She feared that they couldn't tell the difference between vegetables and weeds. They might pull the wrong plants as weeds, or worse yet, they might eat a weed and that might make them sick.

Deana watched from the doorway, afraid to interrupt. But then she saw what her teacher was pulling she couldn't help herself. "Stop!" she screamed, "es verdalaga." She then grabbed one of the weeds from the pile accumulating on the ground and held it up for the teacher to see. "See, mi Abuelita says this is very good to eat, and its good for you too." She was holding one of the sprawling purslanes and before Ms. Claire could respond, Deana had put a sprig of the tender leaves and stems in her mouth.

Ms. Claire screamed at the little girl "STOP!" but it was too late. While the panicked teacher was getting to her feet Deana picked up one of the red leaved amaranths and tried to explain that this was also very good to eat. Ms. Claire grabbed this from her hand and threw it on the ground. Then the little girl saw a couple of the triangle shaped leaves of a lambsquarters, but before she could offer her teacher one as a sample of another "Indian spinach" she was severely scolded a second time. After sending Deana back inside Ms. Claire went to her computer to learn more about this weed, and find out if it was poisonous. She learned a lot more that afternoon than she taught.

This experience taught Ms. Claire a very important lesson. Some of the plants we call weeds have a great deal of food value and were once an important part of the diet of many people in many places. In some places these three "Monsters in the Garden" are still valued. The other important lesson she learned was that not only was she the teacher, she also had the opportunity to learn, that we can all learn from each other. She invited Deana's grandmother into the classroom to talk to the children about these "Wild Things" and it was so interesting that the children decided to grow the weeds as well as the more familiar vegetables in their garden. You too can grow the Wild Things on your windowsill. The following three are not only safe but nutritious and quite tasty. And they will happily grow on your windowsill.

Lambsquarters, *Chenopodium alba* and a multitude of other varieties
This delicious leaf crop is also known as Indian Spinach, wild spinach, Goosefoot, Good King Henry, Red Aztec Spinach. It's a fantastic health food, rich in vitamins, minerals and the micro-nutrients that strengthen the immune system. In fact it is said to produce the most nutritious leaves growing wild in North America.

Varieties of *Chenopodium* are found throughout Europe, every state in the United States, much of Africa and the rest of the planet. There are slim-leaf varieties, red leaf forms, broad-leaf sorts and even one that produces delicious mini-fruits that look like tiny strawberries. There are varieties that thrive in deserts, and others that enjoy the humid tropics. Virtually every climate has either indigenous (or sometimes introduced species) that grow easily and produce both edible leaves, flower buds and seeds. The seeds, known as quinoa, have been used as a favored grain in South America for several thousand years. There is an increasing interest today in this grain, and seeds for some varieties are found in vegetable seed catalogs.

Amaranth, *Amaranthus*, many varieties from all over the world
This is considered a noxious weed in most of the United States but it is a valuable food source for much of the world. Some varieties are called pigweed, while others are referred to as Indian spinach, but both the leaves and the seeds are edible, nutritious and tasty. In the Carribean it's known as *Callaloo*. In Maylasia the leaves are called *bayam* while it is called *lenga lenga* in Central Africa. Amaranth leaves are very high in Vitamin

A, Vitamin C, Calcium, Iron, Magnesium, Manganese, Potassium and many other minerals and vitamins. There are also anti-oxidant compounds in the leaves that serve to strengthen the immune system and are important for overall health. There is no fat, but leaves contain a 12 -19% vegetable protein. Not bad for a "noxious weed." The botanical name Amaranthus is a reference to the fact that the flowers don't fade, in fact they are great in dried flower arrangements. We know these ornamental varieties as Celosia or Cockscomb. Seeds are available almost any place that sells flower and vegetable seeds.

Purslane, *Portulaca oleracea* and many other varieties.

Another "noxious weed," yet it is a delicious and healthy food, containing three times the nutritional value of our common supermarket type spinach. The leaves contain more Omega 3 Fatty Acids than any other vegetable. This is important in controlling the cholesterol level and preventing heart attacks. There are several ornamental varieties of purslane, sometimes called moss rose or yellow eyes. These ornamentals are also edible and seeds are available in most garden centers or seed catalogs.

The tender young leaves of these three wild things can be eaten raw as a snack or in salads. Older leaves can be cooked as you would spinach. They are also a great and flavorful addition to soups, rice, even mashed potatoes. Talk with grandparents or community elders and get some recipes and some good stories about these three plants with an undeserved reputation. Nibble and enjoy.

Warning!

You should never eat any plant you are not familiar with and can not positively identify. Also be very cautious about dining on plants you are familiar with that may have been sprayed with pesticides or have come in contact with pollutants in the soil, water or air.

Materials needed for this project:
Seeds for each of the three Wild Things, young plants you have collected from the wilds of the backyard
A copy of Maurice Sendak's classic children's book, *Where the wild Things Are*.
A cookie tin or other container of your choice
Sufficient potting soil to fill this container
Three colors of decorative sand or stones
Whimsy decorations for your Wild Garden, plastic animals, Fun Meal monsters, etc.
Collect pictures of your favorite monsters from books, movies, cartoon features or comic books
Waterproof glue and sealer
An active imagination, just like Max, the main character in the book

Putting it all together:
➡Learn all you can about these Wild Things you will be growing.
➡Read Maurice Sendak's book, best if shared with friends.
➡Punch holes in the container for drainage.
➡Decorate the tin by gluing the pictures, photos and articles you found around the outside.
➡Seal with the sealer, such as Mod-Podge.
➡Fill the container with the soil.
➡With your index finger draw a free-form pattern on the soil surface, dividing the soil into three parts.
➡Plant the seeds and cover lightly with the colored sand or stones, one color for each section.
➡Choose three favorite "garden monsters" that you can represent the three plants.
➡Place the monsters in your garden, water lightly and place in a sunny windowsill.

➼As the "Wild Things" grow in your garden, nibble, snack and add them to your salad.
➼Share your "Wild Things" with friends and family.

Care and Feeding of Your "Wild Things"

Light: The more light the better. Put your Wild Things in the sunniest window, or move them outdoors after seeds sprout.

Soil: These Garden Monsters are tough. Almost any soil will do, but of course, the better the soil the happier your Wild Things will be.

Water: Keep evenly moist for best growth and tenderest leaves.

Feeding: Your Wild Things don't need encouragement, but if you must, use a half strength solution of Miracle Gro once a month.

Problems: Insufficient light will produce spindly, weak leaves and no flowers. The greatest problem is drying out when they are young seedlings.

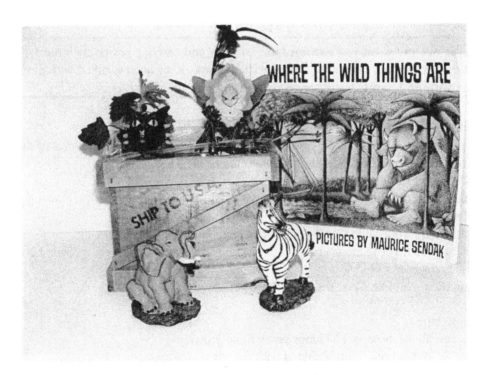

Note:

You can substitute the Troggs great hit *Wild Thing* for Maurice Sendak's book if you prefer. This song was written by Chip Taylor in 1965 and first recorded by The Wild Ones. The Troggs followed with there recording, released by both Fontana and Atco labels. It is the only single to ever simultaneously reach #1 on the Billboard charts for two different companies. Many movies and sporting events have used this song in various versions since its release. *Wild Thing* was the theme song for Rick Vaughn, a rather wild relief pitcher in the 1989 movie *Major League*. The Troggs version was used in the 1992 movie *The Mighty Ducks.*

Part 2

After Dinner Gardening

Gardening projects from pits, peelings and left overs

Avocados are the pits

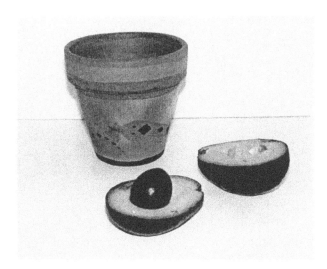

Persea americana (and other species)
Laurel family, *Lauraceae*
Native to tropical America
Also called alligator pear
Safety: Leaves and seeds are mildly toxic and
can also cause allergenic reaction if ingested
 Rating: Very Easy
Time frame: planting to sprouting, 1 to 4 weeks
Life span: If kept happy avocados will grow for
years and reach the ceiling.
Size: Small to medium scale project

Avocados are Good for You
The fruit is rich in dietary fiber and antioxidants. One avocado contains about half the daily fiber recommended by the USDA. This fruit also contains many of the vitamins and minerals we need every day, including Vitamin C. It is low in sodium and cholesterol. While much of a fresh avocado is fat, it isn't the saturated fats that are so bad for us. Avocados are great fresh, in salads, sandwiches or guacamole. You can also find some recipes for other delightful ways to dine on this intriguing fruit, including avocado soup, dips, seafood dishes, even avocado pie. Do a little recipe research and dare to dine as you try one of these recipes you've never tasted before.

Caution
Avocado leaves can cause a rather extreme stomach upset if eaten, and many experience an intense burning sensation in the mouth. The pits are also considered mildly toxic and should not be eaten. Both the leaves and pits can also be toxic to cats, dogs and birds. The fruit is perfectly safe for us and is even used as an oil source for some pet foods.

Avocados are fun
Many tropical fruits have rather large seeds and the avocado seed is one of those that is quite easy to handle, and it has a very good chance of sprouting and growing for you.

Are there children so deprived that they have never stuck toothpicks in an avocado seed and suspended it in a glass of water until they got roots and a couple leaves? We had paid a visit to an elementary school where one class had gone through this childhood ritual with a total, 100% failure. They showed us the plastic cups of water with the seeds suspended from toothpicks. The teacher explained that they had been very careful to keep enough water in the cup to cover about a third of the seed, but still after over a month of anticipation, not a single seed had sprouted. We solved the mystery in a matter of seconds, with one simple observation. Yes, all the seeds had been carefully suspended from the toothpicks, but every last one of them was upside down. It is from the flat end that the root will emerge when the seed sprouts. The second attempt, with new seeds was far more successful.

It may be called Alligator Pear, *Aguacate,* or if you happen to speak Aztec you might call it *ahuacatl.* They are said to have originated in southern Mexico and were being grown along the southern Rio Grande long before Columbus discovered the New World. Legend has it that the first avocado was eaten by a Mayan princess about 300 BC, but they were most likely a popular part of the Mayan diet long before that. Avocados grow on trees ranging from 30 to 60 feet tall with large leaves. It won't get that big on your windowsill, but it will grow quickly and in a year or two it may be three to six feet tall and quite spindly. You can prevent this by pruning out the tip of the shoot. This will encourage the plant to branch, becoming a bushy, beautiful little tree that remains several feet below the ceiling.

Starting your avocado grove, one tree at a time

Materials needed:
3 or more avocados
2 or more friends
1 or more newly discovered recipe(s) for avocados
1 to 3 containers of your choice, equivalent to 4 or 6 inch pots
Sufficient quality potting soil to fill these containers
A sense of adventure
Decor for the container

Putting it all together:
NOTE! We aren't using the glass of water and toothpicks for this one.
1. Combine friendship, sense of adventure and as many smiles as you can locate. Prepare the chosen recipe, rinse, dry & save the avocado pits, dine well, and savor the time with friends.
2. Prepare the container(s) by painting, applying decorative items or simply wiping the dust off of it.
3. Make certain that there is a drainage hole, because avocados don't like soggy soil.
4. Fill the container with the potting mix and firm down so that it is about ½" below the rim.
5. Place the avocado pit, pointed end up, so that it is at least half buried in the soil.
6. Water well and wait.
7. While waiting, try some of the other avocado recipes.

Michael Collier, one of our Green Thumb Club members, chose a large plastic egg left over from an Easter party. He drilled a hole in the bottom and cracked the top with a pair of pliers to make a ragged edge. Then he painted it with a flat white paint, filled it with soil and planted his avocado (alligator pear) seed in it. This was then placed in a shallow basket filled with dried leaves and sphagnum moss. The goal was to create a symbolic alligator's nest where the alligator pear seed would hatch. He finished off the whole project with a plastic toy alligator and entered the newly hatched seedling in a local flower show where he won an honorable mention.

How About a Date?

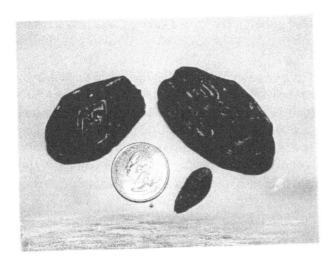
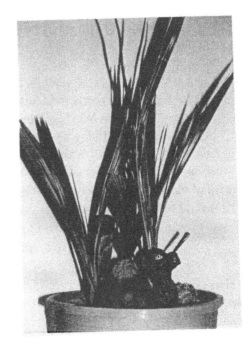

Phoenix dactylifera
Palm family, *Palmae* or *Arecaceae*
Native to Africa, now found in the tropics worldwide
All parts safe
Rating: Very Easy
Time frame: planting to sprouting is about 3 to 6 weeks, sometimes longer
Life span: Date palms will grow slowly for generations
Size: Small scale project, at least for the first couple years.

All you ever wanted to know about dates

The date is the second most well known and widely used of the palms. Only the coconut is more popular. Botanically there are over a dozen species of dates, but most are not grown for food. *Phoenix dactylifera* is the species that we make date bars and candied dates from. There are now several dozen varieties of this species and they are grown in dry, semi-tropical climates all over the world. Commercial date palms will grow from 30 to 100 feet tall, but this takes many years. You can enjoy it for many years before it outgrows your home.

They are native to North Africa and spread into the Holy Land thousands of years ago. The Spanish explorers brought them to the Caribbean and California. Today both Arizona and California have vast date groves with 50 to 100 palms per acre. Iraq and Saudi Arabia are primary global date producers.

There are male and female date palms, and groves are usually planted with one male in the center of a harem of 30 to 50 females. It used to be the practice to cut the stalks of pollen bearing male flowers and tie them into the female flower clusters to assure a large crop of dates. Today the pollen is often collected and dried, then used as needed. The grove keepers use tractor driven dusters to spread the pollen. This dried pollen can be stored for 10 to 14 years.

Dates are started from seed or from the offsets that grow from the base of a mature palm. In some areas male date palms are also grown for the leaves (fronds) that are used on Palm Sunday. They don't remove the leaves from the female because she will need them to produce the fruit.

Dates are a very nutritious food and keep well when they are dried. They are used as a snack food, added to cereals, breads, puddings, cookies, ice cream, juices, alcoholic beverages, jams, and as the source of a sugar solution. In India the seeds are roasted and ground to make a drink similar to coffee. In many parts of Africa the palms are tapped, much like maple trees, for the sap which is used to produce a syrup and palm sugar.

Dates also have a number of traditional medicinal uses. The fruit has been used for thousands of years to treat intestinal upset. A syrup made from boiling the fruit is used to treat sore throats, the common cold, coughs and fever. Dates are used to produce several popular beverages. They are also used to offset the effects of intoxication. The seeds are powdered and also used to treat fever and coughs. Roots are used to treat toothache and sores on the skin. The gum from the tree is used to help control diarrhea and inflammations.

Materials needed:

> Fresh dates, with seeds intact
> Plastic sandwich bags
> Good potting soil
> A sunny windowsill
> Later, a decorative 6" pot

How to start a Date

Enjoy the delicious sweet flavor of three to five fresh dried dates, but save the seeds.

1. Fill a plastic Zip-Loc sandwich bag half full of a good grade potting soil or moist sand.
2. Put the seeds in the moist medium and seal the bag so that there is air space above the soil.
3. Place the bag in the corner of a window, on the surface of a larger potted plant or in the corner somewhere.
4. Now WAIT! But check every few days to see if there are any roots and shoots beginning to grow.
5. When growth starts place the sandwich bag greenhouse on a windowsill where it can get lots of light.
6. After a couple more weeks you should see several roots forming and a single green leaf.
7. Now it's time to transplant them to the 6" pot, or other container of your choice. Use a good sandy cactus or potting soil mix.
8. Keep in a sunny window, or outdoors in warm weather, and keep moist but not soggy.
9. In several months it will produce a second leaf, but it still doesn't look like a palm frond. That won't appear for several more months, or even a year or more. They grow very slowly.
10. Lots of light and slightly moist soil are good. A light feeding with Miracle-Gro or any house-plant fertilizer every two months is also a good idea.
11. This date palm will serve as a beautiful indoor or patio plant for years. It will need to be transplanted to a larger container every two to four years.

for more information on dates go to http://www.hort.purdue.edu/newcrop/morton/Date.html

How Much Do You Know About Garlic?

"To dream that there is garlic in the house is lucky." Richard Folkard in Plant Lore , 1884

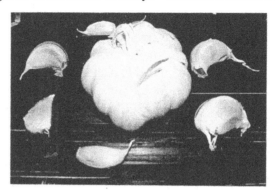

Garlic has been one of our most commonly used culinary herbs for thousands of years. It has also been valued medicinally and used as an element of magic. It has been praised and mocked in literature and on the stage. It has been worshiped and called the food of the devil. Let's see how well you know this famous plant.

1. TRUE or FALSE The Babylonians, Egyptians and Romans believed that garlic would slow the aging process.

2. TRUE or FALSE   The Romans dedicated the garlic plant to Mars, the god of war.

3. TRUE or FALSE   The father of modern medicine, Hippocrates, warned the Greeks against the use of garlic as a medicine.

4. TRUE or FALSE   During the middle ages when Europe was battling the Great Plague thousands of people wore strings of garlic around their neck to protect themselves from the disease.

5. TRUE or FALSE   In some of the rural villages of Mexico garlic was used by teenage girls to attract a potential boyfriend.

6. TRUE or FALSE   Planting garlic in a rose garden will keep some insects away.

7. TRUE or FALSE   In some parts of Africa garlic is used to repel mosquitoes.

8. TRUE or FALSE   Modern medical science is exploring the potential of garlic in the treatment of cancer.

9. TRUE or FALSE   Garlic leaves can be used as a seasoning in much the same way we use the cloves.

10. Gilroy, California calls itself the Garlic Capital of the World and hosts an Annual Garlic Festival

in July. Most of America's garlic crop is grown in the region around Gilroy and the festival attracts over 100,000 people every year. Which American humorist once said of Gilroy, "It's the only town in America where you can marinate a steak by hanging it on the clothesline."
(a) Garrison Keilor,   (b) Bob Hope,   (c) Will Rogers

11. During both WWI and WWII the armies of the Soviet Union used garlic so extensively that it was known as:
(a) The Commie Curse, (b) Russian Penicillin, (c) Russian Breath Mints, (d) The Soviet Secret Weapon

12. In Europe during the Middle Ages it was the custom for a grandmother to hang a braid of garlic on the cradle of a newborn grandchild to:
(a) keep the fairies from stealing the infant, (b) keep snakes away, (c) help the child grow up strong and brave, (d) promote a good appetite.

Answers to the Garlic Quiz

1. TRUE, One source stated that many in these ancient Mediterranean civilizations not only ate garlic as a seasoning, they used garlic oil as a skin cream.
2. TRUE, the Romans were convinced that dining on garlic inspired courage. The juice from garlic was also valued in the treatment of wounds because it helped prevent infection.
3. FALSE, Hippocrates prescribed garlic for everything from leprosy to epilepsy.
4. TRUE, It was strongly advised by the public health authorities of that day that garlic both be consumed and worn to prevent this evil disease of the devil.
5. FALSE, Garlic was used for just the opposite purpose. The young lady would place a clove of garlic on top of a cross made from two twigs, pins or nails in the middle of an intersection of two paths. If she could get the young fellow to step over the garlic clove without noticing it, an unwelcome suitor would loose all interest in her.
6. TRUE, Garlic can be planted in rose gardens, flower beds, vegetable gardens and among berry plants to discourage aphids and Japanese beetles.
7. TRUE, In some regions fresh garlic leaves are woven into necklaces and bracelets. Others eat garlic to repel mosquitoes and there are some cultures that rub garlic juice on their bodies to keep the mosquitoes, flies and other insects away. There are some that also use garlic juice to keep crocodiles and snakes at bay.
8. TRUE, Garlic is known to possess antioxidant and antiseptic properties. It has been used to reduce cholesterol and high blood pressure. While it was part of a popular cure for baldness, the jury is still out on its ability to restore hair.
9. TRUE, Garlic leaves are generally milder but still contain the same healthy compounds and flavor. One herbal described the leaves of garlic as a healthy addition to soup, stew or bread when one is suffering from asthma.
10. (c) Will Rogers made this statement years before Gilroy began hosting their formal Garlic Festival in 1979.
11. (b) Russian penicillin. It was used both in their food and as a antiseptic treatment for wounds.
12. (a) Fairies must have had less socially acceptable habits then than they do today.

Keeping Vampires off the Windowsill

Garlic, *Allium sativum (and many other varieties)*
Lily family, *Liliaceae*
Native to Central Asia, other relatives found around the globe
All parts safe
Rating: Very Easy
Time frame: 1 hour to initiate project. planting to first harvest
will take about two or three months
Size: Small scale project

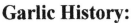

Garlic History:

Garlic is the most popular herb in the world. It has been an important part of both the diet and the pharmacy almost as long as there have been people.

- Garlic was prized by hunter-gatherers before there was agriculture.
- It was said that it originated with the footprints of Satan as he was expelled from Eden. Garlic grew from the left footprints, onions from the right. Another version says it was a gift from the angels to Adam and Eve as they left Eden.
- It was used for barter and trade by the earliest people in the Near East.
- The Egyptians used it as money. Slaves were paid for their labor with a daily ration of garlic bulbs.
- It was valued as a stimulant to ward off fatigue by the Greeks.
- Roman soldiers and athletes were given garlic for strength and health.
- Pliny, the Roman physician recommended garlic for 61 different ailments.
- In Europe's Middle Ages, it was used as a charm against vampires, witches and the tax collector.
- It was universally prescribed for the "plague."
- Culpeper, the British herbalist, recommended it for asthma, internal parasites & dog bites.
- The Chinese and Native Americans valued relatives of it for snakebite and tumors.
- Garlic was added to foods to prevent spoilage. There are anti-bacterial compounds in it.
- In World War I garlic juice was used to clean & disinfect wounds.
- Today research is exploring the anti-cancer properties of garlic.

This most versatile of herbs has been used for:

sunburn	mosquito repellent	heart and circulatory health
Snake bite	rabbit and deer repellent	Hair loss
stomach ulcers	beauty cream	dog & wild animal bites
anti-fungal treatment	athlete's foot	Fire ant bites
stinging nettles, poison ivy	breathing difficulties	almost every culture's menu
garden insect repellent	flea repellent for dogs & cats	Discouraging vampires

---

Garlic was thought to keep vampires at bay. If you are troubled by the miniature vampires that some people call mosquitoes, garlic may be your first line of defense on the windowsill. It is rumored that these pesky little vampires can't stand this valuable herb. If they are a serious problem you might try rubbing garlic on your face and arms.

Materials needed:

1 garlic bulb, actually you will need several cloves, not the entire bulb
1 container, equivalent to a four inch pot. This can be almost any found container that you have on hand
Sufficient good quality potting soil to fill the container.
Paint or decor items to customize your Vampire repellent. Green Thumb Club members have used plastic bats left over from Halloween, clippings from magazines advertising Dracula movies and one very artistic individual constructed a large mosquito out of wire. She then placed it on the container with its mouth piercing a garlic leaf. Is this a sick sense of humor or what?
Your favorite Dracula movie

Putting it all together:

1. With friends, watch the movie, best enjoyed with some fresh, hot garlic bread.
2. Clean and decorate your chosen container.
3. Fill the container with soil.
4. Separate the cloves from the garlic bulb. Do not peel. One Green Thumb Club member refers to these cloves as "garlic mice."
5. Place 3 to 5 cloves in the soil so that only the very tip of the dried garlic skin "mouse's tail" is visible.
6. Place on a sunny windowsill and wait for the vampires to visit.

Care & Feeding of Garlic

There are several kinds of garlic, including elephant garlic, purple garlic, soft neck garlic, garlic chives and society garlic. As the leaves grow you can harvest them for cooking, chewing, discouraging vampires, mosquitoes and unwanted boyfriends. When grown with other plants it helps to keep many insects away.

Light: Garlic can grow in full sun outdoors. Indoors they need to be in a sunny window for best results.
Soil: This is an adaptable plant that will take a wide range of soils, but does will in a quality potting mix. The important thing to remember is that it must be loose and well drained. Some gardeners like to mix some sand with the potting mix for even better results.
Water: This is an adaptable herb. It does best in evenly moist, well drained soil. It will rot out if kept soggy.
Cold: Indoors some garlic will thrive through most of the year, but most varieties will go dormant. The tops will die down in the fall, whether they are chilled or not. When the tops turn brown you know its time to harvest the bulbs. Other varieties will keep producing new leaves for years.
Containers: Garlic can be grown in almost any container where there is good drainage.
Feeding: They do best on a limited diet. Overfeeding can lead to weak growth, or all leaf and no bulb. A weak solution of Miracle-Gro Bloom Booster once every month or two is usually sufficient.
Problems: Very few insects think of the garlic as dinner. Lack of sunlight results in weak growth and no bulb.

Conversations:

This herb generates a great deal of conversation, recipes, and comments. One school group made this a classroom research project and wrote a little book about it. Speaking of books, if you want a good, entertaining and informative book we recommend Stanley Crawford's *Garlic Testament*. It's not just about garlic, it's about life.

195

Gingerbread Friends

A
short story
of the shared joy
and the simple blessings
that can be found in the wishes
of a small child and the wisdom of an old lady

Jessie had reached that point in the afternoon where school was BORING. She had enjoyed the reading class in the morning, and art was always fun. Today she had made a special picture to take home for her mother. But, now Mrs. Olsen seemed to have lost her enthusiasm as well. Last year they would have taken naps, but now they had to learn social studies and math in the afternoon. Jessie had always wondered if teachers took a nap at the same time the kids did. Several times she had tried to stay awake and find out, but she always fell asleep. Now, in first grade, there were no naps.

Today is was really cold outside. Wind whistled around the corners of the school and through the big blue spruce that stood by the flag pole. Jessie suddenly realized that Mrs. Olsen wasn't looking at them, she wasn't even looking at the book she was holding. She was looking out the window! And she was smiling. When she smiled like that it usually meant that the goldfinches and chickadees were having a snack at the sunflowers that had grown from the seeds they all planted last spring.

"Children!" she said. "Do you see what I see?"

Everyone turned their eyes toward the windows. Jessie stared at the sunflowers but couldn't see any birds, just the big seedheads nodding at her in the wind.

"Look closely," Ms. Olsen told them all as she motioned for them to get out of their seats and follow her to the windows.

"IT'S SNOWING!" Tanya shouted.

Everyone of the children strained their eyes to see the first snow of the winter. Next week was Thanksgiving. The snow was late this year. Soon each of them had spotted a flake and followed it to the grass on the lawn, or the sidewalk. In a few minutes the beautiful crystals were appearing so fast that they seemed to be standing on tippy-toe on the blades of grass and the needles of the big old spruce at the corner of the playground. Then they would disappear into mini-puddles of water.

Everyone was hoping that there would be enough snow to do all the fun things we can do with it. Alex was thinking about building a snow fort. Shawna had never seen snow before and was wondering what it felt like to have it melt in your hand. When Carlita closed her eyes she imagined she could feel the wind in her face as she rode her sled down Gourley's hill. Freddie and Tucker had visions of snowball fights. Michelle was trying to remember where she had put her ice skates last spring.

Jessie's joy turned to sadness when she thought about the last time they had snow. It was last spring. She could remember helping her neighbor, Old Mrs. Carter, shovel her walk. Tears formed in her eyes when she thought about her neighbor falling and breaking her hip. She remembered running in the house to call 911. She remembered bringing out blankets and a big old quilt to keep Ms. Carter warm until help came. She remembered them lifting the old lady onto the stretcher and into the ambulance. She remembered that Mrs. Carter never came home. She went back to her seat and got a tissue from her backpack.

Ms. Olsen came over and sat down beside her.

Jessie told her all about how her neighbor had been taken to a hospital, then a nursing home.

"Would you like to visit her?" The teacher asked, as she put her arms around the sadness, giving Jessie a comfortable hug.

"Can I?" Jessie asked in return.

"Of course. I think Mrs. Carter would like to have a visit from you."

The smile returned as Jessie wiped her eyes and tucked the tissue in her pocket. "When can we?"

"The Holly Hill Senior Care Center is only a couple blocks from here. Let's call your mother and see if it's all right for you to go."

Jessie's mother wasn't certain that it would be good for Jessie to see all those old folks at "the home" but finally agreed to let her visit their former neighbor.

By the time school was out there was a soft layer of fresh new snow all over the grass and the trees, but it was all melted on the walkways and the parking lot. There is a magic in the first snow of winter. Jessie had put on her coat and started for the door when she remembered the picture she had drawn for her mother earlier that day. She raced back to her desk and carefully tucked it into her backpack.

When they got to the Holly Hill Senior Care Center, Jessie thought that it looked a lot like a school. There were sidewalks, a parking lot, spruce and holly trees, and there was even a bird feeder right outside the dinning room windows. When they stepped inside she saw several people in wheelchairs, a nurse and several other people who seemed to be very busy. There were bouquets of flowers in the lobby and a big old sandy colored dog keeping an elderly gentleman company down the hall.

"Levenia Carter is in room 143, down this hall and to the right," the lady at the desk said. Then she thought about it for a moment. "Is she expecting you? She doesn't get many visitors."

"We're going to surprise her," Jessie announced. "I even brought her a picture I made today." This piece of artwork had been intended for Jesse's mother but it seemed Mrs. Carter might need it more.

They went down the hall and made a right turn. There was room 143, beside the door was a name plate that said in small red letters "Ms. Levenia Carter." Inside the room was a bed, a night stand, a small table with a TV on it and a rocking chair by the window. That rocking chair was slowly rocking back and forth, but its back was to them so they couldn't see its occupant.

"Mrs. Carter, Ma'am?" Jessie asked as a way of announcing their presence.

197

Slowly the wrinkled dark brown face surrounded by a halo of snow white hair appeared from the side of the rocker. There was a brief moment of pondering, then a smile spread across the entire face and a hand reached for the aluminum walker that waited beside the chair.

"Lord Almighty, if'n you ain't a sight to behold." She stood and grasped the walker with both hands. "Come over here, Child, let me look at you. My how you've growed."

Then she looked at Ms. Olsen and deep lines crossed her forehead. "Who might this be? I know it ain't your Mamma."

Jessie introduced her teacher and they slowly walked down to the end of the hall where there was a sitting room with some comfortable chairs and a window where they could continue to watch the snow falling on the shrubbery and trees outside.

"I remember the last time it snowed. You saved my life when you called them medics." She paused for a long moment, then continued. "Child, I surely do miss you. Come here and give me a hug."

They talked about snow and Thanksgiving and winter and Christmas. Jessie always like to hear Mrs. Carter talk about her childhood in Georgia where she grew up. Her father had been a sharecropper and life was tough. She didn't get to go to school much and didn't learn to read until she moved north with her husband after their farm was sold.

When Jessie gave her the picture she kissed the child and held the colorful drawing of a gingerbread man to her heart. She would pause every few seconds to look at it again.

Soon it was time to go. They walked Mrs. Carter back to her room and put on their coats. After one last hug. Mrs Carter opened the drawer of her night stand and removed a roll of tape. She taped the picture on the wall right beside the window. "There. Now every time I gets lonely I can just look at my Gingerbread Friend." She laughed and everyone hugged again.

Jessie had so many questions she wanted to ask as Ms. Olsen backed out of the parking space and onto the street. She wanted to ask about what it was like to get old. She wanted to ask why everyone seemed so lonely. She wanted to ask why those people had to stay there. She wanted to ask if Ms. Olsen was going to get old and stay there. She wanted to ask if she was going to get old and live there. She wanted to ask why Ms. Carter couldn't come home again. But she held all these questions inside.

It was on the way to her house that the idea came to Jessie. "Ms. Olsen, could we do something?"

"Umm. Maybe. What do you want to do?" She asked as they reached Jessie's driveway.

"Could we come back again? Can we visit Mrs. Carter next week?" Jessie asked hesitantly.

The teacher was quiet for a moment, then answered, "I don't know. Do your think your parents will allow it?"

They did visit the old lady the again, the week after Thanksgiving. Mrs. Carter seemed to have a sparkle in her eyes. Jessie was pleased to see her picture of the "Gingerbread Friend" still taped on the wall where the old lady could see it from anywhere in the room.

They had a nice visit. Mrs. Carter told them about how, when she was just a youngster herself she helped bake gingerbread cookies, because that was all they had to decorate their Christmas tree. "We was too poor to buy ornaments, and us children could eat them cookies when no one was looking."

When they left they walked down the hall passing lonely men and women in chairs and wheelchairs. They all looked so sad, but they smiled when she waved at them and said "Merry Christmas."

"Ms. Olsen, I wish we could do something." Jessie said as they stepped out into the wind and snow that was swirling around the parking lot. "Can we?"

"Well that depends. I think a trip to McDonalds will spoil your dinner. I don't think your parents would like that very much."

"No. That's not what I was thinking." There was a sparkle in her eyes as she spoke. "I wish all of us from school could come over and visit with Mrs. Carter and all the other people here. They all seem so lonely."

"We'll have to talk to the rest of the students, all of your parents and these folks here too." Ms. Olsen was hesitating, not sure this was a good idea, but proud of Jessie for thinking of it.

"But, it was so much fun to hear her tell the story about her Christmas when she made all the gingerbread cookies." Jessie was using her 'please, may I' voice.

An idea was forming in Ms. Olsen's mind. "I think that would be a lot of fun for everyone. Let's find out what we can do."

By the next afternoon Jessie and her friends were on the Internet looking for recipes for gingerbread and Mrs. Olsen had spent her lunch hour with the principle. Jessie's wish was about to come true.

It was Friday afternoon when the bus pulled up to the school and all the children in Ms. Olsen's class piled in, each one carrying cookie cutters, eggs, flour, milk bowls, gingerbread cookie cutters and cookie sheets.

When they arrived at the Holly Hill Senior Center, there was a big Christmas tree in the lobby. Christmas carols were playing and there were dozens of folks with wheelchairs and walkers waiting for them. It seemed like everyone was talking at once as the lady in the blue uniform and Santa hat led them all down the hall to the dining room and kitchen.

They gathered around the tables and started to read recipes, crack eggs, measure milk and flour. Everyone was talking at once and everyone was getting dusty with the flour and sticky with the egg whites, and everyone was having fun. They worked in teams to mix the gingerbread cookie dough, stamp out the shapes with the gingerbread people cookie cutters, put them on the cookie pans, and march them into the kitchen where the chefs would put them in the ovens. Soon the tables were filled with hundreds and hundreds of "Gingerbread Friends."

As soon as they were cool everyone started decorating and trimming them with icing, candy and colored sugar sprinkles. Each table was a mess and every hand had sticky fingers, but everyone was smiling and laughing. Finally it was time to take the cookies out to the empty tree in the lobby.

Trays, and boxes and rolling carts were filled with "Gingerbread Friends." Everyone in a wheelchair had a tray of cookies on their laps as they formed a parade from the dining room to the lobby. The school children were pushing the wheelchairs of their new found grand-friends, and everyone was singing Christmas carols as they paraded down the hall.

Everyone took turns hanging their favorite "Gingerbread Friends" on the tree until that tree was so full of gingerbread ornaments that there wasn't room for even one more "Gingerbread Friend."

But there were still hundreds left, all sizes and shapes of gingerbread men, gingerbread women, gingerbread girls and gingerbread boys.

"Look at all the cookies we have left over," the lady in the blue uniform moaned. "What are we going to do with all of these?"

Mrs. Carter had become quiet, and almost sad as the tree was filled with "Gingerbread Friends." Now she turned to all the people gathered in the lobby. They were all tired, well dusted with flour, dotted with icing in a rainbow of colors. Everyone became quiet while she braced herself against her walker.

"We are all so blessed here today. Look at us. We are warm. We got friends, music and more cookies than we can ever eat."

She paused and shifted to her other foot to ease the pain in her hip. "There's folks out there," she pointed out the window at the swirling snow, "So poor they ain't got Christmas trees, no presents, no warm places to live, so poor they ain't even got a friend."

A big smile crossed her old and wrinkled face. "We can share our blessings. We can share our Gingerbread Friends.

And that's the way it all started. The Gingerbread Friends were boxed up while coats, and scarves, and mittens and hand knitted caps were gathered from each room. Soon they were ready to deliver the Gingerbread Friends to the homeless shelter downtown, and the people who were in the Meals-on-Wheels program, the school for children with developmental disabilities. And other places that got added to the list as they loaded the Holly Hill vans and the school bus.

The next time you eat a gingerbread cookie, or see a gingerbread house, or gingerbread people on a Christmas tree think of the Gingerbread Friends and what grew from a wish made by little Jessie and the vision of an old lady named Levenia. Think of what can happen when we all join together and share our joy, and share our blessings, when we become a blessing to each other.

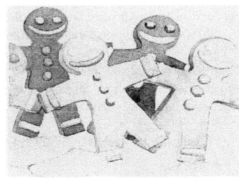

Ginger Gardens

Objective: to grow ginger plants from ginger roots found at the grocery store. Then discuss the fine art of making gingerbread people.

Common ginger, *Zingiber officinale*
Ginger family, *Zingiberaceae*
 Native to the Orient & Pacific Islands
All parts safe
Rating: Easy
Time frame: 1 hour to initiate project, planting to first leaves is 3 to 4 weeks
Size: Medium scale project

A Brief History of Ginger

The ginger family is large and covers the tropics with its flavor and fragrance. This common ginger, *Zingiber officinale* (the one we use as a spice and to make gingerbread friends) is only one member of a big family.

Many gingers get rather tall (four to eight feet), but our common edible ginger only reaches 12 to 24 inches. It produces a three to four inch pine cone shaped flower spike that's green and yellow. These flowers are delightfully fragrant. This ginger will form a clump of tubers that can fill a pot in one short season. These tubers are thick and fleshy, and they are filled with that tangy ginger flavor. The leaves can also be used as a flavoring in many Oriental dishes or to make hot teas or iced drinks. Throughout the Orient ginger root is shaved into bath water and hair rinses to help the bather relax. It is also used in teas to soothe an upset stomach, calm frayed nerves and generally relieve stress.   The dried root is burned as an incense, to produce pleasant dreams, cure a headache, toothache, or scare away the evil spirits of the forest, snakes and tax collectors. We use it to make ginger ale, ginger snaps, and of course, Gingerbread Friends.

Materials needed:
Ginger ale and ginger snaps to share during the project
Ginger antlers (or toes) available in the produce aisle of your favorite supermarket
Container of your choice, at least 6 inches in diameter, best if there are drainage holes
Sufficient good quality potting soil to fill the container
Everyone's favorite recipes for "Gingerbread People" and a copy of the story about the Gingerbread Man

Putting it all together:
★   Enjoy some of the ginger ale and a ginger snap before you get started. It is best if you can share these with friends. At this point you can read the Gingerbread Man story
★   If you wish to paint or decorate the container, do so before planting.
★   Fill almost to the top with soil, making a shallow depression in the middle of the container.
★   Separate the "toes" so that you have about three joints to plant in your ginger garden. Each toe should have a little sprout just waiting to become green leaves.
★   Press your ginger toes (or antlers) into the soil until the only the top is visible.
★   Relax and have some more ginger snaps, you've got some time to wait before anything happens.
★   Keep watered and they should begin to show green sprouts in about 2 to 3 weeks.
★   During the time you are waiting you can test the recipes and bake some gingerbread people.

Care & Feeding of Your Ginger Plant

Light: Indoors any windowsill is acceptable. If the light is too intense on a southern or western exposure there may be some sunburn on the leaves. Outdoors they will thrive in anything from dense shade to almost full sun. The leaves are at their best in light shade.

Soil: Ginger will do well in almost any good organic potting mix. The important thing to remember is that it should be loose and well drained. The better the soil the better the bloom and foliage.

Water: When grown in containers they like to be kept evenly moist but not soggy. In their native habitat they are moderately drought tolerant and can survive without watering for short periods.

Cold: Indoors the common ginger is evergreen. Outdoors the tops will die down if there is a frost, and the entire plant may die if there is a solid freeze.

Containers: Ginger will thrive in almost any well drained container that gives it room to grow. They will do well in community planters with parsley, coleus, Swedish ivy, English ivy and many other plants.

Feeding: A weak solution of Miracle-Gro once a month during the active growing season is usually sufficient. Overfeeding can reduce bloom and turn the leaves a dull green.

Problems: Very few insects dine on this plant and there are no serious diseases that you need to contend with. They will even accept a good deal of abuse, neglect, over watering and under watering.

New plants: Ginger will produce a mass of rhizomes/tubers in a matter of months. These can be left to form a dense clump or divided and potted up as new plants for sharing.

Using fresh ginger

You can harvest a toe, or section of the rhizome, wash and use in cooking or potpourri. A couple thin slices can be used to produce a delightful tea. These toes can also be dried and grated for easy storage in a ginger jar. The fresh ginger slices (or leaves) can be added to rice, tea and fruit drinks to add a spicy ginger flavor. Fish, pork, chicken and vegetables can be wrapped in fresh ginger leaves and baked for a great subtle flavor too. Use your imagination. Try other ways to use ginger, including your bath water or hair rinse.

Digging deeper:

One of our senior gardeners made some gingerbread friends, painted them with waterproof paints then placed them around the young ginger plants. This was a great touch of whimsy, and generated a lot of smiles and giggles from his friends.
A group project at one assisted living community involved making an enormous gingerbread house for the lobby. Use your imagination and see what whimsy you can create.

Conversations:

What is your favorite way to dine on ginger?
Have you ever had a ginger bath or used ginger tea as a hair rinse?
Share stories about gingerbread friends you remember, or make some new gingerbread friends and real people friends.

Pet Grapes

Objective: Start a grape vine from seeds recovered from the dining experience.

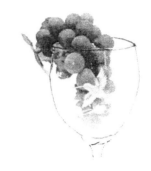

Grapes, *Vitis* varieties
Grape family, *Vitaceae*
Native to most of the world
All parts safe
Rating: Easy
Time frame: 3 to 6 weeks for seeds to sprout
Life span: Years
Size: Small scale project, at least in the beginning

This is a project that starts at the dinner table with your fruit salad. There may be one slight problem though. You will need grape seeds and most of the grapes served at the dinner table these days are of the seedless sort. Once you find some grapes with seeds inside, enjoy the delicious flavor, then wrap the seeds in your napkin and take them to your nearest flower pot or Baggie.

We were introduced to the project by a young gardener, about 7 years of age. It was at Thanksgiving dinner that she discovered grapes with seeds inside. This was quite a discovery because she had never seen anything but seedless grapes. She was curious about how grapes grow and rescued a few of the seeds to plant. They sprouted and grew, and grew, and grew, and grew. By spring she had grape vines almost three feet long climbing around the window. She had been told that the seeds wouldn't grow, but she refused to take her father's word for it. Much to her delight she proved she was right. She was very proud of her "pet grapes."

Materials needed:
A healthy appetite for grapes
Grapes with seeds inside, any color will do
1 cup of good potting soil or soilless mix
A 1 quart Baggie or Zip-Loc plastic bag
A sunny windowsill
1 can of grape juice, brand of your choice

Putting it all together:
- Put the potting mix in the plastic bag and moisten slightly.
- Add seeds and lightly cover with soil, then seal the plastic bag.
- Place in a sunny window and enjoy some refreshing grape juice while you wait for them to sprout.
- While waiting for the seeds to turn into baby plants cut the top from the juice can and punch two or three drainage holes in the bottom.
- When the seedlings have about 4 to 6 leaves transplant into the prepared grape juice can.
- When the grape vine is about 8 to 10 inches you may want to provide a stake or other support.
- By pinching out the top of the vine you can encourage it to grow side branches and look much fuller.

Care & Feeding of a Grape Vine

Light: Provide as much light as possible, they grow best in the sunniest window. Put your 'Grape Pet" outdoors as soon as the weather is warm for best growth.

Soil: Most grapes are tolerant of a wide variety of soils, but when being grown as a container or indoor plant they are at their best in a quality potting mix.

Watering: Keep the soil evenly moist. Your pet grape vine is living in confined quarters and can't develop the extensive root system that it would outdoors in the ground. Each time it dries out it will drop a leaf or two.

Feeding: A snack about once a month with a ½ strength Miracle-Gro solution will keep your pet grape happy.

Containers: After your grape seedling has outgrown its juice can it is time to make a decision. You can turn your pet grape into a very easy and attractive bonsai. It can also be trained as a topiary on a larger scale. This is up to you. Remember, the larger the container the larger the vine will grow.

Digging deeper:

Joyce is the universal grandmother and when they were preparing for an afternoon in the Spring Valley Senior Living Community Garden she was busy. With about twenty children from the Kennedy Elementary School about to descend, she was filling the freezer compartment of her refrigerator with green, red and black grapes. She knew that there was a special delight in frozen grapes.

"Taste better than those freezer pops and make great ice cubes for my pink lemonade," she said smiling broadly.

She was right and since the warm spring afternoon was spent planting five grape vines around the arbor in the garden, it seemed appropriate to serve frozen grapes as a snack. Everyone, elder and child enjoyed this novel treat.

One of our sensory roundtables at an adult day care center focused on sampling three varieties of grapes and voting on the favorite. The small red ones won by a landslide.

Conversations:

What is your favorite way to dine on grapes?
Have you ever had grape pie? What about raisin cookies?
Do you have a favorite variety of grape?
Does anyone in your group know how grapes are grown commercially?

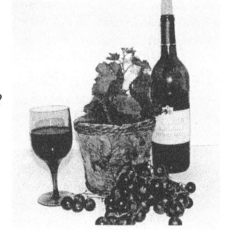

Sunflowers, on My Windowsill?

Objective: to discover and share a delicious
uniquely American vegetable.

Sunchoke, *Helianthus tuberosus*
Sunflower family, *Asteraceae (Compositae)*
AKA Canadian potato, Indian potato & Jerusalem artichoke
Native to North America
All parts safe
Rating: moderately easy
Time factor: 3 to 4 weeks for first shoots to appear
Life span: Sunchokes will grow for years outdoors
Size: Medium to large scale project

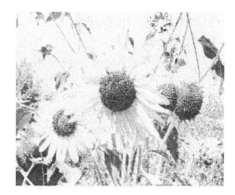

This is that knobby tuber that you can find at the produce counter from autumn to late spring. It is also a proud member of the sunflower family. It will grow vigorously from a piece of that tuber and eventually bloom for you. This grows to be a large plant reaching three of four feet with several stems, each will, in time bear many small bright yellow sunflowers that are great in cut flower bouquets or as a background for your large window or patio garden. Best started on the windowsill, then moved to the sunny outdoors.

History of the "Flower That Follows the Sun"

This was a popular vegetable in North America long before the French and the English arrived on the scene. Early colonial traders carried it back to Europe and it was first cultivated in England in 1617 where it has been a popular garden item since. Although commonly called Jerusalem artichoke, it has nothing to do with Jerusalem. This is a corruption of the French word *Girasola*, which can be loosely translated as 'turning with the sun.' The artichoke in the name refers to the flavor of the cooked tuber.

The Native Americans had enjoyed this delicious tuber for thousands of years and had devised a multitude of ways to store and prepare it. The French explorers took it back to France where it became a popular delicacy and was exported in great quantities from Canada in the 1700's. It is unfortunate that it hasn't become more popular in today's cuisine because it has flavor, versatility and nutritional value.

These tubers can be used raw in a salad, or cooked in a variety of ways. Boiled and served with melted butter they taste very much like artichokes without the effort the true artichoke requires as a part of the dining experience. They can also be baked, batter fried, stir-fried, pickled, added to soups or stews, even mashed. The immature flower buds can be harvested and boiled or added to a stir-fry, open flowers and individual petals can be used as a garnish and tender leaves can be used as a potherb (the flavor is virtually non-existent). The tubers can be roasted and ground to make an almost acceptable coffee substitute. The seeds can be harvested when ripe, shelled and ground as a flavorful flour additive in baking breads and desserts. The seeds can also be pressed for their high quality sunflower oil. The tubers were popular as an inexpensively produced livestock feed at one time.

Because the tuber contains a sugar our body doesn't try to breakdown (much like its cousin the *yacon* from South America) it's a safe and nutritious food for diabetics. These tubers have also been the subject of extensive experimentation as a source of fuel alcohol.

Growing a sunflower on your windowsill is an interesting project for late winter or early spring. We suggest that you start with a trip to your favorite produce market to obtain enough sunchoke tubers for the dinner table and a few extras to plant. You can eat the largest ones; the smaller tubers can go to pot or planter.

Materials needed:

A large windowsill
A 6" or larger pot or container of your choice
Sufficient potting soil to fill your chosen container
Sunflower pictures from last year's seed catalog or empty seed packets, your own sunflower art or photos
glue and waterproof sealer such as Mod-Podge
1 large or 3 small sunchoke tubers

Putting it all together:

- Invite friends over for a "Sunflowers for dinner" party.
- Select a recipe for sunchokes that intrigues you and prepare the meal, using all but a few small tubers.
- After dining on this historic gourmet fair you are ready to garden.
- Start by glueing the photos, seed packets or sunflower pictures on the container of your choice. Then seal with Mod-Podge or other waterproof sealer.
- Next fill the container of your choice about 2/3 full with your favorite potting mix.
- Place two or three small tubers on the soil surface and fill the rest of the way to the rim with the potting mix.
- Water thoroughly and place on a large windowsill or patio.
- In a few weeks you will have stems emerging from the soil. Warning, they grow fast.
- They can be transplanted outdoors after frost danger, or grown as a large container plant, but they need lots of light to do well.
- After growing for about 3 to 5 months the stems will be two to five feet tall and probably have flower buds and a new crop of tubers underground.

Care & Feeding of your Sunchoke

Light: These are sun worshipers. The more light they can get the happier they are. They are best moved outdoors for the summer.

Soil: Any quality potting mix works well. Some experts recommend adding about 1 part play sand to 4 parts soil mix, but this is optional.

Watering: While the sunchoke is quite drought tolerant, it's at its best when kept evenly moist.

Containers: For best results the young plants will need to be transplanted into a container of at least 2 gallon capacity, larger if possible. One of the most beautiful specimens we ever saw was in a bushel basket lined with plastic. Another was growing and blooming in one of the CelluGRO Green Thumb Gardens, where it produced about five pounds of tubers at harvest time.

Feeding: Feeding once a month with Miracle Gro seems to work very well.

Problems: There are very few problems with sunchokes. Lack of light can cause weak spindly growth. Mites can also be a problem if the plants have been neglected or stressed.

Variations on a Sunflower Theme

You can start more traditional sunflower seeds on a sunny windowsill. It's best to use dwarf varieties indoors, but these will need to move outdoors to be happy and bloom well.

You don't need to shell regular sunflower seeds before planting them. You'd be surprised how often we are asked this question.

You can use se the petals from the flowers as a garnish for fresh salads. They also make a great topping for ice cream.

Paint sunflower pictures on the container.

One of our Green Thumb Club members glued smiles and eyes on a bouquet of sunflowers in the lobby of a senior center and caused a lot of smiles. Whimsy is good for all of us.

One classroom planted a small handful of wild bird seed and had a fine crop of sunflowers, millet and some other stuff they couldn't identify.

The sunflower is the official state flower of what state?

Do you know what 20th century presidential candidate used the sunflower as his symbol?

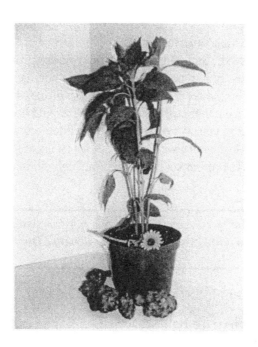

"Put the Lime in the Coconut, and Call Me in the Morning"

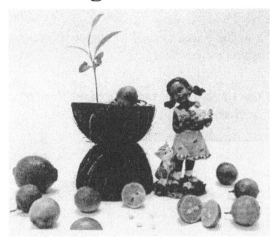

Key Lime, also known as Mexican Lime
Citrus aurantifolia
Rue family, *Rutaceae*
Native to Southeast Asia and Indonesia, now pan-tropical
All parts are non-toxic but they do produce thorns
Time frame: 1 hour to initiate the project; Seeds sprout in about two weeks
Life span: Lime tree will grow and bloom for years
Size: Small to medium scale project

All about limes

Limes are yellow not green when ripe, but most are used before they turn yellow. They are a great addition to many drinks and island dishes. They have an interesting history that begins in the Orient and ends up in the Caribbean. Arab traders brought the lime to the Mediterranean basin. Columbus brought the first lime trees to the Western Hemisphere on his second trip to the Carribean Islands. While we call them Key Limes and enjoy Key Lime Pie, most of the world knows this small fruit as the Mexican Lime. Fortunately for our project they have lots of seeds. Another type of lime, the Persian or Tahitian Lime (*Citrus latifolia*), is larger and almost seedless. It's also almost thornless.

Lime facts:

❀ The seeds of the lime, and most other citrus are poly-embryonic, this means that there may be more than one embryo in each seed. So you may find two or three sprouts from a single seed.
❀ Commercial growers frequently start new trees from seed rather than using grafting because seed grown lime trees tend to live longer and are less likely to contain diseases common to citrus trees.
❀ Limes, and most other citrus, can be trimmed into topiaries and bonsai specimens.
❀ Limes will begin blooming on your windowsill in two or three years, and can be almost everblooming.
❀ British sailors during the 18th century were called 'Limeys" because they received a ration of a lime a day while on the open seas to prevent scurvy. It was the high vitamin C content of limes that prevented this disease.

In the popular song written by Harry Nilsson, a young boy and his sister spend their dimes for a coconut and a lime. They combine the two with unfortunate consequences. Do you recall who are they told to call in the morning?

Materials needed:

A coconut planter from "A Garden on the Half Shell," page 57. You can substitute any 4 inch pot, but the coconut shell planter is more fun.
Sufficient potting soil, or soilless mix with a little sand added, to fill the coconut planter
5 to 10 fresh seeds from a Key Lime, or Persian Lime if you would rather
Your favorite recipe for Key Lime Pie, or a ready made one to share with friends

Putting the lime in the coconut:

1. Fill the coconut planter with the potting soil.
2. Press the seeds into the soil about the depth of a thumb print and make certain they are covered.
3. Place on a windowsill and wait about two to three weeks for the seeds to sprout.
4. Keep the soil moist but never soggy.
5. As the seedlings develop their third and fourth leaves remove or transplant all but 2 or 3 of the seedlings.
6. Sit back and enjoy a piece of key lime pie.

Care & Feeding of a lime tree

Light: The brightest windowsill is best. These are trees that truly enjoy sun bathing. Insufficient light will produce weak spindly growth that insect pests enjoy.

Soil: Any quality potting mix works well, but if you add 1 part coarse sand (even play sand will work) to 4 parts soil mix your lime tree will be even happier.

Watering: Keep evenly moist but never let the soil become soggy. This can seriously damage the root system and encourage the growth of soil fungus and other problems that can affect you as well as the lime trees.

Cold: Limes are very cold sensitive and will suffer serious damage if the temperature drops below freezing for even a short period of time. They will do fine outdoors in the warm months, but get them on the right side of the window before the first frost.

Containers: Any container with drainage holes will work well for your Key Lime as it grows from seedling to tree. We have seen them grow quite well in a wooden orange crate lined with plastic, in decorative pots, galvanized buckets, old wash tubs, and a slightly used charcoal grill.

Feeding: These are acid loving plants and enjoy a periodic feeding with citrus fertilizer or any fertilizer for acid loving plants. Liquid formulas are best used as a half strength solution once a month throughout the year.

Problems: There are a few scale and mite problems but these are usually the consequences of insufficient light or over feeding.

Pruning & Maintenance: Key limes have thorns, long nasty thorns. But when the growth is new and tender these can be trimmed off with scissors or a small pair of pruning shears. Don't be shy about pruning and shaping the tree. Left to its own devices it will be a sprawling shrub. It should be noted that this is an ideal bonsai or topiary subject. A key lime will thrive for years in a container and will bloom and bear, even when kept trimmed to a 2 or 3 foot height.

Digging deeper:

You don't have to limit yourself to limes. Try growing lemons, oranges, grapefruit, even tangerines. All citrus can be started the same way as the lime.

Estele shared a carton of kumquats with her friends at the Rainbow Center. She then had each of the residents plant the seeds in the pots on the windowsill of the lobby. These pots already had African violets growing in them, but she was plotting a surprise for the staff and other residents. Sure enough in about two weeks the first of the seeds sprouted. Estele and her "Secret Gardeners" really struggled to keep from laughing as other residents and staff tried to figure out what was growing. Some wanted to pul them out as weeds, others wanted to wait and see what these seedlings were. Curiosity won and it was weeks before one of the Secret Gardeners let the secret out.

Lychees, a Taste of Heaven

Litchi chinensis
Lychee family, *Sapindaceae*
Common names: Litchi, Lichee, Eyeball Fruit
Native to Southern China
All parts safe
Rating: Moderately easy
Time frame: 1 hour to initiate project, 2 to 4 weeks or seeds to sprout, tree will grow for years
Size: Small to medium scale project.

In the Green Thumb Club we sampled some fresh lychees. You have to eat the fruit to get to the seed. One of the gentlemen in the group commented, "It's sorta like suckin' on an eyeball." Another was shocked at such a coarse comment and replied, "No. I think it's a taste of Heaven." Both comments were accurate. The lychee is a most delicious fruit, and like a peeled grape, it does remind one of an eyeball.

More than you ever wanted to know about lychees

Lychees are the fruit of a handsome tree that can reach forty feet in height but are usually somewhat smaller. The rich green leaves and dense growth habit make it an attractive ornamental as well as a popular fruit tree. The flowers appear in spring in dramatic clusters that range from twenty to thirty inches in length. While each flower is insignificant, the massive clusters are striking. Bees think so as well and the spring honey produced from lychee flowers is in great demand. About four months after flowering the red or pink fruit is ready to harvest.

You can usually find fresh lychees in the produce markets in late summer or early autumn. The grape sized fruit is inside a rough textured papery shell that has to be cut or torn. Inside this shell is the eyeball-like fruit that has such a delightful taste that it was once reserved for royalty. The texture is somewhat like a grape, but the flavor is sweet and delicate with a delightful fragrance. This pulp is really a sack covering a single seed. In the sweetest variety the seeds are atrophied into what are called "chicken tongues." Unfortunately, these won't sprout into a windowsill lychee tree. It should be noted that lychee fruit have a very short shelf life at room temperature, about three days, but they will keep in the refrigerator for a week or two. The fruit can be canned or frozen for later use. It can also be used to make a most delightful juice or wine. Lychee nuts are somewhat like raisins, but they aren't the seeds but the dried flesh of this fine fruit. The Chinese traditionally used the flesh of the lychee to treat the cough and sore throat that accompany the common cold. The seeds are ground into a powder and used to make a tea for headache and general pain relief.

Growing a lychee on the windowsill is easy, but you have to start with fresh seeds. The seed remains viable for only a few days once removed from the fruit.

Materials needed:
We recommend planting about three seeds for best results
Start the seeds in a 4 or 6 inch pot or by using the sandwich bag greenhouse
Sufficient potting soil to fill the container
A few green bean seeds
A sunny windowsill

Putting it all together:

★   If starting in a pot, fill the pot with soil, then place the lychee seeds about ½ inch deep in the soil.

★   Plant three to five bean seeds in the pot. They will sprout first. This will remind you to water.

★   Keep soil evenly moist, but not soggy.

★   If starting the seeds in the sandwich bag mini-greenhouse, you don't need the beans.

★   Place in a sunny window so that the seedlings don't become spindly.

★   Keep the young plants well watered. They should never go dry.

★   The baby lychees will grow quickly to about six inches in height, develop about a half dozen leaves and stop. This pause can last for months. The main effort of the plant is now in root production. Be patient, it will grow in periodic spurts.

★   Lychees are slow growing and can remain in a six inch container for as long as three years.

★   When ready to step up to a larger container you can use a found item with an Oriental look, or customize a pot or planter yourself.

Care & Feeding of a Lychee Tree

Light: They enjoy a sunny window although one of our friends grows them under lights in his basement for the first year. A lack of light will make them weak and spindly.

Soil: Any good, well drained potting mix will work well. Some suggest adding a little sand to promote better root growth, but this is your choice.

Watering: Keep them evenly moist but never soggy. They don't like wet feet.

Cold: Lychees will tolerate a light frost, but when grown as house plants it is best not to expose them to freezing weather.

Containers: Any container will work as long as it has drainage holes in it. An Oriental style planter, or any found container that you can customize into an Oriental theme is fine. Be creative.

Feeding: Feed the seedlings and young trees monthly with an organic plant food or Miracle-Gro for best results.

Problems: Lychees have few problems with insects and disease. Mites and mealy bugs will sometimes attack a weak plant. Biggest problems come from improper watering or over feeding.

Maintenance: This is a slow growing tree that requires little pruning. Remove dead and yellowing leaves. Rotate the tree once a week so that all sides get their day in the sun.

Dancing in the Mango Grove

The mango is a tropical fruit steeped in myth and legend. Poems, songs and prayers have been written to honor it and it's a significant part of the diet in much of the world. It has been called the "Apple of India" and "the King of Fruit" and is found in the dooryard gardens of homes throughout the tropical world. It is said to be the fruit of the gods and the flavor of a tree ripened mango is said to be desired beyond all else. There is a story told in Cambodia of the man who traded his wife for a basket of mangoes. As the family gathers to share the fruit of the mango the following is a story often told to the children.

Many years ago there was a very wealthy, and very selfish old man who had a great mango grove. These trees took the water from the river and the sunshine from the sky and delighted in growing the sweetest mangoes in all of India. This grove was famous for the bright orange color of the fruit, as vivid as the sun itself. But, the owner of these wonderful trees had never tasted a single one of the delicious fruit that his grove produced. All of it was sold to the fruit buyer. This is how he became so wealthy.

The children of the village would often come and play in the shade of these great mango trees. The trees would wave their branches in friendly greeting as the children danced and sang and played. These trees would rustle their leaves to match the music of youth and everyone was happy.

But the selfish owner was afraid that the children would steal his fruit. He would watch from the corner of the wall, or from the gate, or from behind the largest of the mango trees. The children took their delight in the friendly company of the trees and had no intention of stealing any of the fruit. They knew that it wasn't theirs to eat, but thought that the shade was a gift from the trees and belonged to everyone.

The grove owner was so suspicious that he brought his sleeping mat to the grove and even slept under the trees, just in case one of the children would return at night to steal his fruit. He had his servants bring him tea in the morning, and again in the afternoon. This went on for weeks. He grew thinner and thinner. He also grew meaner and meaner, but he would not leave the grove.

Finally, one afternoon, as the children were playing a game of hide and seek around the trunks of these mango trees, a fruit fell from one of the branches. One of the children bent down and picked it up. She was looking for a place to put it where the owner would find it before it spoiled in the summer heat. He watched her carry it to the corner of the grove by the gate and he couldn't hide his anger any longer. He rushed out and seized the little girl, tore the fruit from her hand and screamed at her to never set foot in his mango grove again.

He seized a stick and chased all the children from the shady grove. When they were all gone he stood in the middle of the grove and shouted for his servants to bring all the baskets and boxes and bags. When they arrived he ordered them to pick all of the fruit, and warned them not to eat any of his mangoes. He reminded them that he was watching and the first one to eat one of these mangoes would be fired.

By the time night fell only half of the mango trees had been picked. He ordered the servants to cut branches from the trees to build bonfires so that they could continue to pick the fruit all through the night. By morning the trees were bare. The fruit had been picked and the branches had been burned. There was very little shade indeed. The selfish old man was now happy. Without the fruit and without the shade the children would not return. Now he could rest. The servants were all so exhausted that they fell asleep sitting against the boxes, bags and baskets of mangoes.

The selfish old man saw this and thought to himself, they will eat these mangoes as soon as I go to bed. He roused them from their sleep and ordered them to carry all the mangoes into the storehouse. He then locked all the doors and sent the servants away. After a short nap he went to the fruit buyer. Because the quality of his fruit was well known a good price was offered and it was agreed that the fruit would be picked up the next day.

The next afternoon the fruit buyer arrived with his wagon to haul away the finest mangoes in all of India. He had a large bag of gold coins to pay for this fruit. The very wealthy, and very greedy, grove owner fumbled with his keys as he kept his eyes on the bag of coins. Finally he found the right key and put it in the lock and turned it. He was smiling with pride as he opened the door. But he kept his eyes on the bag of gold coins, so he missed what happened next.

As the door opened there was a great rustle of wings, just like the rustle of leaves in the mango trees. Thousands of bright golden orange birds flew through the doorway and into the bright warm sunshine. Then they began to sing beautiful songs as they flew toward the broken and leafless trees. They continued to sing their beautiful songs as they landed on the trees in such great numbers that they themselves cast shade. The children were so happy to see and hear the birds that they came running from all over the village. They danced around the trees and joined in the songs of the birds. There was so much happiness in the grove of trees that twigs and bright mahogany leaves began to burst from the broken branches.

The greedy grove owner looked inside the door. All that was left were empty boxes, bags and baskets. Each of the mangoes had turned into a beautiful golden bird of happiness. He didn't understand how this could happen. "But, but, where are all my mangoes?" he stammered.

The fruit buyer clutched his bag of gold coins tightly to his chest. "Do you think this is a clever joke?"

The grove owner could only stammer and apologize, "I . . . I'm sorry. I don't now what happened. I . . . think my servants have played a mean trick on me."

"Your joke is not very funny," the fruit buyer said as he turned away. "I will never buy fruit from you again."

The wealthy, greedy grove owner went into the store room and sat down surrounded by the empty boxes, bags and baskets. He found one mango left. He tasted it. This was the first mango from his grove he had ever tasted. With the first taste of this sweet and delicious fruit he smiled. With the second taste he began to dance. He danced all the way to the grove. After the third taste he began to sing. He joined hands with the children as they danced around the trees. The birds joined in the celebration and their singing was so beautiful that they called forth new leaves on all of the mango trees.

By evening every tree was full of beautiful new leaves and clusters of mango flowers were glowing in the light of the full moon. The servants all came back and joined in the singing and dancing. Soon everyone in the village was dancing in the grove, food was brought and shared and everyone was happy. For the first time in his life the wealthy, greedy grove owner had friends. And he was so happy that he declared his mango grove a park where everyone was welcome, and all could enjoy the shade, the songs of the birds, the fruit of the trees and most of all the company of friends. And yes! All the people of the village enjoyed the finest mangoes in all of India as well, and they all helped the grove owner care for the trees, and he had many friends, and he was no longer mean, or greedy. He was still very wealthy, but he now counted his wealth in the number of friends he had, and he had many.

Mangoes, The Sacred Fruit of India

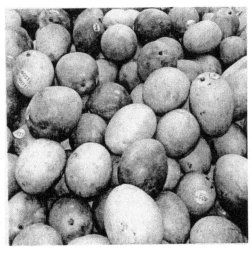

Mango, *Mangifera indica*
Poison ivy family, *Anacardiaceae*
Native to India
Safety factor: Rarely leaves and sap may cause
a mild allergic reaction in some people
Rating: easy to start and grow
Time factor: 1 hour to start, 2 to 6 weeks for the seed to sprout
Life span: Mangoes thrive as a container plant for years
Size: medium size project

Dining on mangoes:

There are hundreds of varieties, some are used when green, others when they are ripe. Even the seed is cooked as a vegetable or ground into a flour that is used in the preparation of many foods. Green mangoes are like green apples, crisp and tart. They are frequently eaten as a snack with salt or chili powder. These unripe fruit are also diced and added to salads or soaked in vinegar. Ripe mangoes are peeled and eaten raw, made into sauces, salsas, chutneys, or juice. The golden fruit is commonly used in cooking chicken, many vegetable dishes and desserts. Dried mangoes will keep for a long time and make a nutritious snack.

The flowers are used to make a sweet tea and the fruit juice can be made into mango beer or wine. Bees make a delightful honey from the nectar of the mango flowers.

There are also a number of medicinal uses for various parts of the mango tree. A mouthwash is made from the bark to ease a sore throat. A tea made from the green fruit is used to treat heat stroke while the ripe fruit is used to cure night blindness. The sap is used in many parts of the world to treat scorpion stings and spider bites.

The ripe fruit is higher in vitamin C than oranges and provides vitamin A, Thiamin, iron and many other nutrients we need.

Growing a mango tree on the windowsill

The mango fruit is delicious, and the young tree is magnificent. New leaves are a rich burgundy, mahogany, bronze or rose color with a tropical look. They start easily from seed and grow well in the average home. There are few pests and problems and it isn't a demanding prima donna plant at all. Some claim that it's actually easier to grow than the ubiquitous avocado.

Materials needed to grow your mango:

1 to 3 mango for the fruit and seeds
Large clear plastic bag, like a freezer bag
1 four to six inch pot, or found container, per seed
Sufficient amount of your favorite potting mix to fill first the plastic bag about half full, later fill the pot
Pruning shears to open the seed coat, if you are planting a naked seed
2 or more friends who will share mango fruit and stories

Putting it all together:

1. A fruit as delicious as a mango is best shared with friends, so the first step is to do just that.
2. After sharing the fruit, scrape as much of the fiber from the seed coat as possible, then wash off and let dry for an hour or two.
3. Fill the plastic bag about half full of the potting mix
4. Use the pruning shears to trim the edge of the seed coat, being careful not to damage the kernel inside.
5. Remove the naked seed and immediately place it in the soil so that it is at least ½ inch deep.
6. Seal the bag and place in a warm place.
7. The seed will sprout in about two weeks and as soon as you see green place it in a sunny windowsill. You may want to open the bag if condensation forms on the inside of the plastic bag.
8. When your seedling has leaves pressing against the sides of the freezer bag open the bag, remove the plant and carefully plant it in the pot.
9. Keep watered. The mango seedling needs to be kept evenly moist, but not soggy.
10. When it has about a dozen leaves it will need to be transplanted into a one gallon size container of your choice.

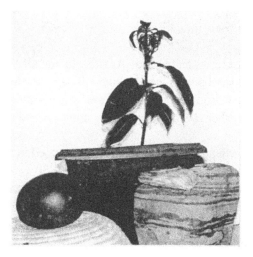

Notes from the field:

Because the young leaves are so rich in color mangoes make an ideal indoor plant. The contrast between the mahogany leaves of youth and rich, deep green leaves of maturity is truly striking. Members of Green Thumb Clubs have decorated the young tree with birds (from the craft store) painted orange. Others have created artistic containers or used Indian brass pots. Use you imagination and make this a distinctive and uniquely yours plant.

Trapped in a Mango Tree, One last mango story.

Ardele was born and raised in south Florida, but now she lived in a nursing home near Orlando. It's sometimes very difficult when your health has declined, you have outlived most of your family and you feel so alone. We were told by the lady at the desk, "The one in the wheelchair by the door, that's Ardele, she's got an attitude problem. Just between you and me, I don't think she's a good candidate for your kids project."

We were starting an intergenerational story swap program at "The Palms" that would involve some children from six to nine and about a dozen seniors. We looked at Ardele, sitting with a scowl on her face. A frown went from forehead to chin as she sat with arms crossed watching the children as they entered the lobby. One of our interns whispered, "Isn't she the sort of person we want to reach?" Of course he was right.

After the introductions, the sharing of names no one would remember and smiles that would be cherished for a lifetime, everyone made their way out to the atrium where there was a fountain and a few trees, some flowers and several dancing butterflies. The first session is always a little difficult, it's the getting acquainted that takes some time, then the magic can begin.

Many of the children had brought books to share and one of the gentlemen from "The Palms" sat clutching a small cassette player with a story told by his great grandson. The shyness soon dissolved into a joyful chaos of people talking, shaking hands, asking questions and becoming friends. One of the elderly ladies pointed to a butterfly and started to tell a story from her childhood about how she rescued a big yellow butterfly from drowning. It seemed that everyone was talking, laughing, and listening as friendships grew. But Ardele sat, still scowling, alone at the corner of all the activity. A young boy was also standing alone watching several bees as they danced around the young mango tree in the planter by Ardele's wheelchair. Finally he pointed to it and smiled a cautious smile as his eyes met Ardele's.

"They make honey from the flowers," she said, as she lifted her head and the frown began to disappear.

The young fellow pondered this for a little bit, then spoke, "How?"

Ardele motioned for him to come closer, and he did. As she told him all about bees and honey and how they visit each flower and then find their way back to the hive and tell the other bees where to fine the nectar. The next time we glanced their way he was sitting on her lap and she was pointing out the deep burgundy new leaves on the young mango tree. Several other children were gravitating toward them, as were some of the elders.

She leaned forward and almost whispered, "Did ya ever get trapped in a mango tree?"

She went on to tell a story from her childhood, when she climbed a mango tree in a neighbor's yard to get one of the fruit, but then was afraid to climb down. She told everyone about all the critters she saw while sitting in that ol' tree, lizards, birds, walking sticks, ants, a racoon walked by in the grass below, several squirrels were racing through the leaves, tasting the mangoes.

The program was to last about thirty minutes, everyone knows the attention span of both children and elders is pretty short. But Ardele continued her story and now everyone was gathered around her. She was a natural storyteller, delivering elements of this adventure with a cadence and voice that drew everyone into that old tree with her. When she pointed to the memory of a snake she had watched slithering under her tree everyone pulled their feet in and took a deep breath. She would point and ask questions, making everyone there a part of the story. It was long past the time when this event was supposed to be over when the activity coordinator came out onto the atrium with a plate heaping with mango slices and a pitcher of lemonade.

Ardele found her place in the universe that afternoon, elders and children made friends and together they made a lifetime of memories. This was possible because we all got out of the way and let it happen. Ardele and the young boy whose name we have forgotten became the model for the rest of them. As the weekly visits continued others felt the freedom and confidence to share stories, make up imaginary adventures and bask in the warmth of new found friends. But, we never did hear how she got out of that mango tree.

Now it's your turn to share a story

Papaya, The Melon Tree

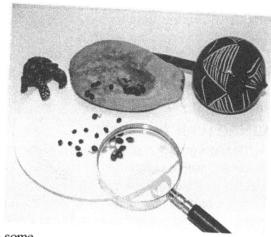

Papaya, *Carica papaya*
Papaya family, *Caricaceae*
Native to Mexico and Central America, now pan-tropical
Safety factor: Milky sap can cause an allergenic reaction in some.
Rating: easy to start and grow
Time Factor: 2 to 3 weeks for germination, grows rapidly after sprouting
Size: small to start, medium size within 3 months

Natural history of papaya

For thousands of years the people of Central America have enjoyed the delightful flavor and high nutritional content of this fruit that is known as papaw, mamao or tree melon. Today there are many varieties grown in many tropical locales. Some, usually called Mexican papayas, produce enormous fruit, sometimes larger than a football. What is usually found in the supermarket is much smaller and are classified as Hawaiian papayas. Both have a delicious flavor and one cup of ripe papaya can provide up to 80% of the daily requirements of Vitamin C, plus many other nutrients. In the tropics papaya juice is a popular sweet drink. The tender young leaves and seedlings are often cooked and eaten as a vegetable. The bark is used to make a tough rope or cord.

Papayas grow on a large plant, ranging from 8' to 20,' that is often referred to as a tree, but in fact it is a large herb. It will grow a single stem with large leaf scars. The flowers and fruit are produced along this stem. The leaves are large and tropical looking, often reaching three feet or more in length. The papaya "trees" are usually either male or female, but some varieties are called solos, meaning that they are capable of self-pollination. The flowers are waxy-white or cream color with a mild, fruity fragrance. This is one of the few fruits that are routinely started from seed rather than cuttings or grafts.

The papaya fruit produces papain, an enzyme that has traditionally been used to aid digestion. Today it is used commercially in meat tenderizers and chewing gum production. It's also a part of the recipe for most of the beers produced in the United States. Papaya extracts can be found in many cosmetics, shampoos and soaps. The people of Central America used the milky sap to remove freckles, corns and warts. Traditionally, the fruit was used to treat tumors and is now being studied for potential anti-cancer properties. There are also studies being done to analyze the potential benefits for diabetics. An extract from the leaves is showing potential in controlling heart rate.

Papayas are easy to grow

They will give you a dramatic tropical looking plant for the patio or large windowsill. Seedlings grow rapidly and in a few months you may have a plant exceeding 2 feet in height. It probably won't grow ten feet tall and bear fruit on your windowsill, but it will certainly give you a tropical conversation piece.

Materials needed:

1 ripe papaya
3 to 6 seeds from this fruit
at least two friends to share the fruit
1 CD of your favorite Latin American music
1 six inch pot or found container that can be painted or decorated in a Latin American theme
Sufficient potting mix to fill the six inch pot

Putting it all together:

1. Invite some friends over and play the music while you eat the fruit. Save some of the seeds.
2. Decorate, paint or customize the container. You can make this a group project.
3. Fill the container with the potting mix.
4. Plant the seeds approximately 1/4" deep and keep moist.
5. Seeds will germinate in 2 to 3 weeks and grow rapidly.
6. Thin to one plant per container, keep moist and give it lots of light.
7. Feed with Miracle-Gro about once a month.

Care & Feeding of your Papaya

Light: Papayas enjoy a sunny windowsill, any exposure seems to work well. We have had great papaya plants in north facing windows. They don't do well back from the window however.

Soil: They thrive in any compost or peat rich potting mix.

Watering: Keep the soil your pet papaya calls home evenly moist and it will reward you with lush tropical growth. If you let it go dry between waterings it will drop leaves and probably attract mites.

Cold: These are tropical plants and the very idea of a frost is enough to make them shiver and drop leaves. Even being too close to the window on a cold winter's night may cause leaf damage.

Containers: Use any container of your choice. After the seedling is on its way to looking like a tree, you will want to transplant it into a container equivalent to a two gallon pot. Feel free to decorate, paint, or customize to make it uniquely yours. You can continue a Mexican or Caribbean theme if you wish.

Feeding: A monthly feeding with Miracle-Gro seems to keep papayas happy. Be cautious about over feeding because this can cause weak growth that some insects seem to enjoy.

Problems: Mites, scale and mealy bug seem to be the most serious problem with papayas kept as house pets. Drying out can stress the plants, and they really don't like a chill.

Maintenance: There is no pruning involved. It is necessary to remove yellowing and fallen leaves. We also advise checking the underside of the leaves frequently for signs of mites or other problems.

Pineapple Plantation, a Quiz

The pineapple is a fruit that carries within its rough textured skin the flavor of the exotic and the lure of a tropical paradise. We have all enjoyed this fruit as a dessert, a juice, a garnish and a snack. Like most fruits and vegetables this plant has a fascinating history and a multitude of myths and legends. Test your pineapple knowledge with this little quiz.

1. TRUE or FALSE   The pineapple originated in the Hawaiian Islands.

2. TRUE or FALSE   Pineapples grow on large sprawling trees.

3. TRUE or FALSE   In colonial America the pineapple was a status symbol.

4. TRUE or FALSE   The name pineapple is derived from the native word for the fruit, *pia-apela*.

5. TRUE or FALSE   Sir Walter Raleigh named it the King Charles Fruit because it was a fruit that wore a crown.

6. TRUE or FALSE   The pineapple is in the same family as Spanish moss.

7. TRUE or FALSE   Pineapple makes a great meat tenderizer because it contains an enzyme called bromeline that digests certain proteins.

8. TRUE or FALSE   When Columbus arrived in the New World he was served pineapple wine.

9. TRUE or FALSE   In some parts of the world people were reluctant to eat pineapple because it was thought to make them sterile.

10. TRUE or FALSE   One variety of pineapple may weigh as much as 20 pounds when ripe.

Answers are on page 222

Apples, Pineapples & Pine Cones

You can share the sensory experience of the exotic pineapple with friends who may have physical or mental limitations, such as Alzheimer's or vision challenges. All you need is a pineapple, an apple and a pine cone.

Feel the texture of each of these botanical objects.

Smell the fragrance of each.

Taste pineapple and apple, either the fruit or juice.

Compare the pineapple and the pine cone. How are they similar? How are they different?

What do pineapples and apples have in common?

Which flavor do you like best? Apples or pineapples?

What is your favorite way to eat pineapples?

Any good pineapple stories you want to share?

Would you like to grow a pineapple?

Pineapples in Your Tropical Paradise

Pineapple, *Ananas lucidas*
Pineapple family, *Bromelidaceae*
Native to South America
All parts safe, some varieties have sharp teeth on leaf edges
Rating: Very Easy
Time frame: 1 hour to 3 days for project initiation, 12 to 18 months from planting to harvest
Size: Medium to large scale project

Pineapple History

- We always associate the pineapple with Hawaii, but it's really native to South America.
- Columbus was served pineapples and pineapple beer (or wine) when he landed in the Caribbean.
- It was carried to the Pacific by other Spanish explorers and traders.
- When King Louis XIV of France was presented with his first pineapple, he graciously accepted the fruit and bit into it without removing the coarse skin. He cut his mouth and cursed the ship captain who brought him the gift.
- Captain James Cook is credited with introducing the pineapple to Hawaii.
- There are several types of pineapples. Some have a sawtooth edge to their leaves, some are variegated, some are quite small and some produce a fruit that exceeds two feet in length.
- Pineapples are a member of the bromeliad family, making them cousins to Spanish moss and the flowering bromeliads that are grown all over the world as house plants.

Pineapple uses

The fruit has been valued because of both the flavor and its nutritional value for thousands of years. The Carib Indians ate it fresh, cooked with it and drank the juice. Many varieties are grown on plantations today, some are used mostly for juice, others for canned pineapple, and others for shipping. They have been a symbol of friendship and hospitality since colonial times. Pineapples carved from wood or cast in iron were a popular part of home decor. The fruit was very expensive and was once considered a status symbol in both Europe and the US.

Growing a Pineapple in 5 Easy Steps

Materials needed:

1 ripe pineapple with a crown of healthy green leaves
1 pot or other container with drainage holes in the bottom, a six inch or one gallon size works well
Sufficient good quality potting soil with sand added. 1 part sand to 3 parts soil mix is a good ratio
A saucer to prevent water damage
A sunny windowsill
One last thing you will need, a CD of your favorite Hawaiian music.

Putting it all together:

You are free to do this project while wearing a traditional Hawaiian lei.
1. Start with a pineapple with a healthy green crown, (that cluster of leaves that are at the top of the fruit). Now seize the pineapple with one hand and the crown with the other and twist.

2. Strip off a few of the small bottom leaves and you will see tiny root primordia just waiting for a chance to grow. You may need to use a magnifying glass to see these baby roots.

3. Planting is easy. Take the crown and place it in a 6 inch pot filled with a good quality potting soil. Make certain that there is good drainage. Press into the soil so that it is firmly in place.

4. Place the newly planted pineapple on a saucer on your windowsill. Now wait. While waiting listen to the Don Ho music and practice your hula dancing. You can drink some pineapple juice too. It's good for you and it tastes good too.

5. When new leaves begin to form you know you have successfully started a pineapple plant.

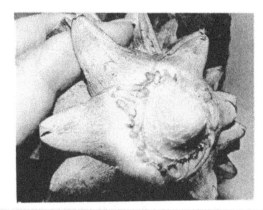

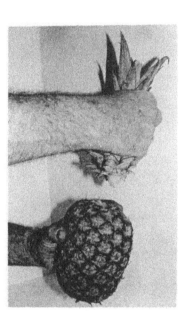

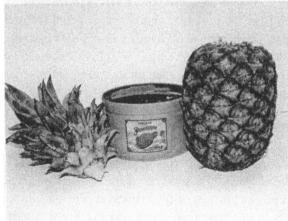

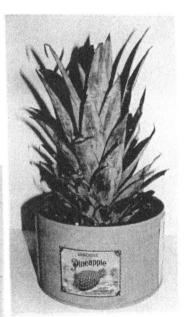

Notes from the field:

A flower stalk will usually form in 12 to 18 months. If the plant is vigorous and looks healthy and mature, but isn't producing a flower stalk from the center of the crown you can encourage it to bloom by placing two or three apple cores at the base of the plant. Cover the plant with a clear plastic bag for a couple days. The ethylene gas that a rotting apple releases will usually initiate flowering.

After blooming the fruit forms. You will know it's ripe when it has a rich golden yellow color throughout. The fruit can be harvested and enjoyed. When harvested ripe the flavor is delightfully sweet. After fruiting the plant will produce side shoots called pups. Then the parent plant usually dies.

Care & Feeding of a Pineapple

Light: It can be grown on any windowsill, or outdoors in full sun to medium shade during warm months.

Soil: This is an adaptable plant that will do well in a wide variety of soils, even sand.

Water: Pineapples are drought tolerant. Giving it a drink once a week is usually sufficient. Generally, they don't like soggy soil, but they can also be started in a glass of water.

Cold: Pineapples are frost sensitive and can be destroyed if they are subjected to temperatures below freezing for more than a few hours.

Containers: They can grow in a six inch pot for the first six months or so, but may need to be stepped up to a two gallon pot before they will develop a full display of leaves and bloom. Many Green Thumb Clubs have had pineapples bloom and bear fruit in their CelluGRO Green Thumb Gardens.

Feeding: Half strength Miracle-Gro once a month or Osmocote twice a year is about all this plant needs. Be careful not to get either fertilizer on the leaves, sometimes called "the vase." This can cause damage to young leaves just forming or the bud stalk.

Problems: Almost no insect or disease problems. Do not use a copper container or watering can. Copper is fatal to almost all bromeliads, including pineapples.

Answers to the Pineapple Quiz

1. FALSE. The pineapple originated in South America and spread to Central America and the Caribbean before the arrival of Columbus. It didn't reach Hawaii until the 19th century.

2. FALSE. Pineapples grow from a rosette type plant with long spike-like leaves that may be up to three feet long. In the Caribbean pineapple plants are planted under windows for security.

3. TRUE. The pineapple was considered the ultimate symbol of success. It was often the most expensive food on the table and pineapples were commonly rented out as an item of decor.

4. FALSE. It was called the pineapple because it looks like a pinecone and is a fruit. Apple was a generic term for almost any fruit. The Spanish word for pineapple is pina, which means pinecone. The Caribbean natives called this fruit *nana* which can be translated "flavor." The botanical name, *Ananas*, means flavor of flavors.

5. FALSE. Sir Walter Raleigh called it "The princess of fruits" but it was called the "King of Fruits" by Father Duerte in 1672. He said it must be the king of fruits because God had placed a crown on its head.

6. TRUE. The pineapple is in the bromeliad family, as are Spanish moss, bromeliads, cryptanthus and tillandsias. This family has a couple thousand members, almost all of them native to the Americas.

7. TRUE. The enzyme, bromelain, is so powerful that it should be used sparingly or it will make the meat fall apart. Pineapple workers usually wear gloves to protect their hands. Prolonged exposure to the bromeline can cause serious irritation.

8. TRUE. Columbus was served both fresh pineapple and pineapple wine, or beer, in 1493 when he landed on the Island of Guadeloupe. In his journal he wrote, "It is shaped like a pine cone, but is twice as large with excellent flavor. So tender that it can be cut with a knife like a turnip." He described the wine as "agreeable."

9. TRUE. Along the coast of South America it was commonly believed that eating too much pineapple would cause women to become sterile and some claimed that it would make men impotent. Other cultures viewed it as an aphrodisiac.

10. TRUE. While most pineapples weigh 3 to 5 pounds, but a variety called *Giant Kiwi* can weigh as much as 20 pounds.

Pomegranate, the Forbidden Fruit

Pomegranate, *Punica granatum*
A family all its own, *Punicaceae*
Native from Iran to India, it became a favorite in
the Mediterranean early in ancient times
All parts safe, including the beautiful flowers
Rating: easy, but slow growing
Time frame: long term
Life span: Pomegranates will thrive on a windowsill for several years
Size: small windowsill project for the first two years

There is also a dwarf pomegranate that will grow and bloom on the windowsill

Pomegranate myth and legend

This delightful fruit is also known as *Granada* in Spanish and *Grenade* in French. It's said to be the model for the hand grenade, and it has a connection with the series of wars between Rome and Carthage that we call the Punic Wars. The pomegranate was known as the Carthage Apple, and Punica was the ancient name of Carthage. There was a grove of these trees within this city and that's how the fruit got its Latin name, *Punica*.

This is a tree, or large shrub, of the deserts where it will grow from 10 to 20 feet or more with glossy green leaves and beautiful scarlet, white or pink globe-shaped flowers. The red fruit range from baseball to softball size. Inside, each seed is packaged in an *aril sack* containing a juicy pulp. This aril sack, with it's tart and tasty flesh, is used as a garnish, great on ice cream, or in baking. The juice of the pomegranate is quite nutritious and delightful to the taste. It's used to make a rich syrup called *Grenadine* and a fine liquor. To obtain the juice you can heat the fruit slightly, then roll it in your hands to soften the contents. Cut a hole in the stem end and set atop a glass. The juice will slowly flow from the fruit, but you can squeeze occasionally to hasten the process.

In the ancient history of this great fruit it was the very symbol of birth, life & death. After all, it is the fruit that bleeds. It was the fruit of Persephone. The Virgin Mary is often seen holding a pomegranate to proclaim her power over death. In one Green myth Side, the wife of Orion is tricked into thinking that she had caused the death of her children. So grief stricken is she that she leaps from a cliff and where her body lands, broken and bloody, the first pomegranate tree sprouted. In Japan the pomegranate was considered a fertility symbol and was consumed by women wanting to bear children.

In many accounts the pomegranate was the forbidden fruit that tempted Eve. There is the story of the wife of a mayor who decided to test her husband's faithfulness by disguising herself as the Forbidden Maiden. When the he spotted her he asked her identity. She told him she could be his for the small price of a pomegranate. The mayor quickly climbed the tree and returned with the largest fruit, plucked from the very top branch. As he handed the price of pleasure to the women she turned around and he discovered that it was his wife. She laughed and told him he had only been tempted by his wife, but he was so filled with guilt and shame that he fasted until death claimed him. For the followers of Islam there was a story proclaiming that from each pomegranate seed would sprout a different fruit from Paradise. In some stories it is the forbidden fruit while others call it the fruit of paradise. The flavor is heavenly and the flowers are beautiful. You can start it easily from seed, but first enjoy the fruit.

Materials to grow your own Forbidden Fruit, or Fruit of Paradise:

1 ripe pomegranate
1 sense of adventure
a dash of curiosity
1 clear plastic sandwich bag with zip top
1 cup of moist potting mix
a warm spot for germination
four inch containers, chosen or decorated to be the permanent home of your Fruit of Paradise
Sufficient potting mix to fill this container

Putting it all together:

1. Either peel part of the fruit to expose the aril sacks and seeds, or prepare juice from it as described above.
2. Enjoy the flavor and take a mental a journey back in time and space to the market place of your favorite exotic Mediterranean city where you can enjoy the music, the dancing, the delightful smells and flavors of the foods, the fine cloth, leather craft, jewelry and delicate perfumes of the vendors.
3. Return to reality and select between three and five seeds for planting.
4. Place the soil in the sandwich bag.
5. Now plant the seeds so that they are barely covered by the soil.
6. The most important part of sprouting pomegranate seeds is next. They must have a temperature above 70 degrees to sprout. This means placing the sandwich bag where it will be constantly warm. We suggest setting it on top of the hot water heater, or near a night light that will keep it warm while you sleep. Light isn't necessary until the seeds begin to sprout, but warmth is vital.
7. As soon as you see the first signs of sprouting, place the bag in a sunny windowsill during the day.
8. As soon as the seedlings have four to six green leaves they are ready to plant into a four or six inch container of your choice. Be very careful not to damage the roots during this process.
9. Now they can stay on the sunny windowsill all the time.
10. It is also important that these seedlings not dry out while they are becoming established.

Care & Feeding of a Pomegranate

Light: They enjoy a bright sunny windowsill to call home. Insufficient light will result in weak spindly growth.
Soil: Any good quality potting mix works well, as long as it is well drained. Some experts recommend adding some coarse sand but this is optional.
Watering: Keep young seedlings evenly moist. In their native habitat they are semi-drought tolerant, but a pot on the windowsill isn't their native habitat.
Cold: They will take a good deal of cold, but will go dormant for the winter. Grown indoors on a sunny windowsill they will be evergreen and probably even bloom throughout most of the year for you.
Containers: Because the pomegranate is so rich in story and myth you can decorate or paint scenes from some of the great folklore and legends that abound concerning this unique fruit.
Feeding: Over feeding can cause weak growth. Green Thumb Club members have been quite successful with a monthly feeding of a ½ strength Miracle-Gro solution once a month.
Problems: These delightful shrubs have few insect and disease problems. The greatest danger for seedlings is drying out. As the plants become more mature they can suffer from wet feet that cause the roots to die back. The leaves should have a healthy, shiny deep green appearance.
Maintenance: There is little maintenance required. Occasionally trim off the shoots that are exceeding your expectations. This keeps the plant compact and busy. It also encourages more bloom. Pomegranates can easily be trained as a very attractive bonsai specimen.

Tomato Soup, a Quiz

The tomato is America's favorite vegetable. Yes, we know, technically, it's a fruit. Regardless of what you call it, it's Number One. In a program that we did once we polled the audience on their favorite way to eat tomatoes. "In a pizza sauce" was by far the first choice. A very close second was "In a salad." Other votes were cast for tomato juice, salsa, ketchup, fresh from the garden and in a Bloody Mary. Perhaps it's because this is such a versatile vegetable (fruit for you purists) that it is our national favorite. Perhaps it's because it tastes good, or is easy to grow. Or is it because it is good for us? No, that couldn't be it.

Whether you like your tomatoes juiced, on a Big Mac or in a soup we thought you might enjoy a little quiz about this delightful food. Let's see how well you know the main ingredient in spaghetti sauce.

1. TRUE or FALSE. The tomato originated in Italy.

2. The tomato is first cousin to:
(a) tobacco, (b) chile peppers, (c) deadly nightshade, (d) all of the above, (e) none of these

3. The first president to grow tomatoes for the table was:
(a) George Washington, (b) Thomas Jefferson, (c) Abraham Lincoln, (d) Theodore Roosevelt, (e) Millard Fillmore

4. The average American eats ___ pounds of processed tomatoes each year:
(a) 25,   (b) 54,   (c) 73,   (d) 107,   (e) 133

5. The community of Bunol in Spain celebrates the world's largest food fight every August. For an hour thousands of people throw thousands of pounds of tomatoes at each other and assorted other targets. What is this festival called?
(a) Festival La Tomatina, (b) Salsa Street Party, (c) Dia Del Loco Tomatillo

6. TRUE or FALSE Tomatoes were long thought to be poisonous.

7. TRUE or FALSE Tomatoes are a great source of Vitamin C.

8. TRUE or FALSE Tomatoes in tin cans were one of the rations provided to both Union and Confederate troops during the Civil War.

9. When the tomato was first introduced to France it was called the:
(a) Stinking apple, (b) Moor's apple, (c) Love apple, (d) Spanish apple.

10. The German name for the tomato inspired its botanical name, *Lycopersicon esculentum*. A translation of the German name means:
(a) Vine with edible fruit, (b) Bitter fruit, (c) Red heart vine, (d) edible wolf peach

Answers to Tomato Soup

1. FALSE, the tomato is native to South America and the Caribbean. It was introduced to Europe by the Spanish in the 1500's where it became a hit in Seville, because it blended so well with olive oil and garlic.

2. (d) all of the above. Tobacco, chile peppers, sweet peppers, eggplant and many popular flowering annuals are in the same family as the tomato. This *Solanaceae* family also hosts nightshade, belladonna and Jimson weed.

3. (b) Thomas Jefferson

4. (C) 73 pounds of processed tomatoes annually, and you can add to that 19 pounds of fresh tomatoes for every man, women and child in the United States.

5. (a) Festival La Tomatina. This festival began in the days of Franco. One source states that the tomatoes were aimed at local politicians. Today it is more of a tourist attraction as a quarter of a million pounds of tomatoes are dumped onto the streets and everyone becomes a target. After one hour of a food fight unrivaled anywhere else in the world everyone hits the showers and high pressure hoses clean the streets.

6. TRUE, the tomato is in the same family as deadly nightshade. Plants, like people are judged by the company they keep, so the tomato was suspect. Still the Spanish, Italians and French appreciated the tomato soon after its introduction to Europe. Spain decreed that tomatoes be planted at all ports of call to provide fruit for their sailors. The incidence of scurvy was much lower on Spanish ships than the English and Dutch. It should be noted that the leaves are toxic and should not be eaten. They contain solanine (a Glycoalkaloid) that can cause severe gastric distress, hallucinations, loss of body functioning and even death.

7. TRUE, tomatoes are very nutritious. Vitamins A & C, iron and lycopene all make this one of those rare combinations of a food that both tastes good and is good for you.

8. TRUE, the canned tomato was a popular part of field rations for both sides. Military campsites often accumulated large garbage dumps filled with empty tin cans. Foods preserved in tin cans were a popular way to store and transport provisions for an army on the march from the Napoleonic expeditions until today.

9. (c) It was called the love apple because of a firm conviction that dining on this fruit could inspire romance. This was in part due to the fact that the bright red fruit symbolized the heart, hence true love. There was a poem written in the mid 1600's that described the tomato as being just like love, delicious, beautiful, and dangerous.

10. (d) It may have been called "wolf peach" because of the hairy leaves that some thought resembled a wolf's ear. Of course the fruit itself does resemble a peach. Carolus Linnaeus adapted this common name when he assigned the botanical nomenclature *Lycopersicon esculentum.*

A Bucket of
Homegrown Tomatoes

The following is a true story reprinted from a collection of short stories inspired by the music, humanitarian work and genuine human compassion of musician, song writer, poet and environmentalist John Denver. This book, *Peace Beyond All Fear, a Tribute to John Denver's Vision*, was written by Hank Bruce and published by Petals & Pages Press. One of John's more popular songs was *Homegrown Tomatoes* written by Guy Clark. Hopefully these stories will inspire you as much as his music has inspired us.

They pushed her into the room just as we were about to begin. She was so frail, with short, straight, pure white hair that was decidedly unkempt. A pink flowered robe about five sizes too large was her attire, along with the with straps that held her upright in the wheelchair. All the aide said when she parked this lady by the table was, "Alzheimer's. Don't respond to nothing." No name, no reason why she had been brought to the room where we were doing our horticultural therapy program.

Perhaps I had better explain. I am a horticultural therapist and my work often takes me to the parts of senior care facilities that are little more than warehouses for the truly forgotten, those with Alzheimer's or other forms of dementia. We use plants, flowers and other botanical items in sensory roundtables for these folks. They often respond to the sensory stimulation of the bright red flowers of a geranium, the scent and texture of a pineapple, or the feel of a ripe red tomato. Sometimes we can trigger a memory or two, sometimes we can even engage in conversation, but the greatest gift is a smile, a gleam in the eye, a moment of enjoyment for these our forgotten elders.

This late arrival was completely unresponsive as we touched pine cones and pineapples, smelled mint and rosemary, remembered great moments with the velvet touch of a bright yellow rose and talked about colors. I was reluctant to disturb her any further as I circulated a small tomato plant and a large home grown tomato among the group. But I stopped and knelt beside her wheelchair, holding the plant and the fruit in front of her. For the first time her eyes struggled to focus, and as she recognized what was before her a smile began to form across the thin lips that quickly turned into a giggle. Before I knew what was happening, she began laughing out loud, laughing so hysterically that she was gasping for breath. Everyone else in the room, sixteen residents and four staff, were caught up in the moment and were all laughing as well. Nothing is more contagious than a good laugh and every person in that room was infected.

Soon, she calmed down and just sat there holding the smooth, warm tomato in her hand. I leaned closer and said, "Wow! You must really like tomatoes."

She starred at me and struggled to find the words. Carefully, ever so slowly she assembled them on her tongue and struggled to release them. "Noooo, ...I . . . .haaate . . . . .to . . . ma . . mat . . . oes." She looked at me with a frown on her face.

I answered her, "Then, you must know a really good story about tomatoes."

At this the laughter came again. This time it wasn't quite as intense, but when she regained control she was smiling broadly and there was a sparkle in her eyes where minutes before there was only a "nobody's home" sign.

She was again searching for the words that she needed to communicate a thought. Finally, she began to slowly put them together with that raspy voice of hers. "I, I . . . .haate . . . .tom . . .atoes. But. . . .Maaaama . . . . useta . . . . . grow . . . .'em." The words came slowly, so slowly that it was difficult to follow her train of thought, albeit, it was on uneven tracks. She paused, then spoke again. Everyone was listening intently as she told her story.

"Maama, . . .she was . . .askeered a . . . . snakes." Her delivery was becoming more cohesive, and was amazingly lucid. "One day . . . she handed me the . . . .bucket. 'Here, Maggie,' . . . she said, 'Go get me some tomatoes.'"

The pause was much briefer as she continued, "So I'm picken' them tomatoes . . . and I sees this little snake. . . . I grabbed it . . . and put it in the bucket. Then I filled it clean full and carried it up to the house. I sat that bucket on the table and tol' her, 'Here, Mama, here's yur tomatoes.' then I turned an ran like HELL!" She was talking so fast by the end of this story that she was almost breathless.

For the third time in less that ten minutes everyone in the room was again laughing. But, this time they knew why. What a great gift Maggie gave to everyone in that room that day; the gift of laughter, the gift of a good story, the gift of a moment of joy. There was another gift as well. Maggie was alert and responsive for a day and a half after relating this story.

For those of us with Alzheimer's the present is all there is. These are the people who truly live in the moment. Here was one of these forgotten people bringing everyone else into that moment as well. We are all capable of sharing gifts. This is the great opportunity we have, and yet we waste the treasure of the wisdom and the stories of our elders. Maggie, an old lady in a wheelchair, who couldn't remember your name, didn't know what she had for breakfast, had forgotten what you call a geranium, gave this gift to thousands of people she never met, because we tell her story in our seminars and programs. The sharing of a good story is an expression of love.

Digging deeper:

Because everyone knows a great tomato story several Green Thumb clubs decided to collect them and write their own "Tomato Book." Esmeralda had been a chef at a bed and breakfast most of her life and when she found herself in an assisted living community she couldn't resist sharing her recipes and giving advice. This soon spread through the community and everyone was talking about their favorites, their memories of regional cuisine and this led to a recipe book. And, we might add, some very good meals for all.

Jack was 93 when the Trevor Lake Adult Day Care center received the gift of a Green Thumb Garden. The folks at this center spent about a week trying to decide what they wanted to grow, but Jack was the elder statesman and the leader of the pack. He convinced everyone that the only thing to grow was tomatoes. Each of the six active gardeners selected their favorite variety of tomato and the race was on. Soon these gardeners were nurturing young seedlings. Next they were staking their green pets. Secret formulas were brought in and the race was on. They decided this was a contest to see who could grow the biggest tomato, the first ripe tomato, the most productive plant, the best tasting tomato and the ugliest tomato.

Rosa was confined to a wheelchair and living in a nursing home when she became the ringleader of a group of elementary school children. She taught them how to plant tomatoes, peppers, chiles and onions. They learned from this little old lady, not only how to grow a garden, but how to make salsa, how to can tomatoes and how to have a lot of fun with home grown tomatoes.

Windowsill Tomato Patch

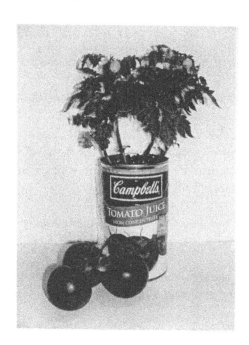

Tomato, *Lycopersican esculentum*
Nightshade family, *Solanaceae*
Native to Central and South America
Warning: leaves and green fruit are toxic
Rating: Moderately easy
Time Frame: 1 hour to initiate project, 3 to 4 months for harvest
Life span: one season
Size: Medium scale project

We are all familiar with the difference in flavor between the fresh "picked from the garden" tomatoes of our youth and the store bought varieties of today. You can enjoy that flavor from yesteryear with a tomato plant growing on your windowsill. In fact, today we even have special tomato varieties bred to grow and produce indoors. Although you can grow almost any variety of tomato on your windowsill there are some that do better than others. Green Thumb Club members have had great success with the following, and these are only suggestions. Feel free to experiment with your favorites, and let us know the results.
Patio,   Yellow pear,   Roma,   Grape, or cherry,   Better Boy

Materials needed:
Seeds for your favorite tomato variety
A large can of tomato juice
Sufficient quality potting mix to fill the can, once you empty it
A sunny windowsill

Putting it all together:
1. Invite friends over and share the tomato juice. It's a party, drink until the can is empty. People who grow tomatoes are a lot like people who fish. They can tell a very good story, and many of those stories are very creative. You can swap tomato garden stories during this phase of the project.
2. Rinse can and punch drainage holes in the bottom.
3. Fill the can with soil and firm so that the soil is about ½ inch below the rim.
4. Place 5 to 10 seeds on the surface and cover lightly with more soil.
5. Water well and place on your brightest windowsill.
6. Keep moist and the seeds should sprout in 7 to 14 days.
7. As the seedlings grow, thin until only the strongest one is left standing. The thinned seedlings can be potted up and shared with friends.

Care & Feeding of a Windowsill Tomato Plant

Light: Tomatoes love sunshine. Placing the seedlings in the brightest light you have available is the best gift you can give them.

Soil: Any quality potting mix will work well. It needs to be well drained and rich in organic material.

Watering: Tomatoes are heavy drinkers. The soil needs to be kept evenly moist for best results.

Cold: Tomatoes are perennial vines in their tropical homeland, but are grown as annual vegetables in our gardens because they don't do frost well. Indoors, if the temperature can be maintained above sixty degrees they will usually thrive and fruit well. You may have to become a surrogate bee using an artist's brush to carry pollen from flower to flower.

Container: You will eventually need to step your tomato plant up to a container equal to a two gallon pot or greater. Green Thumb Club members have grown great tomatoes in their Green Thumb Gardens too.

Feeding: A monthly feeding with Miracle-Gro Bloom Booster is great for encouraging compact, husky plants and abundant blossom and fruit.

Problems: There are few problems with windowsill tomatoes. Insufficient light can cause yellowing leaves and weak growth. Mealy bugs and white fly can be controlled if attacked early with alcohol and a Q-Tip.

Conversations:

Do you have a good tomato story to share?
Is there a favorite kind of tomato?
Why don't tomatoes taste as good today as they used to?
What's your secret for growing the "perfect" tomato?

Part 3

Thinking Like A Plant

Work Is a Four Letter Word,
The Basics of Easy Gardening

Going to Pot

Finding a good home for a new friend

The containers you provide for your plants are 'Home Sweet Home" for them. They can't climb out and run away, or move to a nicer neighborhood, or even drive down to the convenience store for some snacks. Your plants are, in the purest sense of the word, at your mercy. This is why it's important to give them as good a home as you can possibly provide. We have seen plants growing quite happily in everything from old baseball caps to baskets, mason jars to tin cans, coffee mugs to old shoes, and a whole lot more.

The following are a few tips for matching the plant with the planter

★ Size does matter. If the container is too small for the roots the plant will be crowded and growth will be stunted. Neither the plant nor you will be happy with this situation. Plants have a natural proportion between what's hidden in the soil and what you see on top.

★ Construction material is of more significance to you than to most of your plants. The great garden debate over plastic vs clay is something to keep gardeners busy when there's nothing good to watch on TV. It doesn't really matter that much. Commercial growers prefer plastic because it's lighter, doesn't break as easily and is less expensive.

★ Containers that have contained toxic materials, been sprayed with weed killers, or have been infected with fungus diseases or insect eggs that caused the demise of a previous resident can also be a serious problem for the new one. Always wash a used container in soapy water. If in doubt you can sterilize them with a good soaking in a bleach bath (1 part bleach to 10 parts water) for at least 30 minutes.

★ Don't be shy about trying something different, unique or downright weird. In fact, it you have created or used a one-of-a-kind or really original container please drop us an e-mail and tell us about it at **petals_pages@msn.com**

Drainage is critical in keeping your plants happy and healthy

★ Standard, unimaginative clay or plastic pots usually have drainage holes in them. Many people have an irrational fear that all the soil will wash out of this drainage hole. We were told once that this may be a fear related to the universal childhood experience where a toe felt the force of bath water going down the drain. Rather than spending a huge amount of money seeking psychiatric counseling for this fear we offer the "coffee filter solution." Simply place one of those cheap paper coffee filters in the bottom of the pot before adding the potting mix. This will put your mind at ease, and will not stop the flow of water. The filter will deteriorate in a matter of weeks but you feel that you have saved the soil. Some have used broken pottery, stones, pieces of screen or landscape fabric placed in the bottom of the pot.

★ In many of our horticultural therapy projects we use this coffee filter trick as a part of the adventure because it adds an element of coordination.

★ Many tin cans, brass pots, plastic dishes and other weird stuff you have chosen as housing for the plants you love don't have drainage holes but you can solve this problem by drilling, or using a hammer and a punch. The coffee filter is optional with these, it depends on how neat you were with the hole and your mental state at the time.

✿ Glass, porcelain, heavy metal (not the music, the container), coffee cups and many other materials are difficult, and downright dangerous to try to drill into. For these you can use the three step program below.

Three Step Program for containers with only one opening (and that's at the top)

1. Place a small amount of fine gravel in the bottom.
2. Add a teaspoon of crushed aquarium charcoal for each inch of container diameter. (Any charcoal that doesn't have additives to make it burn will do).
3. Fill the container with a quality potting mix, soilless mix or sterile sand, depending on your preference and your new plant's needs.

Now, wasn't that easy?

Where can you find the original, unique and really weird plant containers?

We are often asked where we find the secondhand things that we stuff some of the plants into for our horticultural therapy programs. The answer is that generally, we don't find them, the Green Thumb Club members and participants do. They find them in:

* Closets, attics, under the bed and in the garage, or sometimes in the garbage
* Some of the best finds come from yard sales, flea markets and thrift stores
* Craft items, unfinished craft projects, leftovers from craft activities, woodworking, art and other endeavors can also find their way to the windowsill to adorn your plants.
* Coffee mugs, tea cups, wine glasses, beer steins, old mason jars, can all be found in the kitchen or pantry. One of our Green Thumb Club members turned an old blender into a fern filled terrarium.
* In the kids' closet, if you dare enter, you can also find a wealth of potting resources.
* Don't forget the potential for a truly organic windowsill garden using gourds, coconut shells, sections of bamboo, wooden salad bowls and hollow logs as planters.

Decorating the Pot Can Be at Least Half the Fun

Finding, or creating, a suitable plant container is only the beginning. It is now an opportunity for you to be an artist, be creative, exercise your imagination, even show off your sense of humor. A plain old clay pot is fine as far as the plant is concerned, but many of us need a little more.

* We can use waterproof craft paints or markers to make the container a statement or a work of art.
* One of our horticultural therapy groups collected old buttons, coins and other assorted small treasures from their junk drawers and glued them onto their secondhand Christmas cookie tins. They then sold these planters in the gift shop and helped fund the purchase of some new plants.
* A gentleman who had been a singer and musician for a number of years glued sheet music and pressed flowers on the pots then applied a sealer. These were his gifts to family and friends on his birthday.
* We have seen stamps, photos, newspaper clippings, old maps and pictures from magazines and seed catalogs used very effectively as container decor.
* Others have used ribbons, cord, sewing notions, and pressed leaves, twigs or moss as the trim for otherwise drab containers.
* But one of the best, at least from a whimsy standpoint was the Green Thumb Club that did all of their containers with favorite comic strips from their favorite Sunday paper or comic book.

Dirt 101

After you have selected, decorated, trimmed, customized or otherwise created a distinctive container, it's time to provide your new plants with a growing medium. This is what some call soil, soilless mix, sterile medium, or just plain dirt. Many of the cheaper mixes contain very fine organic matter and hold too much moisture. This is where things can get a little tricky. Different plants have different soil needs, and some will need sand added, or coarse peat, or bark chips. This may seem complex but the good news is that most of the plants we discuss in this book will do quite well in any good quality potting mix.

Here's the class notes for Dirt 101:

Soil is a community of living organisms thriving in a blend of disintegrated rock and decomposed organic matter. It's this thriving, growing assortment of microscopic organisms that makes your garden grow, makes trees grow, even makes the weeds grow. There is a symbiotic partnership between these minute creatures and the roots of your plants on the windowsill as well. But sometimes there are also organisms that may be harmful to us if we are undergoing chemotherapy, have an immune deficiency or even nasty allergies. The good news is that these are usually not a problem in soil that is healthy.

Organic soil is soil that doesn't have chemical fertilizers or pesticides added. It tends to have the healthiest blend of micro-organisms in residence.

Potting soil is usually a packaged blend of organic material and mineral compounds designed to give you the best chance of success with plants being grown in containers. There can be a wide range in the quality of potting or container mixes, but all of them are loose soils that will give better drainage than clay.

Soilless mix is a blend of sphagnum peat moss, perlite, vermiculite, sand and, possibly, other minerals without the actual soil. This was once describes to us as " virtual soil, sort of like watching a cooking show on TV, but not being able to taste the finished product." It lacks many of the organisms that make soil, or topsoil, a healthy growing medium. It generally has a less immediate threat of damping off for seedlings, and less danger of fungi and bacteria that can pose a threat to gardeners. Soilless does not mean sterile.

Dirt is what we sweep under the rug, what lurks under the bed, and what the kids track in just after you have vacuumed the carpets or washed the floors. Dirt is also what we gardeners call the soil that accumulates under our fingernails.

Sand is found in sterile, play, colored and construction forms. Oh, we almost forgot, there is beach sand too, but this usually contains salts that are not good for your plants. The size of the particles can vary from coarse to fine. Sand is easy to wash, clean or sterilize. It is frequently used as a rooting medium for cuttings and some seeds are best stated in sand rather than soil.

Special mixes are often found in the better garden centers. These can range from Orchid Mix to African Violet Mix or Cactus Blends. The coarseness of the organic matter and the amount of sand will vary from blend to blend.

Watering

One of the keys to keeping your windowsill garden happy and healthy lies in the watering. More indoor plants are done in by too much water than too little. But this doesn't mean that they should be dying of thirst before you give them a drink.

➡ We suggest that you use a moisture meter to determine when your plants are thirsty. There are mechanical meters available at most garden centers, but you can also use a 100% organic digital moisture indicator. Some folks call this an index finger (you can also use a thumb). Simply stick you finger in the soil, then analyze the sensory experience. If it's moist you don't need to water, if it's dry, give the plant a drink. The advantage of the mechanical moisture meter is that the probe gets down to where the roots are.

- Smaller containers will dry out faster than larger ones.
- A rootbound plant has less space for water absorption and it will need to be watered more frequently.
- Not all soils absorb the same amount of water, nor do all soils dry out at the same rate. This is why it is difficult to give a basic rule of thumb on watering. We suggest checking the soil every couple days until you are familiar with the rates at which the soil in various containers dries out.
- Watch the plants and they will tell you when they are thirsty. If they start to wilt, check the soil. Plants will also wilt if they are too hot, the air is too dry or if the roots are decaying because the soil is soggy.
- Many plants don't like chlorinated water. For this reason we suggest that you let the water sit overnight. This will allow the chlorine to evaporate from the water.

A Healthy Diet

Plants use energy from the sun, nutrients from the soil and water to grow, produce new leaves, roots and flowers. In the wild, in nature, the soil organisms make food for the plants by turning compost into compounds the roots can absorb and use. In the pots on your windowsill you may have to assume the role of bacteria and fungus and even earthworms. Fortunately modern technology has made this easy for you. There are a multitude of indoor plant foods, some are organic, some are fast release and others are long term. While we prefer organic fertilizers we sometimes use Peters Plant foods, Jack's Classic formulas and Miracle-Gro because they are completely safe and are easy to use. What you use is your decision.

There are, however, several basic rules:
- Don't over feed. There is nothing worse than an obese plant. The weak growth that results from overfeeding is an open invitation to insects and disease organisms. FOLLOW THE DIRECTIONS ON THE PLANT FOOD PACKAGE.
- Don't starve your plants either. If you are using a liquid plant food at the indoor formula rate, once a month is usually sufficient. For many plants this is even more than necessary.
- Because your plants are in a confined area, the pot, there is little opportunity for the leaching away of the chemical salts that are a natural result of plant feeding. When these salts build up they can become toxic to the plants. This is one of the reasons it is advisable to repot and change soil periodically.
- We don't recommend the use of animal manures on indoor plants. There are several reasons for this. There can be an offensive odor, but more significant is the fact that they may harbor bacteria that can be harmful to anyone who has respiratory problems or allergies.

Organic vs chemical fertilizers:
The organic enthusiasts insist that only kelp juice and fish emulsions are worthy of your windowsill landscape. These are good slow release plant foods that also help to condition the soil. These organic plant foods don't build up salts and chemical compounds as rapidly as the chemicals do. It is also more difficult to over feed and burn the plants with organic plant foods.

On the other hand, Osmocote is a slow release fertilizer that can be applied twice a year with great results in most soils. This means that there is a lot less effort required. Remember, W-O-R-K is a four letter word, so make it easy on yourself. The packaged plant foods that you mix with water are also very easy to use, and they give you almost total control, but they are also easy to abuse. Don't make the mix too strong and don't apply too often. Follow the directions. There are special formulas for acid loving (not LSD) plants and other Bloom Booster mixes to encourage flowering and fruit. The choice is yours, but the most important rule to remember is DO NOT OVER FEED.

Thinking Like a Plant

All plants have a few basic needs in common. The problem for us gardeners is that not all plants want these elements in the same proportions. This is why we need to think like a plant. It isn't so much a green thumb that makes some people so successful with plants as it is green wisdom. When you become friends with your plants you get to know them and become familiar with their basic, and individual, needs.

All plants need:
✔   **Light** - The amount of light needed varies with different species of plants. Too much can result in sunburn while too little forces the plant to frantically reach for light. This weak, pale, spindly growth is called etiolation.

✔   **Air** - They use carbon dioxide and add oxygen to the air we breath. It is important for many plants to have the air circulating. Some need a humid atmosphere while others like it dry.

✔   **Water** - Soil needs to be moist, but not soggy, except for the swamp creatures. There are also many plants adapted to desert climes and drying out occasionally isn't traumatic for these rugged individuals.

✔   **Soil or growing medium** - Different plants have different needs, some will even grow in water. Some, like citrus and azaleas, need an acid soil while cacti and many succulents prefer a more alkaline place to put their roots. Some need a sandy soil while others are quite happy with compost.

✔   **Temperature** that is comfortable - Freezing weather doesn't bother and apple tree but oranges don't like it one bit. Again, get to know your plants.

Between Rainforest and Desert is the Windowsill:
Some plants thrive in the high humidity of a rain forest while others are much happier in an indoor desert. It is best to group plants with similar light and humidity requirements together so that the environment can be more easily maintained. If you live in a desert climate and want to grow something at home on the banks of the Amazon, a terrarium may be in order. Placing the containers on a plastic serving tray filled with gravel can also be a way to add humidity to the immediate atmosphere. That is, when you keep the gravel moist.

Air circulation and disease prevention:
Fungus diseases, powdery mildew and other botanical illnesses can result from, or be worsened by, stagnant air. Spacing plants so that they aren't touching is one way to help solve this problem. Providing some air flow is also helpful. We hear all the time from people warning gardeners to keep plants away from air conditioning vents, but actually this can be beneficial for some plants. It may become a far more serious problem when the furnace is running and hot dry air is blowing over your plants. It's also helpful to rotate the plants once every week or so.

Some like it hot:
In the Care and Feeding notes for most of the plants listed we made comments on cold tolerance. This is because people in many of the countries where this book may be used will have some of these plants outdoors at least part of the year. Cold can create problems for some of your plants even without frost or freezing temperatures. Other plants thrive with a cool season so that they can rest. This is why it is important to know as much as you can about your green friends. This is one of the advantages of keeping a journal.

A Haircut and a Shave on the Windowsill Garden:
A pair of pruning shears, or scissors is an essential tool because, like you, the plants need an occasional trim.
❖   Remove old, diseased, or yellowing leaves.
❖   Trim back straggly, spindly, or misshapen twigs and branches.

- ❖ When you trim and prune to shape you can help the plant conform to the space allotted for it in the windowsill community.
- ❖ Pruning back leggy growth encourages more branching and a fuller look
- ❖ When you are growing trees like avocados, mangos or moringa in the house, it may be necessary to pinch out the central leader. This will slow the upward growth and encourage some branching.

Making a Care Plan for your Garden:

If your windowsill collection is only one or two plants then you can probably keep track of when to water, feed and do the other fussing that needs to be done. But if there are many of these plants to care for you might want to get a calendar and write down when to do what.

- ※ Feeding schedule. Note feeding mixes and dates when they need to be applied.
- ※ Make notes of any problems, insects and diseases when they occurred. Note when you will need to do followup treatment.
- ※ Note when to turn the container so that each side of the plant gets its chance at the sunny side of the street.
- ※ It is best to water as needed for the first month or so. After the routine is established you may want to note watering days on the calendar.

Gardens Going to School

At the Roosevelt Elementary School in Bernilillo, New Mexico the enthusiasm of young gardeners was contagious. What a delight to see these students racing to their gardens with their rulers, magnifying glasses, notebooks and sketchpads. They worked in teams to measure growth that had occurred over the weekend, search for bugs and delight in newly sprouted seeds. They were learning about the source of their food, how to work with the soil and partner with nature while they did scientific experiments, kept journals, solved math problems, created art projects and learned how to work together toward a common goal. This is why we wrote *Gardening Projects for the Classroom and Special Learning Programs*.

Lights, Camera, Action!

Take photographs at all stages of each plant's growth, from sowing seeds or striking cuttings to maturity, bloom and fruit. This is a record for you that can be shared. It can also be a resource when you want to paint, sketch, sculpt, write or otherwise be artistic and creative. It can also be proof for you to show the skeptics when they doubt your plant stories and claims. These can be used in your Gardener's Journal, a scrapbook, enlarged and mounted on the wall like a trophy or sent to doubting friends and family.

Increasing the Flock, A Windowsill Nursery

Taking stem cuttings of easy house plants: Begin with clean healthy stock. Check to see that there are no insects, disease or damage problems. Cutting stock shouldn't be wilted or stressed.

Water vs Potting Soil: Many plants will start and grow well in water. If this is the method you choose you can start pothos, philodendron, weeping fig, coleus, sweet potato, avocado, ivy, spider plant and many others.

If you are going to start plants in water:

- Change the water frequently to prevent souring.
- Allow tap water to stand for several hours before using on plants.
- Room temperature water is best.
- You can add small amounts of a liquid houseplant food, but don't overdo it.
- Don't set in direct sun until there are roots.

If you are rooting cuttings in soil:

- Use a good quality potting soil or soilless mix.
- Keep evenly moist but not soggy. Good soil contains more air than water.
- Keep out of bright sun until rooted. New leaves are the best indication that you have roots.
- You don't need to feed until after you have new leaves forming.

Taking stem cuttings:

- Use sharp knife or bypass pruning shears so that you get a clean cut without bruising or crushing.
- Most plants form their roots at the leaf nodes, but some form callus tissue at the base of cutting from which roots will grow.
- Cut leaves from bottom of cutting, don't tear or rip them off.
- Rooting compounds and starter fertilizers can be used but they aren't essential for most of the plants you will be propagating.
- Don't make the cuttings too large. Small cuttings usually root more successfully.
- Succulent plants like geraniums, jade plants, Christmas cactus and orchid cactus need to sit for a day or two to let the cut heal before striking. NO! Don't hit the cutting. This is a term gardeners use that means planting the cutting.
- For most plants it is best to trim flower buds and nip the terminal bud (the tip of the cutting where new leaves are just starting to form) to encourage a fuller plant.
- Use several cuttings in a pot (usually an odd number) to make a fuller plant as it grows.
- Don't start cuttings in too small a container. There is a greater opportunity for them to dry out. Plants, like people, only die of thirst once.
- Succulent plants do, however, prefer soil on the dry side.

Some plants can be started from leaves:

African violets, rex begonias, jade plants, crassulas and kalanchoes are only a few.
Use mature, fresh, healthy leaves, not old, yellowing ones.
Keep the rooting medium lightly moist, but not soggy.
Keep out of direct sun until new leaves are formed, and roots are present.
The use of a deli carton or Zip-Loc bag can increase your chances of success.

Other plants produce offsets: Spider plants, some iris, piggy-back plant, bromeliads, sanserveria, kalanchoes, aloe and many others will produce baby plants, or pups. This is the easiest way to propagate new plants because all you have to do is separate the pup from the mother and pot it up. It is almost failsafe.

Seeds, Life in a Time Capsule

*"If the promise of leaf, flower and fruit lies within the dust-like seed,
then what promise lies within the human heart?"*

Seed Quiz
1. TRUE or FALSE.   Some seeds need to go through a cycle of freezing and thawing before they will sprout.
2. TRUE or FALSE.   Some seeds contain more than one embryo, thus producing more than one seedling.
3. Cilantro leaves are popular in Mexican, Oriental and Mediterranean cooking. The seeds of this plant are also popular but they are known as   (a) anise.   (b) coriander. (c) caraway.
4. TRUE OR FALSE. There are seeds that need to have the seed coat filed or cracked before they will sprout.
5. TRUE OR FALSE.   Most seeds are only viable for one year.

Seed Savvy

Seeds are literally time capsules full of life, held in suspended animation until all the conditions are just right. Each species has its own concept of ideal conditions. Some need a minimum soil temperature over sixty degrees. Others require just the right amount of moisture, the presence of certain fungi, or a raging fire, or a journey through the digestive system of a specific bird or mammal. Some desert plants produce seeds that sprout literally within hours of a rain. Some plants are patient and will wait years for their moment in the sun. There are several pines and other plants that need a forest fire to break the protective seed coat. Some seeds take months, even years, to germinate, others will sprout in days. Some seeds won't sprout unless they are covered with soil, others must have light to trigger the process. Fortunately, most of the seeds we are trying to germinate aren't too demanding.

The process is simple for the seed. The protective coating, the shell or seed coat, is softened by digestive juices, decomposition, freezing and thawing, chemical action, or simply the presence of moisture. As moisture enters the embryo, dormant cells begin to grow. From the hilum (the seed's navel) the infant root emerges and begins its journey downward toward moisture and anchorage for the botanical youngster. Soon the last of the stored food is used to push the seed leaves through the soil and into the sunshine. Then the green leaves can begin to produce the foods needed to build a plant. The "second leaves" soon follow, then more, in a pattern of growth spurts that soon becomes something big enough to be recognized.

Ten Tips for Happy Plants from Seed:
Many get so caught up in following all the rules that growing plants from seed ceases to be fun. Relax and rejoice in the fact that you have a valuable partner in this process. The seed wants to succeed, too.   Just enjoy being a part of nature, even if it's an egg carton of seedlings on your windowsill.

✖ You can start seeds in recycled 3 or 4 inch pots, peat pots, plastic trays, egg cartons or soup cans. Recycling pots is good. But first wash with soap and water, or sterilize these reused pots by soaking them for about 15 minutes in a bleach solution. One part bleach to ten parts water is a good mix. Wear rubber gloves while doing this to prevent damage to your skin.

✖ Use a high quality potting soil or an African violet mix as your seed starting medium. Avoid the temptation to use the cheap stuff that may well contain insect eggs, weed seeds, and disease spores. The soil should not form a crust on the surface if it dries.

✖ Follow the directions on the seed packet. They were put there to help you succeed. The time from sowing to sprouting can often be shortened for some seeds by soaking them overnight in warm water.

- Don't sow the seed too thickly. When they germinate they will crowd each other and general health will decline.
- Don't plant the seeds too deeply. A rule of thumb says that the seed should be covered no more than two or three times the diameter of the seed. This information will be on the seed packet. A light covering of clean sand works well with small seeds.
- Some seed needs to be stratified, a big word that means they want some time to chill out. One of the easiest ways to do this is to wrap the seeds in a slightly moist paper towel. Place the towel and seeds in a plastic bag and store in the refrigerator for a few weeks.
- Keep the soil evenly moist while you're waiting for the seeds to sprout. Some folks cover the pots or trays with a glass or plastic cover. This does retain soil moisture, but it also limits air circulation and that can also encourage fungus problems.
- Once the seedlings begin to germinate, make certain your green infants get enough light. Once they become light starved, weak and spindly, it's difficult to bring them back to good health.
- Keep the seedlings evenly moist, but avoid standing water, soggy soil and poor drainage. This can cause a fungus disease known as damping off.
- Give your seedlings time to develop a good root system before transplanting them into their decorative containers or hanging baskets.

The "Baggie" method of starting larger seeds

You can start many seeds very well by taking several seeds, a little good soil and a 1 or 2 quart Baggie or Zip Top clear plastic bag.

1. Fill the Baggie about ½ full of moist potting soil or medium of your choice.

2. Carefully place the seed or seeds so that they are in the soil.

3. The Baggie can then be placed where the proper temperature can be maintained. Some seeds need a minimum temperature of at least 60° F while others need to be chilled for several weeks before they will even think about sprouting.

4. Light isn't important at this phase of the process, but as soon as they begin to germinate you will need to put them in a windowsill or under Grow Lights while they can develop roots and leaves.

5. As they sprout, you can plant the seedlings in a container of your choice. We have had great success when we placed another, larger Baggie over the newly potted seedlings while they were becoming accustomed to their new environment.

6. Once the new plants have grown from seedling to a junior plant, established and vigorous, the Baggie can be removed.

Answers to Quiz: 1. TRUE, This chilling process is called stratification. 2. TRUE, This is called a polyembrionic seed. Citrus and beets are two examples 3. (b). 4. TRUE. This is called scarification. Lotus seeds are one example. 5. FALSE, many seeds remain viable for decades and there are reports of lotus and date seeds that have sat for hundreds of years then sprouted when given the opportunity.

SAFE & DANGEROUS PLANTS

Safe Plants for Special Gardens

We so often worry about whether a plant is safe or not and even avoid the use of plants in senior care and school settings because of a fear that someone may be harmed. While it is true that some plants, or at least some parts of plants, are toxic, most don't pose a threat. Some plants can cause a skin reaction, such as an inflammation, rash or itching. Others can cause an allergenic reaction for some and not for others. But many of us are allergic to certain medications, foods, pets, etc. Sulfites are used in many foods without any listing on labels, yet many people are violently allergic to these preservatives. As far as poisoning from plants, the risk is far greater from the cleaning compounds found in the bathroom, in the maintenance closet and on easily accessible service carts.

The people-plant connection that Charles Lewis spoke so eloquently about is real. We now understand that many of our children are suffering from "Nature Deficit Disorder." We delight in the garden because we are naturally drawn to the beauty of life itself, the colors, forms and fragrance of flowers and foliage. Being with, and being actively engaged with, plants is good for us physically, mentally, emotionally, socially and spiritually. Horticultural therapists tell us that pending some time gardening can decrease depression, lower blood pressure and reduce anger. It can also increase our sense of self-worth, encourage our instinct for nurturing and foster a general sense of well-being. Even in Alzheimer's and Dementia patients the sensory stimulation and the memory triggering that naturally occurs with plants and flowers is beneficial. For children with developmental disabilities or cognitive limitations, the time spent gardening is rewarding in many ways. Even school children and troubled youths can learn many of life's lessons in the garden.

Still, there are many plants that are generally considered safe, and others that are considered dangerous. The following is a brief list of plants that are usually thought to be safe for most people to handle and pose little threat even if ingested. Having said that, we do need to remind you that people on medications, those suffering from certain illnesses or diseases, our young children and senior citizens may react differently than a healthy adult. In the following list we provide the botanical names of many and notes on others to help you make your best possible decision on whether or not you want to include this plant in your facility's garden. If you have questions, contact your local poison control center or your county extension agent for details. Warning! No matter how safe the plant is, the use of pesticides and some plant foods can render the garden dangerous.

This is by no means a complete list. Thousands of other plants are perfectly safe for use in settings where they might be accidentally consumed. Some of these may cause an allergic reaction or react with medications. Take care and observe closely until certain that there are no problems.

Only the plants you know to be edible should be consumed, and even then, only in limited quantities until you are certain that there isn't going to be any reaction due to health conditions, medications or allergies.

241

SAFE PLANTS: The list

* Indicates plants commonly grown indoors or are suitable for windowsill whimsy projects

Alyssum, sweet
African daisy, *Arctotis*
*African violet, *Saintpaulia*
*Allspice, *Pimenta officinale*
*Aloe vera, safe medicinal herb
*Aluminum plant, *Pilea*
*Amaranth, many types, some with edible leaves and seeds
*Areca palm, *Chrysalidocarpus lutescens*
*Artillery fern, *Pilea microphylla*
Astilbe, Meadow sweet, False spirea, *Astilbe*, many varieties
Bamboo, many varieties
Bachelor's buttons, cornflower, *Centaurea cyanus*, flowers can be eaten
Balloon flower, *Platycodon grandiflorus*
Banana, dwarf or standard, *Musa*
*Basil, edible aromatic herb
*Beets
*Begonias, many types
*Bellflower, *Campanula*, Leaves can be eaten
*Bird's nest fern, *Asplenium nidus*
Black eyed Susan vine, Clock vine, *Thunbergia alata*
Butterfly bush, *Buddleia davidii*
*Boston fern, *Nephrolepis exaltata*
Bottlebrush tree, *Callistemon*
*Bromeliads
*Calendula, flowers are edible
*California poppy, *Eschscholzia californica*
*Calathea, *Calathea*
*Camellia, some of the dwarf varieties will do well indoors, Tea is a camellia
Canna
*Carob tree, St. John's bread, *Ceratonia siliqua*
*Catnip, *Nepeta cataria*
*Chard
*Chives, edible herb
*Christmas cactus
Cleome, Spider flower, *Cleome hasslerana*
Cockscomb, *Celosia*
*Coleus, many varieties
*Coffee, *Coffea arabica*, can be grown in a CelluGro system when young
Coral bells, *Heuchera sanguinea*
Coreopsis, *Coreopsis grandiflora*
*Corn plant, *Dracena*
Cosmos
Crape myrtle
*Cryptanthus, star flower
*Dandelion, *Taraxacum officinale*, edible leaves, flowers and roots

*Dahlia

Daylily, *Hemerocallis*, flowers and roots are edible

*Dianthus, pinks, sweet William, edible flowers

*Dill, edible herb

*Easter lily, *Lilium longifolium*

*English ivy, can cause reaction in some if ingested.

*Fennel, edible herb

*Flame violet, *Episcia*

*Flowering kale, Flowering cabbage, edible leaves

*Flowering maple, *Abutilon*

Fragrant olive, *Osmanthus*, several varieties

*Fuchsia

*Gardenia, *Gardenia jasminoides*

*Geraniums, old fashioned, zonals, scented leaf, ivy and others

*Gerber daisy, cape daisy, *Gerbera jamesonii*

*Ginger, *Zingiber officinale*, edible roots, flowers and young shoots

*Gloxinia

*Green beans

*Goldfish plant, *Columnea*

*Hen & chicks, *Echeveria, Sempervivum*

*Hibiscus, flowers and young leaves are edible

*Holly fern, *Cyrtomium falcatum*

Hosta

*Jerusalem artichoke, (sunchoke) roots are eaten

Job's tears, *Coix lacryma-jobi*

*Joseph's coat, *Alternathera*

*Kalanchoe, many varieties

*Ice plant, several plants, needs full sun to do well

Impatiens, Touch-me-not

*Lambs ears, *Stachys byzantium & lanata*

*Lavender, edible herb

*Lemon grass, *Cymbopogon citratus*, leaves good for tea

*Lettuce

*Lipstick plant, *Aeschynanthus*

Liriope

*Maidenhair fern, *Adiantum*

Magnolia, several varieties

*Marigolds, *Tagetes*, flowers can be eaten or used as a seasoning

*Mint, many varieties

Money plant, *Lunaria annua*

*Moss rose, *Portulaca*, needs full sun

Mulberry, *Morus*, varieties

*Nasturtium, leaves and flowers can be eaten

*Norfolk Island Pine, *Araucaria heterophylla*

*Orchids, most orchids are safe to handle

*Oregano, Greek and Italian, edible herb

*Oregano, Cuban, Mexican or Spanish, edible herb

Palo Verde, *Cercidium*

*Pansy, flowers are edible, short life span indoors
*Parsley, edible herb
*Passionvine, passion flower, *Passiflora*, many varieties
*Peanut, flowers and seeds are edible, some are very allergic to peanuts and the plant
*Peppermint, edible herb
*Petunia
*Piggy-back plant, *Tolmia menziesii*
*Persian violet, *Exicum affine*
*Pineapple, *Ananas* varieties, edible fruit
*Pocketbook plant, pouch flower, *Calceolaria*, short life span
*Polka-dot plant, Hypoestes
*Ponytail palm, *Beaucarnea recurvata*
*Prayer plant, *Maranta*
Purple coneflower, *Echinacea*
*Purslane, *Portulaca,* edible leaves and flowers
*Radish, many types, root, leaves and flowers edible
*Rabbit's foot fern, *Polypodium aureum*
Red hot poker, torch lily, *Kniphofia uvaria*
Rockrose, Scotch broom, *Cistus*
Roses, old-fashioned, shrubs, hybrid teas, climbers and more. Thorns only threat
*Roses, miniature, many colors and varieties, does well on a sunny window
*Rosemary, edible herb
Rose of Sharon, *Hibiscus*
*Sage, common, tricolor, pineapple sage and other varieties *Salvia*, many kinds, edible herb
Snapdragon, *Antirrinum,* flowers are edible
*Spearmint, edible herb
*Spider plant, *Chlorophytum comosum*
*Sunflower, *Helianthus annuus*
*Swedish ivy, *Plectranthus*
Sweet gum, *Liquidambar styraciflua*
*Sweet potato, several ornamental varieties, leaves are edible as well as tubers
*Thyme, edible herb
*Ti plant, Hawaiian ti, *Cordyline terminalis*
*Torenia, Florida pansy, wishbone flower
*Viola, edible flowers
Violet, edible flowers
*Zebra plant, *Aphelandra squarrosa*
Zinnia

Note: Some of these plants are perennials or shrubs and can be started as a windowsill whimsy project but will need to be transplanted to a large container or permanent outdoor site.

Dangerous Plants, an Awareness Guide
for Homes, Schools and Senior Care Facilities

This was not written to frighten anyone wanting to grow plants. In no way do we want to discourage anyone from being a part of the people-plant connection. It is wise for teachers, activity professionals, social workers or community program staff to know which plants need to be used with caution, or avoided by some who might ingest plant parts. Keep in mind also that toxicisty or allergic reaction is not the only way a plant can pose a problem.

There are various ways that a plant can be a threat to an individual.

■ Some, like yucca, prickly pear cactus and roses have thorns, spines or sharp points that can cause puncture wounds. These wounds can be an entry site for infection.

■ Some can cause dermatitis, rashes, or an allergenic reaction. We are all familiar with stinging nettles and poison ivy, but there are others that may cause an uncomfortable to severe problem for some.

■ Often problems can come from common fruits and vegetables. Tomato and potato leaves contain solanine. Onions, horseradish, even chives contain natural chemical compounds that can cause eye inflammation. Mangos and cashews are in the same plant family as poison ivy and some people react to them. Raw cashews are a problem but roasting dissipates the anacardic acid.

■ Many of the plants we commonly cultivate as a part of the landscape or indoor decor can be a problem. Azaleas and mountain laurel, delphiniums and lily-of-the-valley, philodendron and tulips all pose a threat if ingested.

■ Often, a plant, or plant part, that can cause a mild or insignificant reaction in a health adult can cause a serious problem for a child, the frail elderly or someone with chronic health problems.

■ There can also be the danger from a reaction with medications, chemical sensitivity or allergy. The actual number of people adversely reacting to plants considered dangerous is very small.

Fatalities are extremely rare and usually connected with other health problems. Far more people die each year in from insect stings, rattlesnake bites, household chemicals or food poisoning than dangerous plants.

The following is a brief list of common plants that can be considered a threat if ingested. If parts of these plants listed are ingested, immediately contact the nearest poison control center for advice. Assume all parts are a threat unless otherwise noted. It should be noted that many of these plants are commonly used as medicinal herbs and can be beneficial some situations. When we consider the danger we must keep in mind that quantity can be a factor. A whole bottle of aspirin can be dangerous swallowed at one time.

We compiled the following list, not to discourage you from gardening, or even growing these plants, but to inform you of the risk, so that they can be grown where contact can be controlled. We have included botanical names and brief notes to help guide your identification.

DANGEROUS PLANTS: The List

❀ indicates plants commonly used indoors, or suitable for a windowsill whimsy project, when used with caution.

Aconite, Monkshood, *Acomitum,* tubers are the greatest threat, resulting in possible heart damage

❀Aglaonema, *Aglaonema,* can inflame throat and cause suffocation if leaves are eaten

Alamanda

❀Alocasia, *Alocasia,* can inflame throat and cause suffixation if leaves are eaten

❀Amaryllis, *Hippeastrum*

Andromeda

Angels trumpet, Jimson weed, *Brugmansia arborea*

❀Anthurium, (Flamingo flower), *Anthurium,* can cause mild mouth inflammation from eating leaves

Autumn crocus, *Colchicum autumnale* and others, while extracts are used medicinally, deadly

❀Azalea, *Rhododendron*

Balsam pear, cucumber cousin can cause gastric distress

Belladonna, *Atropa belladonna,* while a source of important medicines, the berries can be deadly

Bittersweet, *Celastrus scandens*

Black locust, *Robinia pseudoacacia,* all parts can cause gastric distress

Bleeding heart, *Dicentra*

Blood lily, *Haemanthus*

Bloodroot

❀Boxwood, *Buxus semperens*

Bracken fern

Brazilian pepper tree, *Schinus terebinthifolius*

Buckeye, Horse chestnut, *Aesculus*

Buttercup, *Ranunculus,* many species, all parts can cause skin irritation, inflammation of mouth, vomiting, and in severe cases, respiratory failure.

❀Caladium, *Caladium bicolor* and others

❀Calla lily, *Zantedeschia*

Candelabra tree, (pencil tree), *Euphorbia*

Cardinal flower, *Lobelia cardinalis*

Carolina jasmine, Yellow jasmine, *Gelsemium sempervirens,* all parts dangerous, including nectar from the flowers

Caster bean, *Ricinus comminus,* source of castor oil, the raw beans can be deadly

Cherry tree, Cherry laurel, Chokecherry, *Prunus,* fruit & drying leaves can cause gastric problems

Chinaberry, *Melia azedarach,* eating the berries can result in convulsions or death

❀Chinese evergreen, *Aglonemia*

Chinese lantern, *Physalis alkekengi* & others, roots and leaves are poisonous

Christmas rose, *Helleborus niger*

Clematis, *Clematis* spp.

Columbine, *Aquilegia,* many varieties, can cause cramps and breathing difficulties

Coral plant, *Jatropha* spp.

Coral tree, *Erythrina* spp.

Cotton

Cowslip

Crinum lily, *Crinum* spp.

❀Cyclamen, *Cyclamen* spp.

❀Daffodil, Narcissus, jonquil, *Narcissus* spp.

Daphne, *Daphne odorata* and others, all parts can cause breathing difficulty & kidney damage

Death camas
Delphinium, *Delphinium*
Dipladenia
❀Dumb cane, *Dieffenbachia*, can inflame throat and cause suffixation if leaves are eaten
Dutchman's breeches, *Dicentra*, several species, contains poisonous alkaloids, gastric distress
Dutchman's pipe, *Aristolochia*
Elderberry, Sambucus spp. (Ripe berries are both safe and delicious in pies)
Elephant ears, *Alocasia, Colocasia & Xanthosoma* spp.
Euonymus, Spindle tree, many landscape shrubs, all parts can cause severe abdominal pain
❀Fishtail palm, *Caryota* spp.
Flowering tobacco, *Nicotiana glauca*, nicotine poisoning can result from eating leaves or flowers
Four O'clock, *Mirabilis jalapa*, gastric distress
Foxglove, *Digitalis purpurea*, leaves most dangerous, can cause cardiac arrest
Glorisa lily, Climbing lily, Glory lily, *Gloriosa*
Golden rain tree, *Laburnum anagyroides,& others*, seeds can cause vomiting & delirium
Ground cherry, nightshade, *Physalis*
Ground ivy, *Glechoma hederacea*
Heather, Scottish heather, *Calluna vulgaris*
Heliotrope, *Heliotropum arborescens* and others
❀Holly berries and raw leaves, *Ilex*
Horse nettle, nightshade, *Physalis*
❀Hyacinth, *Hyacinthus orientalis*
❀Hydrangea, *Hydrangea*
Iris, *Iris*
Jack-in-the-pulpit, Indian turnip, *Arisaema triphyllum*
Jasmine, *Cestrum*
Jerusalem cherry, *Solanum pseudocapsicum*
Jimson weed, *Datura stramonium*
❀Lantana, *Lantana camera*
Larkspur, *Delphimium*
❀Ligustrum, privet, *Ligustrum*
❀Lily-of-the-valley, *Convallaria majalis*, all parts, if ingested, can cause cardiac arrest
Lupine, Lupinus, many varieties, can case respiratory distress and digestive disorders
Mandavilla
Marsh marigold, *Caltha palustris*, not deadly, more an irritant
Mayapple, *Podophyllum peltatum*, The roots are the problem, not the above ground parts
Mexican flame vine
Mistletoe, Viscum album, and others, all parts poisonous, damages red blood cells
❀Narcissus
Nightshade, common, *Solanum nigrum*
Oleander, *Nerium oleander*, all parts poisonous, can case cardiac arrest
Oriental poppy, *Papaver orientalis*, source of Opium, Codeine & Morphine
❀Peace lily, *Spathiphyllum*
Peony, *Paeonia officinalis*
Pelican flower, *Aristilochia*
Periwinkle, *Vinca major, V. Rosea*, all parts can cause minor digestive upset, now used for both cancer treatment and to control blood pressure
❀Philodendron, many varieties, all can cause inflammation of mouth & throat even suffixation

Pieris japonica

Poinciana

Poison hemlock, *Conium maculatum,* not the tree but a bog plant similar to Queen Anne's Lace

Poison ivy, oak & sumac, both topical and internal reactions, can be serious

❀Potato leaves & green potatoes, contains solanins that can cause vomiting & discomfort

❀Pothos, *Epipremmum aureum,* can inflame throat and cause suffixation if leaves are eaten

Precatory bean, rosary peas, rosary bean, *Arbrus precatorius*

Primrose, *Primula species,* some can cause skin irritation, others severe gastric discomfort

Privet, *Ligustrum, species*

Rain lily, Zephyr lily, Fairy lily, *Zephyranthus*

Ranunculus, Buttercup, *Ranunculus,* many species, all parts can cause skin irritation, inflammation of mouth, vomiting, and in severe cases, respiratory failure.

Rhododendron, all parts toxic

Rhubarb, leaves, leaves contain oxalic acid but stems are safe

Rosary pea, Crab's eye, *Abrus precatorius,* beautiful red & black seeds can be deadly

Star anise, Japanese star anise, *Illicium anisatum,* not the related culinary spice (*Illicium verum*)

String of pearls, rosary vine, *Senecio,* disorientation, gastric discomfort

❀Sweet pea, all parts can cause gastric distress

Thornapple, see nightshade

Tobacco, *Nicotiana tabacum,* nicotine is such a potent insecticide that is has been banned from use in many states.

❀Tomato, the leaves and green tomatoes are toxic and can cause gastric distress & hallucinations

Tree of Heaven, *Ailanthus altissima*

❀Tulip, the bulb contains alkaloids

Vetch, common or hairy, all parts can cause minor gastric distress

Water lettuce, *Pistia stratiotes,* can cause severe mouth & throat irritation if eaten raw

❀Windflower, *Anemone*

Wisteria, *Wisteria sinensis,* seeds are toxic

Yews, *Taxus,* many varieties, the both leaves & seeds are toxic

Rashes and inflamations

The following are only a few of the plants may cause contact dermatitis, rash or skin inflammation if handled. There are many other plants that can cause an allergenic reaction in those sensitive to compounds contained in these plants.

African milk tree, *Euphorbia*

Century plant, *Agave,* sap can cause a reaction in some

Dumbcane, *Diffenbachia,* can inflame throat and cause suffixation if leaves are eaten

Moses in a boat

Pencil cactus, *Euphorbia*

Purple Passion Plant, *Senecio*

Poinsettia, may cause a reaction in some, but modern varieties are considered safe for most people

Poison ivy, oak & sumac, *Toxicodendron*

Stinging nettle

Wandering Jew

The Last Word

Hi, It's Me Again.
People-Plant Connection Indeed.

Tomi and Hank have spent a lot of words telling you about this people-plant connection, an idea made popular by my good friend, a true visionary beyond his time and an inspiration to generations, the late Charles Lewis. Now it's my turn. By the way, I prefer to call it the plant-people connection, but if it makes people feel better about themselves that's ok. Anyway, I wanted to set the record straight. This is a matter of science and history so bear with me.

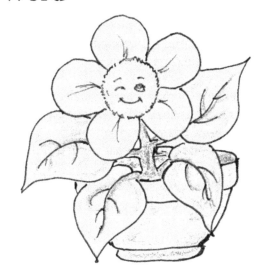

Remember, we were here first. People and plants have been living, working and playing together for a long time. To be honest, you guys couldn't exist without us plants. That's why there's an instinctive need within most of you to be with us. Hey! You can't live without the oxygen that us plants put into the atmosphere. Nor can you survive without the food plants produce that sustains you.

But this connection goes deeper, deep into your psyche. We play with your mind. We inspire you with our beauty. You lust after our naked flowers, glory in our green leaves, and take delight in the perfume of our fruits. You are dwarfed by the glory of our trees, intrigued by our Alpine cousins, frightened by our deadly nightshades and poison ivies, held in awe by our desert dwelling kin. You are comforted by the shade we create, the birds and animals we shelter and feed. When we green your cities they heal, when you place us in planned communities, you call them gardens and parks, you know real joy. But, remember, we were here first.

Us plants are generous though.

We gave you people your first clothing, the *fig leaf.* Cotton and silk have been around since the dawn of history, long before the washing machine. Yeah, I know, silk is from silkworms, but what do you think they ate to live long enough to spin the silk?

We sheltered you from the beasts, the elements and other people with our wood, straw, leaves and twigs, even sod. Now green roofs and rooftop gardens are a part of a sustainable response to global warming and air pollution, problems you caused but us plants can solve.

Plants provide a majority of the medicines, salves, ointments, bandages, tonics and insect controls for most of you people around this green globe we call home. We feed you, cloth you, protect and shelter you. It's ok to go out and hug a tree, say thanks to the flowers and talk to our cousins on the windowsill. I kinda like this plant-people connection. Don't you? We do work, play ,and grow well together, don't we?

That's why we like the idea of a *Green Thumb Club* that can be an informal support group helping both us plants and you people. It feels good to get your hands dirty, watch seeds you planted sprout, see new leaves unfurl or flowers appear and know you are a part of making this happen. It's a joy to feel the texture of our leaves, seeds or bark. For you it's just plain fun. For us it's a matter of survival.

249

Be honest now. Isn't holding and smelling a rose a lot more fun than just looking at the picture of one in a book? Petting a rosemary plant is a pleasant experience, for both of us. And what compares to eating a vine ripened tomato that you grew? Or eating the flowers from a lablab bean? Or playing with a sensitive plant or snapdragon flower? We provide cheap entertainment. In reality it's all a trick. If we can entice you into planting and nurturing us, we survive. When we thrive in your care, we can be happy in the knowledge that our grandchildren will carry on long after we have become mulch.

As a card carrying, chlorophyl producing member of the plant kingdom, I offer this suggestion to you. This is a way to benefit us both. Why not start a *Green Thumb Club*? This can be a club with both plant and people members. Since this will be your club you have the right to call it whatever you wish. It is also up to you to include plants and activities that are of specific interest to each of your members.

Warning: These sessions are most rewarding and successful when the professionals, teachers and activity directors step back and "let things happen." When you stop being in control us plants can empower the gardeners, making them smile, guiding them to learn new stuff, helping them succeed, encouraging them to tell stories (some may even be true), and empowering by letting them make the decisions and discoveries.

What the people participants can gain from a Green Thumb Club
- Socialization & communication
- Mental & Physical stimulation
- Memory stimulation
- A garden; something to nurture, experience and share
- An enjoyable experience
- A sense of worth and value to the community

What US plants can gain from a Green Thumb Club:
- Be in a place where someone cares about us, maybe even talks to us
- Be protected from the cold, the bugs, drought and starvation
- See hope for our future generations
- A safe home where we can put down roots
- Good music, the smell of coffee in the morning and all the oxygen we need

Each meeting can have a combination of these elements.
- A "take home" or "windowsill" project
- Reminisce experiences, memories triggered
- Story telling & creative expression
- Show & Tell with something weird & wonderful, or simply playful
- Sharing sensory experiences, sight, touch, scents, tastes, colors and sounds. Members can taste foods, discover exotic plants, feel bark textures, observe insects, unusual flowers, leaves or seeds.
- Discussion and socialization about the plants, gardening and whatever topics arise
- Gardening with a higher purpose projects to benefit others

These sessions should be subject to change. Be aware of the needs of the plants you are adopting and make certain to accommodate the skill levels and interests of the participants. The objective is to make this a pleasant and stimulating experience, for both you and us. This plant-people connection is an opportunity for us to be nurtured, and you to nurture. While we bask in the sun and dream of tropical isles you can engage in a social activity, gain some much needed physical exercise and stimulate your mind a little bit. It won't hurt you kids to do something besides those silly video games. And you seniors out there, there's more to life than Bingo. Come on, grow with us.

Notes to staff or faculty:

1. Getting your hands dirty is half the fun. The projects discussed in this book are only the beginning. Our Green Thumb Clubs can take field trips, plant butterfly gardens, do landscaping projects, grow trees for Arbor Day, or be a part of the preservation of heritage flowers and vegetables.

2. It's vital that the club members do the work. A horticultural therapy program isn't implemented to provide more work opportunities for the staff or faculty.

3. The staff should be involved in the Green Thumb Club as members. When staff share in the gardening experience there is a common bond and topics of conversation that can make the benefits of the program extend far beyond the garden or the few hours spent with a club meeting.

4. The members of the Green Thumb Club should meet at least weekly and each meeting should contain elements from those listed above.

5. Problems need to be addressed as soon as possible. Often the solution can be found among the participants, but it not, contact a horticultural therapist or master gardener before the problems become serious.

6. Everyone needs to know that not all plants are going to survive. Some of us are called annuals because we were were born to bloom once. Others of us will fall victim to neglect, or be "fussed to death." For you people, this can be a learning experience, an opportunity to try something else; for us it's fodder for the compost pile.

7. Be aware of my kin who can be dangerous or even toxic. It's also important to avoid the use of pesticides because they can pose a threat to both you and me.

Now Some Notes to Green Thumb Club Members:

1. I am putting my family in your care. They are your responsibility. It's up to you to plan, prepare, plant and nurture. You will have to water, trim, feed and maintain the plants that you choose to grow.

2. Since this is your garden we suggest that you make decisions, set the agenda and share responsibilities. You can also share the joy.

3. If you are willing to share your wisdom, knowledge, experiences and thoughts about some of us plants that you choose to grow on your windowsill, or in the landscape, you can enrich other people's lives and make them better gardeners.

4. You can research information on those of us you choose to grow in books, magazines, catalogs, the Internet and by asking others. You should never stop learning. This is part of the joy of living. Besides, there's a lot you have to learn about us plants.

5. You can propagate our offspring to give as gifts, share or plant in the landscape for the benefit of others. You can share the vegetables and herbs that you grow with the kitchen, visitors or a food pantry.

6. We suggest that the human Green Thumb Club members keep a gardener's journal . Fill it with information on the plants you grow are sharing your windowsill with, planting times, notes on growth, any problems and most important, photographs. This can be shared. You can sing to us, or even write even a song. We do like music.

7. Use the garden as inspiration for art and poetry. The communion with living plants is inspirational. This can be a very personal expression of your thoughts or feelings, or it can be a creative work to share. Don't worry about rules and technique; creativity is best when it comes from the heart.

8. Visit your plants friends every day, because every day there will be a new discovery. We work hard to prepare surprises for you. It might be a new leaf, a flower bud opening, or a seed sprouting. This visit can be done with friends or alone, but the discoveries are best when shared.

9. Approach the garden and us plants with a sense of adventure, not as a chore. This is an opportunity, not an obligation. Relax and enjoy the plant-people connection.

10. Enjoy our company. Give us a smile, talk to us, all we want is to be friends.

There, I had the last word in this book. Thank you for reading and using it. Thanks also for hearing my side of the story.

Oh, by the way, if you enjoyed this book, or found it helpful I wanted to let you know that Tomi & Hank have written several other books. For the senior crowd they wrote *Gardening Projects for Horticultural Therpay Programs*. It has a bunch of projects and activities that put my family and friends to work. It features the CelluGRO Green Thumb Garden, a neat portable, wheelchair friendly, indoor-outdoor garden.

For the students they wrote *Garden Projects for the Classroom and Special Learning Programs*. It makes us plants the heroes in all the school subjects, from science and history to language arts, music and math. My kin are sort of teachers in this book filled with projects. It also features the CelluGRO Green Thumb Garden, that neat portable, wheelchair friendly, indoor-outdoor garden that let's the kids grow green friends all winter long.

They also wrote *Gardens for the Senses, Gardening as Therapy* as a why to garden book rather than a how to guide. This is an introduction to horticultural therapy, one of the neatest jobs us plants can have.

And, in spite of what Kermit sings about being green, I think it's quite easy, and I don't think I would want it any other way.

Resources for Seeds, Plants and Tools

The following are only a few of the reliable, dedicated suppliers of the tools, plants, ect that we all need for our horticultural therapy programs.

ACF Environmental, CelluGRO Div. Cardwell Road, Richmond, VA 23234, Phone: 800-448-3636 www.cellugro.com Manufacturer of the popular portable, indoor-outdoor Green Thumb Garden and other CelluGRO gardening systems.

American Horticultural Therapy Association, 201 East Main Street, Suite 1405, Lexington, KY 4050. Phone 859-514-9177, www.ahta.org The ultimate resource for information on horticultural therapy.

Banana Tree, Inc. 715 Northampton St., Easton PA, 18042, USA
Phone: 610-253-9589 www.banana-tree.com   Reliable source for exotic seeds and plants.

Charley's Greenhouse Supply, Great source for tools and gardening accessories.
17979 State Route 536, Mount Vernon, WA 98273-3269 www.charleysgreenhouse.com

ECHO (Educational Concerns for Hunger Organization), 17430 Durrance Rd., North Fort Myers, FL 33917-2239, USA, Phone: 941-543-3246, www.echonet.org Excellent organization, reliable source for significant seeds such as moringa & lablab bean.

Evergreen Y. H. Enterprises, PO Box 17538, Anaheim, CA 92817, USA, Phone: 714-637-5769 www.evergreenseeds.com   A great resource for Oriental vegetables

Fiskars Tools, premier source for specialized and ergonomic tools.   780 Carolina St., Sauk City WI 53583, Phone: 800-500-4849 www.fiskars.com

Flaghouse, 601 Flaghouse Dr., Hasbrouck Heights, NJ 07604-3116, www.flaghouse.com Source for the CelluGRO Green Thumb Garden and many other materials for special needs populations.

Gardeners Supply Company, 128 Intervale Road, Burlington, VT 05401, 888-833-1412 www.gardeners.com Great selection of tools and materials for every gardener.

The Glasshouse Works, P.O. Box 97, Church Street, Stewart, OH 45778-0097, USA, Phone: 740-662-2142, www.glasshouseworks.com Super source for truly unusual plants.

Logee's Greenhouses LTD, 141 North St., Danielson, CT 06239-1939, USA, Phone: 888-330-8038 www.logees.com   Great source for unusual tropicals and houseplants.

NASCO - Fort Atkinson, 901 Janesville Ave., PO Box 901, Fort Atkinson, WI 53538-0901 Phone: 800-558-9595 www.enasco.com A source for the CelluGRO Green Thumb Gardens, other adaptive garden tools and a multitude of other materials for seniors and special populations.

Native Seeds SEARCH, 526 N. 4th Ave., Tuscon, AZ 85705, USA, Phone: 866-622-5561 www.nativeseeds.org A non-profit organization dedicated to preservation of Native American food plants and native species.

Nichols Garden Nursery, 1190 North Pacific Highway, Albany, OR 97321, Phone: 541-928-9280 www.nicholsgardennursery.com

Pinetree Seeds, PO Box 300, New Gloucester, ME 04260, Phone: 207-926-3400 www.superseeds.com A great and reliable source of seeds, books and supplies for gardening and horticultural therapy programs.

Richters, Goodwood, Ontario, LOC 1AO Canada,   Phone: 1-905-640-6677, inquiry@richters.com Reliable source for familiar and uncommon herbs and spices, both plants and seeds.

Seeds of Change, P.O. Box 15700, Santa Fe, NM 87506, USA

Phone: 888-762-7333 www.seedsofchange.com Wonderful source for vegetables, flowers and herbs.

S & S Worldwide, 75 Mill Street, Colchester, CT 06415, Phone: 800-288-9941   www.ssww.com They offer a wide range of materials for people of all ages with special needs.

South Paw Enterprises, PO Box 1047, Dayton, OH 45401, Phone: 800-288-1698 www.southpawenterprises.com Dedicated to serving children with special needs.

Thompson & Morgan Seed Company, P.O. Box 1308, Jackson, NJ 08527-0308, USA

Phone: 800-274-7333 www.thompson-morgan.com Excellent source for flower, herb and vegetable seeds.

Tropiflora, 3530 Tallevest Road, Sarasota, FL 34247, USA, Phone: 941-351-2267, www.tropiflora.com Source for uncommon tropicals, exotics and rare plants.

PETALS & PAGES PRESS

860 Polaris Blvd SE
Rio Rancho, NM 87124
petals_pages@msn.com

More books available from Petals & Pages Press

Non-fiction:

Gardens for the Senses, Gardening as Therapy, by Hank Bruce an intro to the field of horticultural therapy, a "why to" garden book with helpful lists of edible flowers and safe and dangerous plants. ISBN 0-932855-57-1 $14.95

Garden Projects for Horticultural Therapy Programs, by Hank Bruce & Tomi Jill Folk, is more "how to" as well as "why to." Great collection of gardening activities for senior care facilities. ISBN # 0-97059-620-0 $18.95

Garden Projects for the Classroom and Special Learning Programs, by Hank Bruce & Tomi Jill Folk, a guide for the integration of diverse subject disciplines; great for classroom, special needs students and home school settings. ISBN 0-9705962-1-9 $25.95

Global Gardening, by Hank Bruce & Tomi Jill Folk, explores the causes of hunger and how we can all be a part of the solution, included information on over 200 underused vegetable resources from all over the world. ISBN 0-932855-74-1 $19.95

The Courage to Create, a Writer's Workbook, by Hank Bruce has been used as a text for seminars and by creative individuals. ISBN 1-883114-14-4 $15.95

The Family Caregiver's Journal: A Guide to Facing the Terminal Illness of a Loved One, by Hank Bruce & Tomi Jill Folk, uses facts, stories, & poetry along with journal space to explore feelings and help the caregiver through this difficult and rewarding time. ISBN 0-7880-1434-X $14.95

Cue Tips; A Stage Management Handbook for High School Theatre, by Elizabeth D. Ward, a textbook and terrific organizational tool. ISBN 978-0-9797057-2-4 $15.95

Visits with the Old Indian Storyteller, Stories with universal themes that use a wide range of objects from corn husk dolls to spirit blankets, walking sticks, and cracked pots. Retold by Tomi Jill Folk ISBN 978-0-9797057-1-7 $19.95

Fiction:

Oblivion, A Novel Place to Live, An artist and a poet bring new life to a New Mexico ghost town & create an eco-friendly community. ISBN 978-0-9797057-0-0 $19.95

Peace Beyond All Fear: A Tribute to John Denver's Vision, 15 short stories dealing with peace, the environment, hunger, refugees, love and eagles, all inspired by the work of John Denver. ISBN 978-0-9797057-3-1 $19.95

About the Authors

Hank Bruce & Tomi Jill Folk are a husband and wife team residing in New Mexico. They follow an active schedule, speaking with groups all over the United States on hunger, horticultural therapy, environmental and peace issues. Together they have written over 20 books and hundreds of articles and information sheets on hunger, family gardening, diabetes, school and community gardens and more. They initiated a horticultural therapy showcase, the Opportunity Garden, as a part of the annual International Flower & Garden Festival at EPCOT in 1999 and spoke at EPCOT from 1999-2002 on horticultural therapy.

Brief Biography of Tomi Jill Folk, M. Div.

Tomi is the owner of Petals & Pages Press, an activist working with hunger and peace issues, writer, a poet and a former Lutheran minister. She is the president of Hunger Grow Away, a non-profit food security organization focused on the elimination of hunger and malnutrition by promoting family food production, mainly in Native American communities of the Southwestern United States, but also in Haiti, Mexico, Uganda, and Kenya . Her recent work has involved the prevention of renewed uranium mining in New Mexico because of the dangers involved to the miners and their families, along with the environment for all of us.

In 2007 Tomi released *Visits with the Old Indian Storyteller*, a collection of stories from a ten year friendship with a Native American elder. She uses storytelling both as a learning tool and as a pathway to healing.

Brief Biography of Hank Bruce

Hank is a writer and the Program Director of Hunger Grow Away. Hank is also a food security advocate and has done extensive research on micro-intensive gardening systems, home grown nutrition programs and global food resource diversity. Current projects include research into underused vegetables for arid lands, family gardens as a means of improving nutrition, dietary disease prevention and control and the cultivation and use of indigenous resources for today's dinner table. He has taught courses at the University of New Mexico Con-Ed Dept. on Horticultural Therapy, Hunger Solutions and Writing. He was awarded the American Horticultural Therapy Association's Humanitarian of the Year Award in 1999, and the Florida chapter's Lifetime Achievement Award in 2007.

He had two fiction works published in 2007, *Oblivion, a Novel Place to Live* is his first fictional work. It involves a new concept in community building focused on creativity rather than control and environmentally friendly lifestyles rather than consumption and waste. *Peace Beyond All Fear, a Tribute to John Denver's Vision* , is a collection of 15 short stories dealing with HIV/AIDS in Kenya to Darfur refugees, veterans with PTSD to children planting flowers on a former bombing range, alcoholism to Alzheimer's.

CPSIA information can be obtained
at www.ICGtesting.com
Printed in the USA
LVHW101532230120
644587LV00004B/413